Social Anxiety and Phobia in Adolescents

Klaus Ranta • Annette M. La Greca
Luis-Joaquin Garcia-Lopez
Mauri Marttunen
Editors

Social Anxiety and Phobia in Adolescents

Development, Manifestation and Intervention Strategies

Springer

Editors
Klaus Ranta
Department of Adolescent Psychiatry
Helsinki University Central Hospital
Helsinki
Finland

Department of Psychology
University of Turku
Turku
Finland

Annette M. La Greca
University of Miami
Coral Gables, FL
USA

Luis-Joaquin Garcia-Lopez
Department of Psychology
University of Jaen
Jaen
Spain

Mauri Marttunen
Department of Mental Health and
Substance Abuse
National Institute for Health and Welfare
Helsinki
Finland

Department of Psychiatry
University of Helsinki
Helsinki
Finland

ISBN 978-3-319-16702-2 ISBN 978-3-319-16703-9 (eBook)
DOI 10.1007/978-3-319-16703-9

Library of Congress Control Number: 2015943504

Springer Cham Heidelberg New York Dordrecht London

Printed on acid-free paper

Springer International Publishing AG Switzerland is part of Springer Science+Business Media (www.springer.com)

Preface

We hope that this book will prove valuable to a number of audiences. First and foremost, professionals and clinicians working with youth aged from 12 to 20 years of age will readily acknowledge the need for a volume concentrating on social anxiety and phobia in adolescents. This is the case for mental health nurses, specialist teachers, or counsellors working in schools, as well as for clinical psychologists, therapists, or psychiatrists in primary/secondary healthcare services or private sector. All such professionals are likely to repeatedly encounter adolescents who withdraw from peers, display shyness and inhibition in their social contacts, and struggle hard to raise their hand or speak in class. When referred for clinical treatment, often these youth have already begun to miss important peer group gatherings or activities due to their social avoidance. Clinicians who treat adolescents will often witness that the youths' primary anxiety symptoms are social-related fears, even among youth with no prior treatment history.

In addition to professional interest, we believe that advanced students in the fields of clinical psychology and psychiatry also will find a volume that focuses on social anxiety in youth to be important. A developmental psychopathology perspective is important to understanding the etiology, course, and outcome of social anxiety disorder prior to adulthood. The focus on the adolescent period highlights the relevance of the multilevel, pervasive changes in biological, cognitive, affective, and social functioning that occur and are associated with adolescent social anxiety.

Finally, we believe that developmental researchers who are interested in identifying pathways leading to the clinical syndrome of social anxiety disorder also will be served well by the up-to-date reviews on adolescent social anxiety and phobia, written by recognized international experts, which are contained in this volume. We believe that such a developmentally tailored presentation can be useful in the formation of new clinical hypotheses, for example, as well as in the refinement of clinical methodology for the advanced study of the etiology, epidemiology, phenomenology, assessment, and treatment of adolescent social anxiety and phobia.

Adolescents differ from children (and adults) in many key ways. Take, for example, the paramount changes in adolescents' peer relationships, the way anxiety is manifested and related to changes and problems in these relationships, and even the assessment methods used for detecting social phobia – each of which differs for adolescents relative to children. Internationally, a growing interest in age-appropriate treatment is mirrored in the growing number of developmentally sensitive treatment programs for adolescents with social anxiety. As a result, we believe that there is a strong need for a volume that brings together findings from basic developmental research, clinical research, assessment methodology, epidemiology, and psychosocial and biological treatments that focus on adolescent social anxiety and phobia. We hope the present volume lives up to these important areas of need.

Helsinki, Finland — Klaus Ranta, MD, PhD
Coral Gables, FL, USA — Annette M. La Greca, PhD, ABPP
Jaen, Spain — Luis Joaquin Garcia-Lopez, PhD
Helsinki, Finland — Mauri Marttunen, MD, PhD

Contents

Contributors

Anne Marie Albano, PhD, ABPP Department of Psychiatry, Columbia University Clinic for Anxiety and Related Disorders, New York Presbyterian Hospital/Columbia University Medical Center, New York, NY, USA

Candice A. Alfano, PhD Department of Psychology, University of Houston, Houston, TX, USA

Deborah C. Beidel, PhD Department of Psychology, University of Central Florida, Orlando, FL, USA

Anke W. Blöte, PhD Developmental & Educational Psychology Unit, Institute of Psychology, Faculty of Social and Behavioural Sciences, Leiden University, Leiden, The Netherlands

Chad Brice, PhD Cognitive and Behavioral Consultants, White Plains, NY, USA

Daniela Colognori, PsyD Department of Advanced Studies in Psychology, Kean University, Union, NJ, USA

Cathy Creswell, BA (Ox) Hons, D Clin Psy, PhD School of Psychology and Clinical Language Sciences, University of Reading, Reading, Berkshire, UK

Joanne Davila, PhD Department of Psychology, Stony Brook University, Stony Brook, NY, USA

Andres De Los Reyes, PhD Department of Psychology, University of Maryland at College Park, College Park, MD, USA

Jill Ehrenreich-May, PhD Department of Psychology, University of Miami, Coral Gables, FL, USA

Luis-Joaquin Garcia-Lopez, PhD Department of Psychology, University of Jaen, Jaen, Spain

John D. Guerry, PhD Department of Child and Adolescent Psychiatry and Behavioral Sciences, The Children's Hospital of Philadelphia, Philadelphia, PA, USA

James Hambrick, PhD Department of Psychiatry, Columbia University Clinic for Anxiety and Related Disorders, Columbia University Medical Center, New York, NY, USA

David A. Heyne, BA, Dip Ed Psych, M Psych, PhD Developmental & Educational Psychology Unit, Institute of Psychology, Faculty of Social and Behavioural Sciences, Leiden University, Leiden, The Netherlands

Jennifer L. Hudson, MClinPsych, PhD Department of Psychology, Centre for Emotional Health, Macquarie University, Sydney, NSW, Australia

Susanne Knappe Institute of Clinical Psychology and Psychotherapy, Technische Universität Dresden, Dresden, Germany

Annette M. La Greca, PhD, ABPP Department of Psychology, University of Miami, Coral Gables, FL, USA

Chloe Lau Department of Psychiatry and Behavioural Neurosciences, McMaster University, MacAnxiety Research Centre, Hamilton, ON, Canada

Thien-An Le Department of Psychology, University of Central Florida, Orlando, FL, USA

Mauri Marttunen, MD, PhD Department of Mental Health and Substance Abuse, National Institute for Health and Welfare, Helsinki, Finland

Department of Psychiatry, University of Helsinki, Helsinki, Finland

Lauren F. McLellan, PhD Department of Psychology, Centre for Emotional Health, Macquarie University, Sydney, NSW, Australia

Franklin Mesa, MS Department of Psychology, University of Central Florida, Orlando, FL, USA

Anne C. Miers, PhD Developmental & Educational Psychology Unit, Institute of Psychology, Faculty of Social and Behavioural Sciences, Leiden University, Leiden, The Netherlands

Laura Mufson, PhD Department of Psychiatry, College of Physicians and Surgeons and New York State Psychiatric Institute, CUMC, Columbia University, New York, NY, USA

Beth Patterson, MSc, BEd Department of Psychiatry and Behavioural Neurosciences, McMaster University, MacAnxiety Research Centre, Hamilton, ON, Canada

Klaus Ranta, MD, PhD Department of Adolescent Psychiatry, Helsinki University Central Hospital, Helsinki, Finland

Department of Psychology, University of Turku, Turku, Finland

Ronald M. Rapee, AM, PhD, MSc (Psych) Department of Psychology, Centre for Emotional Health, Macquarie University, Sydney, NSW, Australia

Maria do Ceu Salvador, PhD Department of Psychology, University of Coimbra, Coimbra, Portugal

Amanda Sanchez, BA Department of Child and Adolescent Psychiatry, NYU Langone Medical Center, New York, NY, USA

Satoko Sasagawa, PhD Faculty of Human Sciences, Mejiro University, Tokyo, Japan

Lisa R. Starr, PhD Department of Clinical and Social Sciences in Psychology, University of Rochester, Rochester, NY, USA

Maria Tillfors, PhD Department of Law, Psychology and Social Work, Örebro University, Örebro, Sweden

Jasmine Turna, BSc Department of Psychiatry and Behavioural Neurosciences, McMaster University, MacAnxiety Research Centre, Hamilton, ON, Canada

Michael Van Ameringen, MD, FRCPC Department of Psychiatry and Behavioural Neurosciences, McMaster University, MacAnxiety Research Centre, Hamilton, ON, Canada

Nejra Van Zalk, PhD Department of Law, Psychology, and Social Work, Örebro University, Örebro, Sweden

Carrie Masia Warner, PhD Department of Psychology, William Paterson University, Wayne, NJ, USA

Nathan Kline Institute for Psychatric Research, Orangeburg, NY, USA

Department of Child and Adolescent Psychiatry, NYU Langone Medical Center, New York, NY, USA

P. Michiel Westenberg, PhD Developmental & Educational Psychology Unit, Institute of Psychology, Faculty of Social and Behavioural Sciences, Leiden University, Leiden, The Netherlands

Quincy J.J. Wong, PhD/MPsychol (Clinical) Department of Psychology, Centre for Emotional Health, Macquarie University, Sydney, NSW, Australia

Jami F. Young, PhD Graduate School of Applied and Professional Psychology, Rutgers University, Piscataway, New Brunswick, NJ, USA

Introduction 1

Klaus Ranta, Annette M. La Greca, Luis-Joaquin Garcia-Lopez, and Mauri Marttunen

Introduction

In the middle of the first talk before the class in his new high school, a presentation about a novel, James halted. He sensed an acute feeling of shortness of breath and noted that he suddenly lost all words. Always being one who remained in the outer circle of peers in school gatherings, socializing usually with just few good friends, James panicked. Already at the very outset of the term, he had worried that he might convey a negative image of himself to new students, having recollections of feeling unpopular and odd in middle school, recognizing only too well his slight tendency for stuttering. Preparing for this talk had been a 2-week period of increasing tension and worry. James had difficulties falling asleep each night, and he had memorized word for word over and over again the main punch lines he was going

K. Ranta, MD, PhD (✉)
Department of Adolescent Psychiatry, Helsinki University Central Hospital, Helsinki, Finland

Department of Psychology, University of Turku, Turku, Finland
e-mail: klaus.ranta@hus.fi

A.M. La Greca, PhD, ABPP
Department of Psychology, University of Miami, Coral Gables, FL, USA

L.-J. Garcia-Lopez, PhD
Department of Psychology, University of Jaen, Jaen, Spain

M. Marttunen, MD, PhD
Department of Mental Health and Substance Abuse, National Institute for Health and Welfare, Helsinki, Finland

Department of Psychiatry, University of Helsinki, Helsinki, Finland

K. Ranta et al. (eds.), *Social Anxiety and Phobia in Adolescents: Development, Manifestation and Intervention Strategies*, DOI 10.1007/978-3-319-16703-9_1

to say. Now, in the moment, as the sudden pause becoming longer and longer, visual images of himself as a red, speechless, and clumsy idiot rushed to his mind, with everybody else's eyes on him, looking astonished and amused. Unable to stand it, James froze and just stood there for a while; then he walked out of class.

For any of us observing and witnessing adolescents' interactions with their peers, as parents, as therapists, as researchers, we see the tremendous, almost magnetic pull of peer relationships. Youth seem to long for and seek peers' companionship, opinion, and approval and sometimes conform to even ill-advised peer advice. Yet, in other types of circumstances, for example, observing 13–15-year-olds in formal adult-type performance situations or as the center of attention of larger audiences or authority figures, we may catch a glimpse of a different kind of uncertainty. Adolescents commonly report fears of negative evaluation in anonymous surveys, yet adolescents will rarely openly disclose such fears to their friends.

Our own recollections of our adolescent years might provide an inside perspective of the urgent need to fit in, of the fear of being picked on, and sometimes of the feeling of terror for saying something stupid that would single us out as "odd" or "a loser." In some inexplicable way, we were embarrassed by the mere presence of our parents in situations where peers were also present, feeling some kind of vague shame of being too childlike, wanting to get rid of our parents as quickly as possible. And we may remember our confused and fearful feelings when we were expected to find our way to chemistry class in the midst of unknown students and meet the new teacher, to speak with an adult to make a request for something we did not totally grasp, or to act as lecturer in front of the whole class.

So, there is something very familiar in the self-conscious teen. However, in the clinic and in schools, we also encounter young, shy preschool and elementary school children who do not appear self-conscious, but who seem more like they are functioning in an energy-saving mode. They are almost totally silent, and when they do talk, they speak in a barely audible voice; these children have few if any friends and are almost invisible in the classroom. These children may be picked on, teased, or bullied, be unable to articulate feelings of shame, and seem to act as if they are disinterested in socializing.

These phenomenological variations of social anxiety and its clinical form, social anxiety disorder (SAD), among children and adolescents resemble each other, yet are different. What in childhood is manifested, or perhaps just communicated, as more of a pure fear and related social avoidance, transforms in adolescence into a vivid inner experience characterized by self-centeredness, worries of being different, and feelings of inferiority and shame. The increasing cognitive capacity of adolescents, along with the increased importance of peer comparisons and peer relations, undoubtedly influences adolescents' perspective.

Fears of social situations, of negative evaluation, and of embarrassment – all primary symptoms of SAD – go hand in hand during childhood and adolescence. For approximately 3–9 % of adolescents, the severity of these symptoms reaches the point where they cause significant suffering or functional impairment and thus meet criteria for a clinical disorder. However, we also know that there often is variation or fluctuation in symptom severity among youth who are above or below clinical cutoffs at any given time. Nevertheless, a general tendency to develop a stable and chronic course of symptomatology is observed among those with SAD, and it is likely that increasing demands for independent social functioning contribute to the worsening of adolescents' symptoms. By that time, the typical maintaining factors of social anxiety, such as avoidance of social situations or dysfunctional safety behaviors, are likely to be present.

Developmental transitions occurring during childhood and adolescence also affect youths' experience of social anxiety: not only do adults require greater independence in youths' social functioning, but also peers require standing up and speaking for oneself, and avoidant or shy behavior may be poorly tolerated. So, the social milieu in which adolescents develop changes markedly and permanently.

Given the developmental variations in social functioning and the normative rise in social fears and social anxiety from childhood to adolescence, no wonder it has been a challenging task for researchers and clinicians to reach a consensus as to what developmentally constitutes a disorder; what the relationship is between inhibited childhood temperament, childhood shyness, and social phobia; and how best to distinguish between normative social anxiety and a social anxiety disorder. Not surprisingly, definitions of SAD have varied across the successive editions of the DSM and the ICD classification systems (APA 2013; WHO 2014). Although efforts have focused on developing common diagnostic criteria for SAD across age groups, developmental specifications have been added to account for symptom variation across individuals of different ages. In fact, with the recent DSM-5, six developmental specifiers (e.g., crying, tantrums, freezing, clinging, shrinking, or failing to speak) have been added to describe young children's socially anxious behavior (APA 2013). Such specifiers are not as relevant for adolescents or adults.

The key DSM-5 criteria state that the individual with SAD almost without exception experiences marked fear or anxiety in one or more social situations (e.g., social interactions, being observed, performing in front of others), experiences fear of negative evaluation (either resulting from the individual's own behavior or from showing anxiety symptoms) in these situations, and either avoids or endures them with intense anxiety. DSM-5 further specifies that the fear must be disproportionately intense (with regard to the actual threat posed by the situation or to the sociocultural context), that it persists for longer than 6 months, is not due to the physiological effects of a substance, a medical condition, or another mental disorder, and that it leads to clinically significant distress or impairment in important areas of functioning. Moreover, DSM-5 specifies a performance-limited SAD subtype when the fear is restricted to speaking or performing in public (APA 2013).

However, empirical evidence is controversial with regard to the actual prevalence of such performance -limited SAD is in clinical contexts (Kerns et al. 2013; Garcia-Lopez et al. (in press); Garcia-Lopez and Moore, 2015).

The ICD-11 criteria (to be published by WHO in 2015) are largely identical with regard to the clinical manifestation of SAD, proposing that "Social anxiety disorder is characterized by marked and excessive fear or anxiety that consistently occurs in one or more social situations such as social interactions (e.g., having a conversation), being observed (e.g., eating or drinking), or performing in front of others (e.g., giving a speech). The individual is concerned that he or she will act in a way, or show anxiety symptoms, that will be negatively evaluated by others. The social situations are avoided or else endured with intense fear or anxiety." However, in ICD-11, the duration criterion is defined more loosely: "The fear, anxiety, or avoidance persists for at least several months and result in significant distress or significant impairment in personal, family, social, educational, occupational or other important areas of functioning" (WHO 2014).

Thus, currently both of the two major mental health disorder classifications recognize the need to define both a condition where the excessive anxiety is experienced in the context of one social situation (being a performance situation in the majority of cases) and the excessive anxiety tied to several social situations under the term social anxiety disorder. However, the proposed ICD-11 classification scheme at the present stage no longer includes different categories and criteria for adult- and childhood-/adolescent-onset anxiety disorders, which the preceding ICD-10 did (WHO 1992), distinguishing between social phobia and social anxiety disorder of childhood.

In this volume, *Social Anxiety and Phobia in Adolescents: Development, Manifestation and Intervention Strategies*, we aim to fill a gap in the literature on the developmental aspects of social anxiety and SAD. Specifically, we review empirical research on the developmental etiological and risk factors for social anxiety and SAD, we describe epidemiological and clinical manifestations of social anxiety and SAD in adolescence, and we present an up-to-date selection of available treatment strategies for this age group.

The first section of the book covers background and theoretical accounts of the study of social anxiety and phobia in adolescents. The opening chapter by Quincy Wong and Ron Rapee presents a comprehensive review of suggested etiological factors (innate, distal, and proximal) implicated in the onset of SAD in adolescence. Studies of genetic, temperamental, and biological risk factors are first addressed, followed by the role of environmental and psychological etiological factors. For each proposed etiological factor, the authors present the theoretical explanatory models describing how the factor is thought to have its effect and then review empirical research supporting or contradicting the models. Finally, the authors present a synthesis of the findings within a developmental framework.

In the next chapter, Susanne Knappe, Satoko Sasagawa, and Kathy Creswell provide an overview of the literature on the epidemiology of social anxiety in adolescents. The authors report on the prevalence and risk factors for the onset and course of social anxiety in adolescents. This chapter is notable for the integration of biological, behavioral, and environmental factors that contribute to the development and maintenance of the disorder, providing the reader with a heuristic framework for the epidemiology of SAD.

In Chapter 4, Maria Tillfors and Nejra van Zalk present a neurobiological and developmental explanatory model of SAD in which the advanced development of the subcortical brain regions in combination with the late maturation of the prefrontal cortical regions contributes to increases in emotionally driven behavior that are difficult to control in adolescence. They hypothesize that adolescents with poor peer and parent relationships will have a larger developmental gap between these regions compared to adolescents with supportive peer and parent relationships and may therefore be at higher risk for developing social anxiety.

Chapter 5 by Annette La Greca and Klaus Ranta reviews the literature on how the common developmental transitions of adolescence may contribute to or exacerbate adolescents' symptoms of social anxiety and SAD. This chapter specifically covers school transitions, changes in peer and romantic relationships, pubertal and body morphological changes, and changes in family relationships that occur during the adolescent period. Central findings are discussed along with gaps in research that suggest potential avenues for future studies.

Moving on to the second main section of the volume, *Recognition and Manifestations of Adolescent Social Anxiety and Phobia in Diverse Settings*, Chapter 6 by Luis-Joaquin Garcia-Lopez (Spain), Ceu Salvador (Portugal), and Andres De Los Reyes (USA) presents an extremely thorough review of the literature on the assessment of social anxiety disorder in youth. The authors review clinical assessment procedures, including multi-informant and context-sensitive clinical assessment, physiological assessment methods, and observational and role-play procedures. The need for having a screening protocol to increase the awareness and detection of social anxiety in adolescents is emphasized. This is an important issue given the elevated number of misclassified cases, resulting in poor treatment outcome.

In Chapter 7, Anke Blöte, Anne Miers, David Heyne, and Michiel Westenberg focus on the different facets of social anxiety with regard to how it presents in the school environment, and how the interpersonal peer group processes in the school context might interact with the development and maintenance of the symptoms. Additionally, school absenteeism related to social anxiety is discussed. A significant body of research performed at Leiden University supports the chapter contents. The authors close their review with a model of how social anxiety is initiated and maintained in new, emerging, and established peer relationships and with suggestions for prevention.

Chapter 8 by Joanne Davila and Lisa Starr focuses on how social anxiety might influence the development of romantic relationships. Starting with a review of how social anxiety limits functioning in peer groups thus reducing opportunities for engaging with youth of the opposite sex, they proceed to review impairments in the initiation of romantic relationships (shown as dating anxiety) and finally review dysfunctional behavior patterns of socially anxious adolescents within the relationships they have managed to initiate. The authors close with identifying key research gaps, which include a call for studies of developmental trajectories of romantic relationship in socially anxious adolescents as well as for studies of mediators and/or moderators in the social anxiety – romantic involvement link.

In Chapter 9, John Guerry, James Hambrick, and Anne Marie Albano present a developmentally informed account of the presentation and assessment of socially anxious adolescents in a clinic setting. They provide rich and practical clinical descriptions and guidelines. The authors also discuss how biological risk factors, family psychopathology, interpersonal contributing factors, and conditioning experiences should be taken into consideration in treatment planning for adolescent SAD. Furthermore, the authors present a description of a novel developmental treatment model for emerging adults with SAD built on the cognitive behavioral group treatment model.

The third part of the volume focuses specifically on *intervention strategies*. It begins with Chapter 10 by Lauren McLellan, Candice Alfano, and Jennifer Hudson who review the way cognitive interventions are used for adolescents with SAD. The authors first cover cognitive assessment and then review how cognitive techniques are woven into cognitive behavior therapy (CBT). Finally, the authors present a rich clinical example of treating an adolescent male with individual CBT.

In Chapter 11, Laura Mufson, Annette La Greca, Jami Young, and Jill Ehrenreich-May present the application of interpersonal psychotherapy (IPT) for socially anxious adolescents. The authors first review the relevance of interpersonal theory and intervention for adolescent emotional disorders, such as depression and SAD. They also discuss modifications to IPT that have been developed with adult populations to tailor IPT to the treatment of SAD. The authors then discuss the relevance of IPT for the treatment and prevention of adolescent SAD and describe preliminary findings of a preventive school-based intervention (IPT-AST/Peer Version) that takes a transdiagnostic approach to preventing both SAD and depression among at-risk adolescents who are experiencing interpersonal peer victimization.

In Chapter 12, Carrie Masia Warner, Daniela Colognori, Chad Brice, and Amanda Sanchez review issues in treating social anxiety in school settings. School interventions are receiving considerable empirical attention given that few socially anxious adolescents seek clinical treatment. After reviewing existing school-based interventions for SAD, the authors detail a specific treatment protocol and highlight areas to be addressed by future research. Finally, the authors stress the importance of conducting evidence-based treatments in community settings such as schools and describe school strategies (e.g., training school counselors) that are important for achieving sustainable school-based programs.

Franklin Mesa, Thien-An Le, and Deborah Beidel provide an overview of treatments for SAD, including social skills training, in Chapter 13. In an attempt to highlight gaps in interventions for adolescents with SAD, the authors describe current social skill-based interventions and future directions for research. In particular, the authors provide information on challenges to be faced in treating adolescent SAD. Preliminary data from their lab are presented on the use of a virtual environment-based intervention along with directions for future study.

In the final chapter, Chapter 14, Michael van Ameringen, Jasmine Turna, Beth Patterson, and Chloe Lau present a comprehensive review of the psychopharmacological treatment for adolescent SAD. Compared with literature on adult SAD, psychopharmacological treatment of youthful SAD is much less studied, and many studies have included several anxiety disorders instead of studying "pure SAD." Based on the extant literature, the first-line pharmacological treatment for adolescent SAD is selective serotonin reuptake inhibitors, although evidence is emerging also for the serotonin noradrenalin reuptake inhibitors (SNRIs).

We hope this volume will be of use for readers and researchers working in professional areas such as developmental psychology and psychiatry, as well as for clinicians and counselors working in schools, primary healthcare services, and child and adolescent psychiatric services. We are deeply indebted to our adolescent patients who, by their distressing symptoms, have taught us something essential about the developmental phase of adolescence: bringing forth how the need to belong, to be accepted, and to be free from criticism can evolve into self-maintaining vicious cycles and worsening pathways in the inherently insecure social milieu around them. We hope this book will contribute to a continuing interest in the research on social anxiety and phobia in adolescents and to the further development of developmentally sensitive methods for early recognition, assessment, and treatment.

References

American Psychiatric Association (APA) (2013) Diagnostic and statistical manual of mental disorders, 5th edn. American Psychiatric Publishing, Arlington

Garcia-Lopez LJ, Moore H (2015) The Mini-Social Phobia Inventory: psychometric properties in an adolescent general and clinical population. PLOS One (in press)

Garcia-Lopez LJ, Saez-Castillo A, Beidel DC, La Greca AM (in press). Brief measures to screen for social anxiety in Spanish adolescents. J Dev Behav Pediatr

Kerns CE, Comer JS, Pincus DB, Hofmann SG (2013). Evaluation of the proposed social anxiety disorder specifier change for DSM-5 in a treatment-seeking sample of anxious youth. Depress Anxiety 30:709–715

World Health Organization (WHO) (1992) The ICD-10. Classification of mental and behavioral disorders. World Health Organization, Geneva

World Health Organization (WHO) (2014) ICD-11 Beta draft. Mental and behavioral disorders. Retrieved from http://apps.who.int/classifications/icd11/browse/l-m/en

Part I

Background/Theoretical Accounts

The Developmental Psychopathology of Social Anxiety and Phobia in Adolescents

2

Quincy J.J. Wong and Ronald M. Rapee

The Aetiology of Social Anxiety Disorder

Social anxiety is a common experience that occurs in response to the perceived threat of evaluation from others before, during, or after social situations. For some individuals, the level of social anxiety experienced is sufficiently high to negatively impact their functioning and cause distress in which case a diagnosis of social anxiety disorder (SAD; also known as social phobia) is warranted. Current research indicates that the highest incidence rates for SAD occur during the period from late childhood to early adulthood (between 10 and 20 years of age; Beesdo et al. 2007; Wittchen et al. 1999). Over the last 20 years, there has been a rise in the number of aetiological models and reviews of aetiological factors for SAD (e.g. Hofmann and Barlow 2002; Kimbrel 2008; Morris 2001; Rapee and Spence 2004), and a number of these models and reviews have specifically focused on the childhood and adolescent periods (e.g. Higa-McMillan and Ebesutani 2011; Kashdan and Herbert 2001; Kearney 2005; Ollendick and Benoit 2012; Ollendick and Hirshfeld-Becker 2002; Velting and Albano 2001). In all of these papers, a number of biological, psychological, and social factors have been proposed that increase risk for the development of SAD. Although most papers have been descriptive (i.e. they have summarised proposed aetiological factors and evidence for them), some of the papers have offered a greater level of explanation (i.e. they have proposed how aetiological factors operate and interact to produce SAD; e.g. Higa-McMillan and Ebesutani 2011; Hofmann and Barlow 2002; Kearney 2005; Kimbrel 2008; Morris 2001; Rapee and Spence 2004). In this chapter, we review from a theoretical perspective proposed aetiological factors that have the potential to contribute to the

Q.J.J. Wong, PhD/MPsychol (Clinical) (✉) • R.M. Rapee, AM, PhD, MSc (Psych)
Department of Psychology, Centre for Emotional Health, Macquarie University, Sydney, NSW 2109, Australia
e-mail: quincy.wong@mq.edu.au; ron.rapee@mq.edu.au

K. Ranta et al. (eds.), *Social Anxiety and Phobia in Adolescents: Development, Manifestation and Intervention Strategies*, DOI 10.1007/978-3-319-16703-9_2

development of SAD in adolescence. We then examine relevant evidence for these factors in the existing literature and highlight important directions for future research.

Genes

Theory

Most theoretical accounts point to a strongly heritable component to SAD. Some researchers have proposed that genes may provide a general predisposition to anxiety and mood disorders, rather than a specific vulnerability to SAD (e.g. Eley 1997; Hofmann and Barlow 2002). Researchers have also highlighted that even with a genetic vulnerability to SAD, environmental factors can influence the expression of genes and therefore need to be taken into account (e.g. Kearney 2005). Some researchers have proposed that SAD as a construct is too complex and that genetic links to endophenotypes or intermediate phenotypes of SAD (e.g. attentional biases towards social threat, behavioural inhibition) are more likely to be found than genetic links to SAD itself (e.g. Smoller et al. 2003; see also Lenzenweger 2013). Given the importance of a genetic basis to the aetiology of SAD, it is likely that particular genes will contribute risk to SAD onset in the adolescent period. However, there is no indication in the literature at this stage that any genetic influence is specific to the adolescent period.

Research

The existing literature has focused on (a) the heritability of SAD and constructs related to the disorder and (b) specific genes that are associated with a diagnosis of SAD and SAD-related constructs. In relation to heritability, twin studies have provided evidence of the heritability of SAD (see Scaini et al. 2014 for a meta-analysis). The majority of studies have shown that the concordance for SAD in monozygotic (MZ) twins is higher than that for dizygotic (DZ) twins in adult twin samples (e.g. Kendler et al. 1992, 2001) and child twin samples (e.g. Eley et al. 2008), although some studies have not found evidence for this relationship (Skre et al. 1993). Estimates of the heritability of SAD range from 14 to 55 % across child and adult twin samples (e.g. Czajkowski et al. 2011; Eley et al. 2008; Kendler et al. 1992, 1999, 2001; Scaini et al. 2014), which suggest that SAD has moderate heritability. Interestingly, Scaini et al. (2014) have found that the heritability of social anxiety decreases with age, suggesting that genetic influences play more of a role in SAD vulnerability for youth than for adults. Some studies with adult twin samples have indicated that the genetic contribution to SAD is comprised of a combination of genetic factors specific to the disorder and genetic factors common to anxiety disorders (Hettema et al. 2006b; Kendler et al. 1992, 2001). For example, Kendler et al. (1992) reported that the proportion of variance in vulnerability to SAD that was due to genetic factors specific to the disorder was 21 % with a further 10 % of the variance due to genetic factors common to the anxiety disorders analysed in the study. Other twin studies have suggested that it is not SAD that is specifically inherited but rather a more general disposition towards social anxiety. For example, twin studies have demonstrated the heritability of constructs such as fear of negative evaluation, shyness, behavioural inhibition, and social concern across child and adult twin samples (Beatty et al. 2002; Dilalla et al. 1994; Eley et al. 2003; Stein et al. 2002; Warren et al. 1999).

Several studies have found relationships between specific genes and SAD in child and adult samples (e.g. Donner et al. 2008; Gelernter et al. 2004; Lochner et al. 2007; Reinelt et al. 2013; Rowe et al. 1998; Sipilä et al. 2010). For example, Donner et al. (2008) found single nucleotide polymorphisms in two genes (ALAD and CDH2) and a haplotype in the EPB41L4A gene were associated with SAD. Some studies, however, have not found associations between particular genes and SAD, including studies of dopamine system genes (Kennedy et al. 2001) and genes for the serotonin transporter protein and the serotonin type 2A receptor (Stein et al. 1998). Other studies with child and adult samples have indicated that specific genes, while not directly associated with SAD, are associated with constructs that may be considered to be intermediate phenotypes of SAD, such as introversion (Stein et al. 2004), neuroticism (Hettema et al. 2006a), behavioural inhibition (Smoller et al. 2003, 2005; Fox et al. 2005), and shyness (Arbelle et al. 2003). For example, Stein et al. (2004) showed that a functional variant of the β_1 adrenergic receptor gene was associated with introversion (low extraversion). Another line of study into specific genes has examined the link between genes and the neurobiology of adults with SAD (e.g. Furmark et al. 2004, 2009; Klumpp et al. 2014). For example, in individuals with SAD, the presence of specific genes has been linked to enhanced amygdala activation in response to social-evaluative stimuli (e.g. angry faces or speech task; Furmark et al. 2004, 2009). One important limitation of gene association studies is that they have recruited individuals already diagnosed with SAD. By recruiting such individuals, it is not possible to examine in a prospective manner whether the presence of specific genes increases the risk for the onset of SAD. Once research has identified reliable gene-SAD associations, the next step will be to test whether the identified genes can prospectively predict SAD onset.

Overall, the study of genes and SAD suggests that there is likely to be a genetic component that can increase risk for the development of SAD in adolescence. However, this risk may be conveyed by broad genetic factors that increase vulnerability to general emotional difficulties, specific genetic factors that increase vulnerability to SAD or intermediate phenotypes of SAD, or a combination of these genetic factors.

Temperament

Theory

There is theoretical agreement that a child's temperament can play a role in the development of SAD, and there is the suggestion in the field that temperament as a fundamental way of interacting with the world is largely genetically determined (e.g. Kagan 1989; Rothbart et al. 2000). As such, temperament is assumed to be more influential during childhood in contributing vulnerability to SAD, and the extent that temperament contributes vulnerability at later developmental stages is not clearly explicated in theoretical accounts. There is the proposal in the literature that temperament can elicit particular environmental responses that in turn can independently contribute vulnerability to SAD as well as modify temperament (e.g. certain temperaments may elicit particular parenting styles or influence peer interactions; Kearney 2005; Ollendick and Benoit 2012; see also sections "Parent factors" and "Peer experiences"). Specific temperamental constructs (e.g. behavioural inhibition) have also been conceptualised as early manifestations of what is later labelled as SAD (e.g. Rapee and Coplan 2010), suggesting that those temperamental constructs cannot contribute independent risk for SAD because the temperament and SAD constructs are one and the same. Overall, applying current theorising to the onset of SAD in adolescence, temperament is viewed as an independent risk factor but is more likely to contribute risk for SAD onset in childhood than in adolescence. It should be noted though that temperamental influences during childhood on particular environmental factors may lead to environmental effects in childhood that last into adolescence that then confer risk for SAD onset during adolescence (e.g. a child's behaviourally inhibited temperament might elicit negative peer interactions in childhood that sets the foundation for the way they interact with peers as they get older; see also section "Peer experiences").

Research

Behavioural inhibition has been the most widely studied temperamental style in relation to the development of SAD. Cross-sectional studies have demonstrated an association between behavioural inhibition and SAD in children, adolescents, and adults (e.g. Ballespi et al. 2012; Biederman et al. 2001; Mick and Telch 1998; Wittchen et al. 1999). Prospective longitudinal studies (see Clauss and Blackford 2012 for a meta-analysis) have demonstrated a positive association between childhood behavioural inhibition and either social anxiety or a diagnosis of SAD in later childhood (Hirshfeld-Becker et al. 2007; Hudson et al. 2011; Muris et al. 2011) and adolescence (Bohlin and Hagekull 2009; Chronis-Toscano et al. 2009; Hayward et al. 1998; Rapee 2014; Schwartz et al. 1999). From this literature, there is evidence to suggest that behavioural inhibition plays a role in the development of social anxiety and SAD in adolescence. Additionally, there is some evidence that this longitudinal relationship between behavioural inhibition and social anxiety/SAD may be specific to the more generalised form of social anxiety rather than social anxiety that is limited to performance situations (e.g. Schwartz et al. 1999; it is noteworthy though that the *Diagnostic and Statistical Manual of Mental Disorders*, 5th Edition, has removed the "generalised" specifier for SAD). Future research will need to examine the factors that might moderate the longitudinal relationship between behavioural inhibition and social anxiety or SAD in adolescence (e.g. attentional biases to social-evaluative threat; Pérez-Edgar et al. 2010).

Biological Factors

Theory

There is support for the proposal that biology plays a role in the development of SAD with the emphasis placed mainly on neurobiology (e.g. Higa-McMillan and Ebesutani 2011; Kimbrel 2008). Accounts of proposed biological factors that confer risk for SAD vary in detail and level of explanation (e.g. emphasis on neurotransmitter systems; Higa-McMillan and Ebesutani 2011; emphasis on brain structures; Kimbrel 2008). For some of these accounts, it is unclear from a theoretical perspective as to how specified biological factors at certain levels of explanation (e.g. neurotransmitters) can contribute vulnerability to SAD. It is also unclear from existing accounts as to the developmental timeframe during which particular biological factors might exert an influence to convey risk for the onset of SAD. For example, certain neurobiological developments are more likely to occur during adolescence (e.g. significant development in the prefrontal cortex) which in turn allows the emergence of processes that convey risk for the development of SAD (e.g. prefrontal cortex development allows improved metacognitive and self-evaluative capabilities; e.g. Schmitz et al. 2004; Steinberg 2005). Thus, it appears that current theorising on the role of biological factors that convey risk for SAD in adolescence will need to be expanded to indicate the developmental timeframes for the emergence of proposed biological factors and when these factors can convey risk for SAD onset (see Chap. 3).

Research

Existing studies on biological factors associated with SAD have mainly focused on neurobiology. Specifically, a line of research has investigated the activation of brain regions to threat-related stimuli in adults with SAD (see Fouche et al. 2013; Freitas-Ferrari et al. 2010; Shin and Liberzon 2010 for reviews; see Hattingh et al. 2013 for a meta-analysis). This line of research has consistently implicated the involvement of the amygdala. For example, fMRI studies have shown that compared to non-anxious controls, adults already diagnosed with SAD exhibited greater amygdala activation in social-evaluative situations or when viewing stimuli related to social-evaluative threat (e.g. faces displaying negative emotions, critical comments referring to the self; see, e.g., Freitas-Ferrari et al. 2010). Other fMRI studies employing adults with SAD and non-anxious controls have found that SAD is associated with a range of other aberrant brain activity, including: dysfunctional prefrontal cortex activity (Blair et al. 2008, 2010, 2011; Ding et al. 2011), dysfunctional connectivity of the amygdala (Pannekoek et al. 2013), dysfunctional connectivity between frontal and limbic areas (Baur et al. 2013), and dysfunctional activity in other brain regions (e.g. anterior cingulate cortex; Amir et al. 2005; insula; Klumpp et al. 2012; precuneus and posterior cingulate regions; Gentili et al. 2009; striatal structures; Sareen et al. 2007). The primary limitation to these fMRI studies is the use of cross-sectional designs that utilise adults already diagnosed with SAD. It is unclear whether the demonstrated aberrant brain activity in these studies is evident prior to the onset of SAD. In relation to SAD onset in adolescence, future studies will need a prospective longitudinal design to examine whether the presence of aberrant brain activity during childhood predicts a later diagnosis of SAD in the adolescent period. Such studies would provide better evidence to evaluate the aetiological role of aberrant brain activity for SAD in adolescence. Besides the potential for aberrant brain activity during childhood to contribute to SAD vulnerability in adolescence, there is the possibility that new and qualitatively different brain processes associated with brain maturation in adolescence also contribute to the development of SAD (e.g. changes in striatal activity in the context of structural and functional reorganisation in the brain during adolescence; see Caouette and Guyer 2014).

Another line of research has examined neurobiological factors at the neurotransmitter level in relation to SAD. Compared to non-anxious controls, adults with SAD have been shown to have a smaller number of striatal dopamine reuptake sites (Tiihonen et al. 1997), reduced dopamine D_2 receptor binding potential (Schneier et al. 2000), reduced serotonin-1A receptor binding potential in several brain areas including the amygdala (Lanzenberger et al. 2007), higher binding potentials for the serotonin transporter in the thalamus and the dopamine transporter in the striatum (van der Wee et al. 2008), and higher glutamate levels in specific brain regions (Phan et al. 2005) and at the whole brain level (Pollack et al. 2008). Again, these studies of neurotransmitters are cross-sectional and have utilised adults already diagnosed with SAD as participants. Future research will need to examine whether the obtained neurotransmitter differences in the previous studies are evident prior to SAD onset and if so, whether the differences relate to SAD onset in particular during adolescence.

In terms of neurobiology, there are also cross-sectional electrophysiological studies that have examined the brain responses of adults with SAD via event-related potentials. For example, compared to non-anxious controls, adults with SAD have been shown to have larger P1 amplitudes in identification tasks involving emotional schematic faces (Kolassa et al. 2007, 2009), larger P1 amplitudes in response to angry faces relative to happy faces in a modified dot-probe task (Mueller et al. 2009), and larger N170 amplitudes over the right hemisphere in response to angry faces during an emotion identification task (Kolassa and Miltner 2006). These studies cannot be used to evaluate the aetiological significance of the identified electrophysiological indices because of their cross-sectional designs and recruitment of individuals already diagnosed with SAD. In contrast, a recent longitudinal study has provided preliminary evidence that the N400 amplitude in response to the processing of angry faces in childhood prospectively predicted SAD symptoms in adolescence (Battaglia et al. 2012).

A line of research has also investigated the autonomic nervous system (ANS) and cortisol response of individuals with SAD. Cross-sectional studies have shown that compared to non-anxious controls, adults with SAD exhibit elevated indices of ANS functioning in response to social-evaluative tasks (e.g. Davidson et al. 2000). However, some studies have not demonstrated this elevated ANS response in adults with SAD (Edelman and Baker 2002) or children with SAD (Krämer et al. 2012). Other cross-sectional studies have demonstrated that adults with SAD exhibit a greater rise in cortisol compared to non-anxious controls in response to a social-evaluative task (e.g. Condren et al. 2002). In contrast, some studies have not demonstrated this rise in cortisol in youth with SAD (e.g. Krämer et al. 2012; Martel et al. 1999). Further studies in this line of research are needed to clarify the inconsistencies in findings. Prospective longitudinal studies may subsequently be carried out to investigate whether the aforementioned biological indices can predict a later diagnosis of SAD during adolescence.

In summary, the majority of studies on biological factors related to SAD have utilised adults already diagnosed with the disorder. There is a need for future researchers to use prospective longitudinal designs to evaluate biological factors that both precede and relate to SAD onset, particularly for an onset that occurs during the adolescent period.

Cognitive Factors

Theory

Although cognitive factors are commonly considered from a theoretical perspective to contribute vulnerability to SAD (e.g. Hofmann and Barlow 2002; Kearney 2005), the nature and number of specific cognitive factors that have been proposed vary. For example, some researchers have proposed a single cognitive process that contributes to the development of SAD (e.g. self-focus; Hofmann and Barlow 2002), while other researchers have proposed multiple cognitive processes (e.g. different cognitive biases such as negative self-evaluations of social performance and attention towards social threat cues; Morris 2001). In the cases where multiple cognitive processes have been proposed, researchers have provided different accounts of how the processes are proposed to interact. For example, Higa-McMillan and Ebesutani (2011) proposed self-focus as the main cognitive process leading to SAD onset. However, they also noted that cognitive biases, while playing mainly a maintenance role for SAD, could also influence SAD development. Furthermore, Higa-McMillan and Ebesutani (2011) suggested that the increase in metacognitive ability (i.e. ability to consider own thoughts as well as the thoughts and perceptions of other people) during adolescence increases the risk of SAD onset across that developmental period. It is unclear though as to the point where normative developmental increases in self-centredness and metacognitive ability during adolescence (see Steinberg 2010) contribute to the experience of social anxiety and the emergence of the aberrant self-focused processing style that is relevant to SAD. More generally, it is also unclear from current theorising on cognitive factors that convey risk for SAD as to when proposed cognitive constructs emerge during development and influence SAD onset. Nonetheless, it appears from a theoretical perspective that cognitive maturation in general over childhood and adolescence makes it possible for proposed cognitive factors to emerge and convey risk for SAD onset in adolescence. Current theorising on cognitive factors and SAD vulnerability in adolescence would benefit from an integration of findings on the development of relevant cognitive processes in adolescence (e.g. perspective taking; Blakemore and Choudhury 2006).

Research

Currently, a number of cross-sectional studies have demonstrated that various cognitive constructs such as social-evaluative cognitions (e.g. beliefs), cognitive biases (e.g. threat interpretations, predictions of performance), and other relevant cognitive processes (e.g. self-focus, ruminative thinking and selective intentional forgetting) are all positively associated with SAD in samples of youth (e.g. Alfano et al. 2006; Cederlund and Öst 2011; Gomez-Ariza et al., 2013; Kley et al. 2012; Schmitz et al. 2010; Ranta et al. 2014; Rheingold et al. 2003; Spence et al. 1999; Tuschen-Caffier et al. 2011; see Miers et al. 2011 for a review) and adults (e.g. Abbott and Rapee 2004; Gros and Sarver 2014; Voncken and Bögels 2008; Wong et al. 2014). However, it is unclear in these studies whether the examined cognitive factors were present before the onset of SAD. Additionally, based on the cross-sectional nature of these studies, it is not possible to use them to evaluate the aetiological role of cognitive factors for SAD in adolescence. In contrast to the cross-sectional studies, one recent longitudinal study has examined whether particular cognitive factors may increase vulnerability to social anxiety during adolescence. Miers, Blöte, de Rooij, Bokhorst, and Westenberg (2013) identified three groups of nonclinical youth with different trajectories of social anxiety over the adolescent period: a high and changing trajectory, a moderate and decreasing trajectory, and a low and decreasing trajectory. Although there were both increases and decreases in social anxiety within the high and changing trajectory, the high trajectory was nonetheless maintained relative to the other identified trajectories. Relative to the moderate and decreasing trajectory group, those characterised by a high and changing trajectory showed higher levels of biased interpretation of ambiguous social situations and self-focus (during a speech task) at initial assessment. This result suggests that biased interpretations and self-focus may play more of a maintaining role for social anxiety, rather than an aetiological role. Overall, based on the current literature, it is evident that more longitudinal studies that provide a test of whether specific cognitive factors increase vulnerability to SAD are required. Studies of this sort, particular with their endpoint in the adolescent period, will be valuable for the evaluation of the aetiological significance of specific cognitive factors for SAD onset in adolescence.

Parent Factors

Theory

There is general support for the role of parent behaviours in the development of SAD (e.g. Kearney 2005; Rapee and Spence 2004). However, a variety of parenting behaviours have been proposed. For example, particular parenting styles (e.g. parenting characterised by overprotection, overcontrol, low warmth, or rejection) and certain parent-child attachment styles (e.g. insecure attachment) have been emphasised as factors that can increase vulnerability for SAD. However, such broad parent factors do not by themselves provide sufficient detail to indicate how they can convey risk for SAD. In contrast, parent-related learning mechanisms (e.g. modelling, information transfer) have been highlighted as important for the specific development of social-evaluative cognitions and behaviour and hence for increasing vulnerability to SAD (e.g. Kearney 2005; Rapee and Spence 2004). For example, parents can provide the basis for their child to acquire social-evaluative concerns (e.g. parents emphasise the opinions of others, parents express social-evaluative thoughts) and behaviours aimed to avoid social-evaluative situations (e.g. parents themselves engage in social avoidance, parents suggest avoidance as a solution to social problems). Based on current theorising on the role of parents in the development of SAD, it is assumed that risk for SAD is conveyed to a child as long as they are exposed to the types of parent factors discussed. Since adolescence is characterised by increasing independence from parents (Steinberg 2010), exposure to these parental factors may confer the most risk for the development of SAD during childhood with declining risk throughout adolescence. It should be noted that although parent behaviours that convey risk for SAD may be most influential during childhood, these behaviours may have effects in childhood that last into adolescence and confer risk for SAD onset during this period despite decreased exposure to parents (e.g. parental modelling of social avoidance for a child leads the child to avoid social situations as an adolescent despite reduced exposure to the parental modelling during adolescence).

Research

Existing studies on parent factors that convey risk for SAD has mainly examined broad parent factors (e.g. parenting style characterised by overprotection, overcontrol, low warmth, or rejection; insecure parent-child attachment), and there is less research that has examined specific parent-related learning mechanisms (e.g. information transfer, modelling). It is worthwhile to note though that parent-related learning mechanisms that convey specific risk for SAD may be an extension of broad parent factors. For example, one aspect of an overprotective and overcontrolling parenting style may manifest in a parent as specific behaviour that decreases their child's opportunities for social interaction, resulting in the modelling of social avoidance. In relation to broad parent factors, existing cross-sectional studies have shown that adolescents and adults with SAD retrospectively report that their parents were overprotective, controlling, rejecting, lacked emotional warmth, and critical (Antony et al. 1998; Arrindell et al. 1989; Bruch and Heimberg 1994; Juster et al. 1996; Knappe et al. 2009, 2012; Lieb et al. 2000; Rapee and Melville 1997; Taylor and Alden 2006) (For more details, see Chap. 3). Notably, these studies are based on retrospective reports of individuals already diagnosed with SAD and as such may be influenced by memory biases. Cross-sectional observational studies have been conducted though and have demonstrated that parents of socially anxious children were more negative and more controlling in their interactions with their children compared to parents of nonsocially anxious children (Greco and Morris 2002; Hummel and Gross 2001). One cross-sectional study with child participants has also demonstrated that secure attachment in childhood was negatively associated with social anxiety, while insecure attachment (specifically the disorganised type) in childhood was positively associated with social anxiety (Brumariu and Kerns 2010).

Importantly, in addition to the aforementioned cross-sectional studies, longitudinal studies exist in this area of research. One recent study has demonstrated that the association between consistently high behavioural inhibition in childhood and later social anxiety in the teen years was moderated by maternal parenting style characterised by overcontrol. That is, consistently high behavioural inhibition predicted higher social anxiety over time but only in the presence of high maternal overcontrol (Lewis-Morrarty et al. 2012). Other longitudinal studies have shown that relative to insecure parent-child attachment styles, secure attachment in early childhood predicted better social functioning and a tendency to experience lower levels of social anxiety in later childhood (Bar-Haim et al. 2007; Bohlin et al. 2000; Brumariu and Kerns 2008). Emotional overinvolvement, hostility and criticism are part of expressed emotion (EE) construct. Garcia-Lopez et al. (2009) found that parents with high levels of EE play a role in treatment outcome of social anxious adolescents. Last year, Garcia-Lopez et al. (2014) have found that the inclusion of parent training to reduce EE in a treatment program designed to address social anxiety in adolescents had a positive effect on their improvement, particularly when the parents' EE status changed from high to low expressed emotion after treatment.

In relation to parent-related learning mechanisms, cross-sectional studies have demonstrated that relative to non-anxious controls, adults with SAD reported that when they were growing up, their parents were more controlling of their socialisation experiences, were less encouraging of the family's sociability with others, were more concerned with the opinions of others, and engaged in less socialising themselves (Bruch and Heimberg 1994; Rapee and Melville 1997). Again, these studies are limited because they are based on retrospective reports of adults already diagnosed with SAD. In addition to these studies, there are longitudinal and experimental studies that have demonstrated that the expressed anxiety of mothers during an interaction with a stranger predicts child avoidance of the stranger (de Rosnay et al. 2006; Murray et al. 2008).

In sum, the longitudinal and experimental studies in this section provide evidence that exposure to certain parent factors is likely to lead a child to have higher levels of social anxiety later in time, such as during adolescence. Future studies with prospective longitudinal designs will need to further investigate whether exposure to these specific parent factors predicts a later diagnosis of SAD particularly during the adolescent period.

Life Events

Theory

Several theories propose that negative or traumatic life events, particularly those of a social nature (e.g. exposure to interpersonal conflict in the family; physical, emotional, or sexual abuse), can increase vulnerability to SAD (e.g. Hofmann and Barlow 2002; Kimbrel 2008). Such experiences may provide circumstances for the learning of social-evaluative fears and may include specific events (e.g. loss of a loved one) or events that occur over time (e.g. parental psychopathology). There is the suggestion in the literature that negative or traumatic life events may not convey a specific risk for SAD but may convey risk for psychopathology more generally (e.g. Rapee and Spence 2004). Life events that have the potential to convey risk for SAD are assumed to occur at any time during an individual's life.

Research

There are currently only cross-sectional studies that have examined negative or traumatic life events in relation to SAD. These studies have demonstrated a positive association between the self-reported experience of negative or traumatic life events and a diagnosis of SAD in samples of youth (Tiet et al. 2001) and adults (e.g. Chartier et al. 2001; Kuo et al. 2011; Magee 1999). However, these studies are limited in that they were based on retrospective reports of individuals already diagnosed with SAD, which may be subject to memory biases as well as interpretation biases characteristic of SAD (e.g. Gilboa-Schechtman et al. 2000; Voncken et al. 2003). Furthermore, these studies lacked a prospective longitudinal design which would allow an examination of whether negative or traumatic life events experienced actually predict later onset of SAD. For the study of SAD onset in adolescence, future research will need to conduct the sort of longitudinal study described with the study's endpoint during adolescence. We note that negative or traumatic experiences related to peers (e.g. bullying) will be discussed in the next section.

Peer Experiences

Theory

There is support for the proposal that negative peer experiences (e.g. ostracism, teasing, bullying) can contribute risk for the development of SAD (e.g. Garcia-Lopez et al. 2011; Kearney 2005; Morris 2001; Ranta et al. 2009, 2013). Similar to negative or traumatic life events, negative peer experiences theoretically provide the elements needed for the direct conditioning of social-evaluative fears. There is some suggestion in the literature that negative peer experiences are part of a vicious cycle that increases risk for SAD (e.g. Rapee and Spence 2004). For example, a child with a shy or behaviourally inhibited temperament is likely to appear withdrawn and socially anxious to their peers which in turn can lead to negative peer experiences. Experiences may include being isolated by peers or being teased by peers. The former isolating type of experience can prevent the child from experiencing habituating social experiences, while the latter type of social-evaluative experience can lead to the conditioning of social-evaluative fears. Ultimately, each type of negative peer experience contributes risk for SAD. Current theorising on the role of peer experiences in the development of SAD has emphasised peer experiences during childhood and adolescence. These developmental periods are associated with an increase in exposure to peers and new social settings (e.g. starting school during childhood, starting high school during adolescence, starting a job in adolescence, access to more social activities in adolescence; Steinberg 2010), and this provides opportunities for negative peer experiences to occur. From a theoretical perspective, adolescence is thus a developmental period where there is a greater likelihood for negative peer experiences to contribute risk for the onset of SAD. While theory has emphasised peer experiences in childhood and adolescence as being relevant to the development of SAD, it is unclear whether negative peer experiences during other life periods would also be similarly influential.

Research

Cross-sectional studies have demonstrated that SAD is associated with poor peer relationships. For example, studies have shown that children with SAD initiate and engage in fewer peer interactions (Beidel et al. 1999; Spence et al. 1999), while adults with SAD retrospectively report having fewer friends in childhood compared to nonclinical controls (Rapee and Melville 1997). Notably, there have been a larger number of cross-sectional studies that have looked at peer relationships in relation to social anxiety levels in nonclinical samples of youth. These studies have shown that higher levels of social anxiety are associated with having fewer friends, less intimate friendships, lower levels of peer acceptance, more negative peer and classmate interactions, increased peer- and self-reported victimisation, and higher levels of social withdrawal (Blöte et al. 2010; Blöte and Westenberg 2007; Erath et al. 2007; Garcia-Lopez, Irurtia, Caballo, and Diaz-Castela 2011; Greco and Morris 2005; La Greca and Harrison 2005; La Greca and Lopez 1998; Ranta et al. 2009, 2013). In prospective longitudinal studies of youth, negative peer experiences (such as relational victimisation [e.g. exclusion from peer experiences], overt victimisation [e.g. physical or verbal assault], and low peer acceptance) have been shown to predict higher levels of social anxiety over time (Loukas and Pasch 2013; Ranta et al. 2013; Siegel et al. 2009; Storch et al. 2005; Tillfors et al. 2012; Vernberg et al. 1992). These longitudinal studies provide evidence to support the suggestion that negative peer experiences can lead to later elevated social anxiety during adolescence. Future studies with prospective longitudinal designs will be required to examine whether exposure to negative peer experiences predicts a later diagnosis of SAD.

Performance Deficits

Theory

There is support for the proposal that performance deficits in social situations play an aetiological role for SAD (e.g. Kearney 2005; Rapee and Spence 2004). Most theoretical accounts highlight that such deficits may be due to state anxiety interfering with behaviour or due to a lack of age-appropriate social skills or knowledge. Performance deficits are thought to contribute to the development of SAD because the deficits can result in negative evaluation from other people, which provide circumstances for the conditioning of social-evaluative fears. This in turn contributes vulnerability for SAD. On the basis of existing theoretical accounts that discuss the role of performance deficits, it is unclear as to the causes of the state anxiety or lack of age-appropriate social skills/knowledge that are proposed to lead to the performance deficits. Nonetheless, potential causes for the state anxiety that interferes with social performance may include the stigmata of existing physical or health difficulties (e.g. stuttering, obesity, etc.) and potential causes for a lack of age-appropriate social skills or knowledge may include decreased exposure to social situations (e.g. due to overprotective parenting). Based on current theorising on the aetiological role of performance deficits for SAD onset, it is assumed that such deficits can occur at any time during an individual's life, and there is no suggestion that there is a greater likelihood of performance deficits occurring during adolescence compared with other developmental periods. However, the transition from childhood to adolescence is typically associated with an increase in social demands (e.g. from peers) and an increase in access to various new social environments (e.g. recreational, educational, and vocational settings; Steinberg 2010). Given the social pressures and novelty in these contexts, the transition to adolescence may be associated with a greater likelihood of performance deficits as well as potential for subsequent negative evaluation from others and thus a greater risk of SAD onset.

Research

Compared to non-anxious controls, youth with SAD exhibit poorer observer-rated performance on role-play, conversation, and speech/reading tasks (Alfano et al. 2006; Beidel et al. 1999, 2014; Inderbitzen-Nolan et al. 2007; Spence et al. 1999), although there are some exceptions (Tuschen-Caffier et al. 2011). The finding of performance deficits exhibited by individuals with SAD relative to controls has also been demonstrated in adult samples (Baker and Edelman 2002; Voncken and Bögels 2008). Notably, in the studies that have demonstrated performance deficits, it is unclear as to whether the relatively poor performance of individuals with SAD was due to interference from state anxiety or due to a lack of social skill or knowledge for the task at hand. Furthermore, it is unclear as to whether the individuals in the studies had experienced performance deficits in social-evaluative situations prior to the onset of SAD. Hence, it is difficult to tell from these studies whether performance deficits are a cause or consequence of social anxiety. Future studies will need prospective longitudinal designs to obtain better evidence to evaluate the aetiological role of performance deficits for SAD in adolescence.

General Learning Mechanisms

Theory

Although the emphasis in the literature is on parent-related learning mechanisms that convey risk for SAD (see section "Parent factors"), there is support for the role of learning mechanisms more generally that increase vulnerability for the disorder (e.g. Hofmann and Barlow 2002; Kearney 2005). These mechanisms include direct and indirect conditioning experiences. Examples of direct conditioning experiences that can convey risk for the development of SAD have already been discussed (see sections "Life events", "Peer experiences", and "Performance deficits"). Indirect conditioning experiences that convey risk for the development of SAD involve the acquisition of social fears via another person, such as through observation of their fear response (e.g. modelling; adolescent sees a peer who is being bullied) or through verbal communication (e.g. information transfer; adolescent listens to negative experience of peer being bullied). The learning processes specified are assumed to have the potential to occur at any time in one's life via different experiences (e.g. parenting, life events, peer experiences, performance deficits). Relevant to SAD onset in adolescence, it appears that greater independence from parents and increased exposure to peers and new social environments (e.g. recreational, educational, vocational) during this period (Steinberg 2010) may mean that parent-related learning processes are less likely to occur, while learning processes associated with peer experiences and performance deficits may be more likely to occur and convey risk for SAD onset.

Research

Besides research that has already been discussed in relation to learning processes (e.g. parent-related learning mechanisms; de Rosnay et al. 2006), there are conditioning studies that have directly examined the learning processes of individuals with SAD. Relative to healthy controls, adults with SAD exhibited a greater fear response to neutral faces that were conditioned with critical facial expressions and insults (Lissek et al. 2008). This finding suggests that SAD is associated with enhanced fear conditioning when socially relevant unconditioned stimuli are involved. However, the findings of this study contrast with other experimental studies that have not been able to demonstrate enhanced fear conditioning for adults with SAD, either when socially irrelevant unconditioned stimuli (Hermann et al. 2002; Schneider et al. 1999) or socially relevant unconditioned stimuli (Tinoco-González et al. 2014) are involved. In relation to these conditioning studies, future research will first need to clarify the inconsistent findings. Should evidence of reliable conditioning processes that are relevant to the aetiology of SAD emerge, prospective longitudinal studies will then need to be conducted to investigate whether such processes can predict a later diagnosis of SAD, particularly during adolescence.

Cultural Factors

Theory

Although culture has been proposed to contribute to the development of SAD (Rapee and Spence 2004), it is not a widely supported aetiological factor from a theoretical perspective. Rapee and Spence (2004) proposed that cultural norms can influence how social anxiety is expressed, the associated consequences, and the level of expressed social anxiety that is deemed as problematic and interfering with one's life. It is unclear from current theorising as to when cultural factors might exert their influence to affect the risk of SAD onset. However, given that cultural influences are present from birth and also affect the ways in which parents handle a child, it is likely that this influence begins relatively early. In relation to SAD onset in adolescence, there is currently no indication in the literature as to whether the risk of SAD onset during adolescence due to cultural factors would be any different from the risk of SAD onset from cultural factors during other developmental periods.

Research

There are currently only cross-sectional studies that have demonstrated an association between cultural factors and a diagnosis of SAD. One line of research (see Brockveld et al. 2014; Hofmann et al. 2010 for reviews) has demonstrated that the lifetime prevalence estimates of SAD are generally higher in Western regions of the world (e.g. 5.0–12.1 % in the USA, Grant et al. 2005; Kessler et al. 2005; 6.65 % in Europe, Fehm et al. 2005) compared to Middle Eastern countries (e.g. 0.82 %; Mohammadi et al. 2006) and Asian countries (e.g. 0.5 %; Lee et al. 1990). There are also cross-sectional studies that have looked specifically at ethnicity and SAD. These studies have shown that White Americans are more likely to be diagnosed with SAD compared to Asian Americans, Hispanic Americans, and African Americans (Asnaani et al. 2010; Breslau et al. 2006; Grant et al. 2005). One suggestion is that these cultural differences in diagnosis reflect differences in the life impact of social reticence, thereby influencing the assignment of a disorder (Rapee et al. 2011). For example, it has been found that a more positive attitude towards socially reticent behaviour among Eastern compared with Western populations is already applied from childhood (Chen et al. 1998, 2009). Overall, given the studies that have linked cultural factors (e.g. living in Western regions of the world, endorsing a Caucasian ethnicity) to SAD are cross-sectional in nature and have recruited individuals already with a diagnosis of SAD, it is difficult to tell whether the presence of these cultural factors contributes risk for the development of SAD. Future studies will need to employ prospective longitudinal designs to test whether the presence of certain cultural factors leads to later elevated social anxiety levels or a diagnosis of SAD. In relation to the onset of SAD in adolescence, longitudinal studies of the sort described will need to have their endpoint during the adolescent period.

Limitations of Existing Research on the Aetiology of SAD and Directions for Future Research

Several limitations of the existing research base on the aetiology of SAD have already been highlighted in previous sections. These limitations, together with some additional ones, will be summarised in this section. Based on the limitations of existing studies, directions for future research will be proposed with particular emphasis on issues relevant to the onset of SAD during adolescence.

Based on the current research reviewed in this chapter, it is evident that certain proposed aetiological factors for SAD have generally been more heavily studied (e.g. biological factors) compared with other factors (e.g. cultural factors). A more serious limitation is that the majority of research into proposed aetiological factors has utilised cross-sectional designs. Only half of the number of described factors have been studied using prospective longitudinal studies, and these types of studies have been in the minority. Temperament, parent factors, and peer experiences are the factors most commonly studied prospectively. Longitudinal studies have shown that childhood behavioural inhibition predicts higher social anxiety levels and a diagnosis of SAD both in later childhood and in adolescence (e.g. Clauss and Blackford 2012). Additionally, several parent factors including both parenting style (e.g. characterised by overcontrol or expressed anxiety) and parent-child attachment (e.g. insecure attachment) have been shown to play a role in the prediction of higher levels of later social anxiety and treatment outcome in youth (e.g. Bar-Haim et al. 2007;

Garcia-Lopez et al. 2009, 2014; Lewis-Morrarty et al. 2012). Finally, negative peer experiences during youth (e.g. relational or overt victimisation, low peer acceptance) have been shown to predict future increases in social anxiety (e.g. Ranta et al. 2013). At least two further longitudinal studies have evaluated the prediction of social anxiety in adolescence from cognitive factors (interpretation bias, self-focus; Miers et al. 2013) and a biological factor (event-related potentials; Battaglia et al. 2012), respectively. Longitudinal studies are of particular importance to evaluate whether the presence of a factor predicts future levels of social anxiety or a diagnosis of SAD. Hence, there is a need for future studies to recruit individuals without high levels of social anxiety or a diagnosis of SAD in order to test the predictive nature of proposed factors. Of course, ultimate conclusions about causality can only follow experimental manipulation of particular variables, a design that is especially difficult to apply to theories of the development of disorder. However, a variation of the experimental design, the use of highly targeted intervention, can help to indicate the causal status of variables especially when combined with longitudinal designs.

Based on the theoretical accounts of risk factors for SAD reviewed in this chapter, it is evident that most accounts point to the importance of interactions between relevant factors in the development of SAD (e.g. Higa-McMillan and Ebesutani 2011; Morris 2001; Rapee and Spence 2004). Indeed, there may be some factors that are more likely to interact with others. For example, in childhood, temperament may be more likely to interact with parent factors (e.g. Kiff et al. 2011; Lengua and Kovacs 2005; Rubin et al. 1999) and peer experiences (e.g. Sanson et al. 2004; Van Hecke et al. 2007) as opposed to other proposed aetiological factors. In relation to SAD onset in adolescence, significant developments in cognition and neurobiology during adolescence, together with increased exposure to peers and novel social environments (e.g. recreational, educational, vocational; Blakemore 2008; Blakemore and Choudhury 2006; Steinberg 2010) may mean that interactions between cognitive factors, biological factors, peer experiences, and performance deficits may be more likely. In addition, given the higher heritability of social anxiety in youth compared to adults (Scaini et al. 2014) and the substantial changes in social environments during adolescence that have been referred to, there may be an increased likelihood of gene-environment interactions that influence the onset of SAD during the adolescent period (see also Caspi and Moffitt 2006).

There are some existing longitudinal studies that have already demonstrated interactions between key variables. For example, as previously noted in relation to temperament and parent factors, Lewis-Morrarty and colleagues (2012) showed a significant link between consistently high behavioural inhibition during childhood and higher levels of social anxiety during adolescence in the presence of high maternal overcontrol, while there was no such link between behavioural inhibition and later social anxiety levels in the presence of low maternal overcontrol. As another example in relation to temperament and cognitive factors, although not specific to the prediction of social anxiety, Pérez-Edgar et al. (2010) demonstrated a link between consistently high behavioural inhibition during childhood and higher levels of later social withdrawal during adolescence but only for adolescents with an attentional bias towards social threat. Clearly, future research will need to take potentially complex interactions into account. On a related point, there is a lack of consideration of the role of protective factors in most current theories of the aetiology of SAD. This may be the case because protective factors are assumed to be the reverse of proposed risk factors. For example, avoidance of social-evaluative situations (e.g. due to parental modelling or encouragement) has been proposed to convey risk for SAD, and in contrast, exposure to such situations has been discussed as a protective factor for SAD (e.g. Kearney 2005; Kimbrel 2008). However, there may be protective factors that are not simply the reverse of proposed risk factors for SAD. To illustrate with an example in the context of peer experiences, there is evidence that the impact of peer victimisation is decreased when children have a close friendship (e.g. Hodges et al. 1999). In general, future longitudinal studies should take protective factors and their potential interactions with proposed aetiological factors into account.

As is evident in previous sections of this chapter, the timing of occurrence of proposed aetiological factors is important to consider. However, current theoretical accounts of proposed aetiological factors rarely provide a timeframe of influence for the factors. For example, although temperament is currently theorised to convey the most risk for SAD during childhood, it is unclear as to the developmental timeframe during which biological factors exert their influence on the risk of SAD. Besides the timing of the occurrence of aetiological factors, two other dimensions that the factors can vary on are duration and intensity (e.g. Higa-McMillan and Ebesutani 2011; Rapee and Spence 2004). Future longitudinal studies should take these dimensions into account from both a theoretical and empirical perspective (e.g. how will a factor's duration and intensity be operationalised?) when they examine aetiological factors.

Conclusions

SAD is a relatively common disorder with high societal and personal burden. Improved understanding of factors that maintain and provide risk for this disorder is critical to help reduce its impact. The development of a number of valuable models of the maintenance of SAD (e.g. Clark and Wells 1995; Rapee and Heimberg 1997) led to improved treatments that have increased effect sizes for the established disorder (Clark et al. 2006; Rapee et al. 2009). In a similar fashion, an understanding of the factors and their interactions that promote risk for SAD would help to develop efficacious intervention and prevention strategies. Existing theoretical accounts of the aetiology of SAD have highlighted several potential risk factors for the disorder. However, while there is evidence to suggest that the more commonly studied risk factors such as temperament, parent factors, and peer experiences play a role in the onset of SAD during adolescence, evidence to evaluate the aetiological role of the other proposed risk factors for SAD onset in adolescence has been lacking. Given the early age of onset and the chronic course of SAD, it is vital that the required research is conducted to enable a greater understanding of critical risk factors and the developmental stages at which they are most influential so that intervention and prevention strategies can be developed and enhanced. There are still many pieces of the puzzle to uncover.

We are still a long way from recognising all relevant risk and protective factors and especially their likely very complex interactions. With continued research, this complicated puzzle will begin to emerge.

References

Abbott MJ, Rapee RM (2004) Post-event rumination and negative self-appraisal in social phobia before and after treatment. J Abnorm Psychol 113:136–144. doi:10.1037/0021-843X.113.1.136

Alfano CA, Beidel DC, Turner SM (2006) Cognitive correlates of social phobia among children and adolescents. J Abnorm Child Psychol 34:189–201. doi:10.1007/s10802-005-9012-9

Amir N, Klumpp H, Elias J, Bedwell JS, Yanasak N, Miller LS (2005) Increased activation of the anterior cingulated cortex during processing of disgust faces in individuals with social phobia. Biol Psychiatry 57:975–981. doi:10.1016/j.biopsych.2005.01.044

Antony MM, Purdon CL, Huta V, Swinson RP (1998) Dimensions of perfectionism across the anxiety disorders. Behav Res Ther 36:1143–1154. doi:10.1016/S0005-7967(98)00083-7

Arbelle S, Benjamin J, Golin M, Kremer I, Belmaker RH, Ebstein RP (2003) Relation of shyness in grade school children to the genotype for the long form of the serotonin transporter promoter region polymorphism. Am J Psychiatry 160:671–676. doi:10.1176/appi.ajp.160.4.671

Arrindell WA, Kwee MG, Methorst GJ, van der Ende J, Pol E, Moritz BJ (1989) Perceived parental rearing styles of agoraphobic and socially phobic in-patients. Br J Psychiatry 155:526–535. doi:10.1192/bjp.155.4.526

Asnaani A, Richey JA, Dimaite R, Hinton DE, Hofmann SG (2010) A cross-ethnic comparison of lifetime prevalence rates of anxiety disorders. J Nerv Ment Dis 198:551–555. doi:10.1097/NMD.0b013e3181ea169f

Baker SR, Edelman RJ (2002) Is social phobia related to lack of social skills? Duration of skill-related behaviours and ratings of behavioural adequacy. Br J Clin Psychol 41:243–257. doi:10.1348/014466502760379118

Ballespi S, Jané MC, Riba MD (2012) Parent and Teacher Ratings of Temperamental Disposition to Social Anxiety: The BIS 3–6, J Personal Assess 94:164–174

Bar-Haim Y, Dan O, Eshel Y, Sagi-Schwartz A (2007) Predicting children's anxiety from early attachment relationships. J Anxiety Disord 21:1061–1068. doi:10.1016/j.janxdis.2006.10.013

Battaglia M, Zanoni A, Taddei M, Giorda R, Bertoletti E, Lampis V, Tettamanti M (2012) Cerebral responses to emotional expressions and the development of social anxiety disorder: a preliminary longitudinal study. Depress Anxiety 29:54–61. doi:10.1002/da.20896

Baur V, Brühl AB, Herwig U, Eberle T, Rufer M, Delsignore A, Jäncke L, Hänggi J (2013) Evidence of frontotemporal structural hypoconnectivity in social anxiety disorder: a quantitative fiber tractography study. Hum Brain Mapp 34:437–446. doi:10.1002/hbm.21447

Beatty MJ, Heisel AD, Hall AE, Levine TR, La France BH (2002) What can we learn from the study of twins about genetic and environmental influences on interpersonal affiliation, aggressiveness, and social anxiety?: a meta-analytic study. Commun Monogr 69:1–18. doi:10.1080/03637750216534

Beesdo K, Bittner A, Pine DS, Stein MB, Höfler M, Lieb R, Wittchen HU (2007) Incidence of social anxiety disorder and the consistent risk for secondary depression in the first three decades of life. Arch Gen Psychiatry 64:903–912. doi:10.1001/archpsyc.64.8.903

Beidel DC, Turner SM, Morris TL (1999) Psychopathology of childhood social phobia. J Am Acad Child Adolesc Psychiatry 38:643–650. doi:10.1097/00004583-199906000-00010

Beidel DC, Alfano CA, Kofler MJ, Rao, PA, Scharfstein L, Sarver, NW (2014). The impact of social skills training for social anxiety disorder: A randomized controlled trial. J Anxiety Disord 28:908–918

Biederman JA, Hirshfeld-Becker DR, Rosenbaum JF, Herot C, Friedman D, Snidman N, Kagan J, Faraone SV (2001) Further evidence of association between behavioural inhibition and social anxiety in children. Am J Psychiatry 158:1673–1679. doi:10.1176/appi.ajp.158.10.1673

Blair K, Geraci M, Devido J, McCaffrey D, Chen G, Vythilingam M, Ng P, Hollon N, Jones M, Blair RJ, Pine DS (2008) Neural response to self- and other referential praise and criticism in generalized social phobia. Arch Gen Psychiatry 65:1176–1184. doi:10.1001/archpsyc.65.10.1176

Blair KS, Geraci M, Hollon N, Otero M, DeVido J, Majestic C, Jacobs M, Blair RJ, Pine DS (2010) Social norm processing in adult social phobia: atypically increased ventromedial frontal cortex responsiveness to unintentional (embarrassing) transgressions. Am J Psychiatry 167:1526–1532. doi:10.1176/appi.ajp.2010.09121797

Blair KS, Geraci M, Otero M, Majestic K, Odenheimer S, Jacobs M, Blair RJ, Pine DS (2011) Atypical modulation of medial prefrontal cortex to self-referential comments in generalized social phobia. Psychiatry Res: Neuroimaging 193:38–45. doi:10.1016/j.pscychresns.2010.12.016

Blakemore S-J (2008) The social brain in adolescence. Nat Rev Neurosci 9:267–277. doi:10.1038/nrn2353

Blakemore S-J, Choudhury S (2006) Development of the adolescent brain: implications for executive function and social cognition. J Child Psychol Psychiatry 47:296–312. doi:10.1111/j.1469-7610.2006.01611.x

Blöte AW, Westenberg PM (2007) Socially anxious adolescents' perception of treatment by classmates. Behav Res Ther 45:189–198. doi:10.1016/j.brat.2006.02.002

Blöte AW, Duvekot J, Schalk RDF, Tuinenburg EM, Westenberg PM (2010) Nervousness and performance characteristics as predictors of peer behavior towards socially anxious adolescents. J Youth Adolesc 39:1498–1507. doi:10.1007/s10964-009-9463-3

Bohlin G, Hagekull B (2009) Socio-emotional development: from infancy to young adulthood. Scand J Psychol 50:592–601. doi:10.1111/j.1467-9450.2009.00787.x

Bohlin G, Hagekull B, Rydell AM (2000) Attachment and social functioning: a longitudinal study from infancy to middle childhood. Soc Dev 9:24–39. doi:10.1111/1467-9507.00109

Breslau J, Aguilar-Gaxiola S, Kendler KS, Su M, Williams D, Kessler RC (2006) Specifying race-ethnic differences in risk for psychiatric disorder in a USA national sample. Psychol Med 36:57–68. doi:10.1017/S0033291705006161

Brockveld KC, Perini SJ, Rapee RM (2014) Social anxiety and social anxiety disorder across cultures. In: Hofmann SG, DiBartolo PM (eds) Social anxiety: clinical, developmental, and social perspectives, 3rd edn. Elsevier, New York, pp 141–158

Bruch MA, Heimberg RG (1994) Differences in perceptions of parental and personal characteristics between generalized and nongeneralized social phobics. J Anxiety Disord 8:155–168. doi:10.1016/0887-6185(94)90013-2

Brumariu LE, Kerns KA (2008) Mother-child attachment and social anxiety symptoms in middle childhood. J Appl Dev Psychol 29:393–402. doi:10.1016/j.appdev.2008.06.002

Brumariu LE, Kerns KA (2010) Mother-child attachment patterns and different types of anxiety symptoms: is there specificity of relations? Child Psychiatry Hum Dev 41:663–674. doi:10.1007/s10578-010-0195-0

Caouette JD, Guyer AE (2014) Gaining insight into adolescent vulnerability for social anxiety from developmental cognitive neuroscience. Dev Cogn Neurosci 8:65–76. doi:10.1016/j.dcn.2013.10.003

Caspi A, Moffitt TE (2006) Gene-environment interactions in psychiatry: joining forces with neuroscience. Nat Rev Neurosci 7:583–590. doi:10.1038/nrn1925

Cederlund R, Öst LG (2011) Perception of threat in children with social phobia: comparison to nonsocially anxious children before and after treatment. J Clin Child Adolesc Psychol 40:855–863. doi:10.1080/15374416.2011.618448

Chartier MJ, Walker JR, Stein MB (2001) Social phobia and potential childhood risk factors in a community sample. Psychol Med 31:307–315. doi:10.1017/S0033291701003348

Chen X, Hastings PD, Rubin KH, Chen H, Cen G, Stewart SL (1998) Child-rearing attitudes and behavioral inhibition in Chinese and Canadian toddlers: a cross-cultural study. Dev Psychol 34:677–686. doi:10.1037/0012-1649.34.4.677

Chen X, Chen H, Li D, Wang L (2009) Early childhood behavioral inhibition and social and school adjustment in Chinese children: a 5-year longitudinal study. Child Dev 80:1692–1704. doi:10.1111/j.1467-8624.2009.01362.x

Chronis-Toscano A, Degnan KA, Pine DS, Perez-Edgar K, Henderson HA, Diaz Y, Raggi VL, Fox NA (2009) Stable early maternal report of behavioral inhibition predicts lifetime social anxiety disorder in adolescence. J Am Acad Child Adolesc Psychiatry 48:928–935. doi:10.1097/CHI.0b013e3181ae09df

Clark DM, Wells A (1995) A cognitive model of social phobia. In: Heimberg RG, Liebowitz MR, Hope DA, Schneier FR (eds) Social phobia: diagnosis, assessment, and treatment. The Guilford Press, New York, pp 69–93

Clark DM, Ehlers A, Hackmann A, McManus F, Fennell M, Grey N, Wild J (2006) Cognitive therapy versus exposure and applied relaxation in social phobia: a randomized controlled trial. J Consult Clin Psychol 74:568–578. doi:10.1037/0022-006X.74.3.568

Clauss JA, Blackford JU (2012) Behavioral inhibition and risk for developing social anxiety disorder: a meta-analytic study. J Am Acad Child Adolesc Psychiatry 51:1066–1075. doi:10.1016/j.jaac.2012.08.002

Condren RM, O'Neill A, Ryan MCM, Barrett P, Thakore JH (2002) HPA axis response to a psychological stressor in generalised social phobia. Psychoneuroendocrinology 27:693–703. doi:10.1016/S0306-4530(01)00070-1

Czajkowski N, Kendler KS, Tambs K, Røysamb E, Reichborn-Kjennerud T (2011) The structure of genetic and environmental risk factors for phobias in women. Psychol Med 41:1987–1995. doi:10.1017/S0033291710002436

Davidson RJ, Marshall JR, Tomarken AJ, Henriques JB (2000) While a phobic waits: regional brain electrical and autonomic activity in social phobics during anticipation of public speaking. Biol Psychiatry 47:85–95. doi:10.1016/S0006-3223(99)00222-X

de Rosnay M, Cooper PJ, Tsigaras N, Murray L (2006) Transmission of social anxiety from mother to infant: an experimental study using a social referencing paradigm. Behav Res Ther 44:1165–1175. doi:10.1016/j.brat.2005.09.003

Dilalla LF, Kagan J, Reznick JS (1994) Genetic etiology of behavioural inhibition among 2-year-old children. Infant Behav Dev 17:405–412. doi:10.1016/0163-6383(94)90032-9

Ding J, Chen H, Qiu C, Liao W, Warwick JM, Duan X, Zhang W, Gong Q (2011) Disrupted functional connectivity in social anxiety disorder: a resting-state fMRI study. Magn Reson Imaging 29:701–711. doi:10.1016/j.mri.2011.02.013

Donner J, Pirkola S, Silander K, Kananen L, Terwilliger JD, Lönnqvist J, Peltonen L, Hovatta I (2008) An association analysis of murine anxiety genes in humans implicates novel candidate genes for anxiety disorders. Biol Psychiatry 64:672–680. doi:10.1016/j.biopsych.2008.06.002

Edelman RJ, Baker SR (2002) Self-reported and actual physiological responses in social phobia. Br J Clin Psychol 41:1–14. doi:10.1348/014466502163732

Eley TC (1997) General genes: a new theme in developmental psychopathology. Curr Direct Psychol Sci 6:90–95. doi:10.1111/1467-8721.ep11512831

Eley TC, Bolton D, O'Connor TG, Perrin S, Smith P, Plomin R (2003) A twin study of anxiety-related behaviours in pre-school children. J Child Psychol Psychiatry 44:945–960. doi:10.1111/1469-7610.00179

Eley TC, Rijsdijk FV, Perrin S, O'Connor TG, Bolton D (2008) A multivariate genetic analysis of specific phobia, separation anxiety and social phobia in early childhood. J Abnorm Child Psychol 36:839–848. doi:10.1007/s10802-008-9216-x

Erath SA, Flanagan KS, Bierman KL (2007) Social anxiety and peer relations in early adolescence: behavioral and cognitive factors. J Abnorm Child Psychol 35:405–416. doi:10.1007/s10802-007-9099-2

Fehm L, Pelissolo A, Furmark T, Wittchen HU (2005) Size and burden of social phobia in Europe. Eur Neuropsychopharmacol 15:453–462. doi:10.1016/j.euroneuro.2005.04.002

Fouche J-P, van Der Wee NJA, Roelofs K, Stein DJ (2013) Recent advances in the brain imaging of social anxiety disorder. Hum Psychopharmacol: Clin Exp 28:102–105. doi:10.1002/hup.2281

Fox NA, Nichols KE, Henderson HA, Rubin K, Schmidt L, Hamer D, Ernst M, Pine DS (2005) Evidence for a gene-environment interaction in predicting behavioural inhibition in middle childhood. Psychol Sci 16:921–926. doi:10.1111/j.1467-9280.2005.01637.x

Freitas-Ferrari MC, Hallak JEC, Trzesniak C, Filho AS, Machado-de-Sousa JP, Chagas MHN, Nardi AE, Crippa JAS (2010) Neuroimaging in social anxiety disorder: a systematic review of the literature. Prog Neuropsychopharmacol Biol Psychiatry 34:565–580. doi:10.1016/j.pnpbp.2010.02.028

Furmark T, Tillfors M, Garpenstrand H, Marteinsdottir I, Långström B, Oreland L, Fredrikson M (2004) Serotonin transporter polymorphism related to amygdala excitability and symptom severity in patients with social phobia. Neurosci Lett 362:189–192. doi:10.1016/j.neulet.2004.02.070

Furmark T, Henningsson S, Appel L, Åhs F, Linnman C, Pissiota A, Faria V, Oreland L, Bani M, Pich EM, Eriksson E, Fredrikson M (2009) Genotype over-diagnosis in amygdala responsiveness: affective processing in social anxiety disorder. J Psychiatry Neurosci 34:30–40. Retrieved from http://www.cma.ca/publications/jpn

Garcia-Lopez LJ, Muela JA, Espinosa-Fernández L, Diaz-Castela MM (2009) Exploring the relevance of expressed emotion to the treatment of social anxiety disorder in adolescence. J Adolesc 32:1371–1376

Garcia-Lopez LJ, Irurtia MJ, Caballo VE, and Diaz-Castela MM (2011) Ansiedad social y abuso psicológico [Social anxiety and psychological abuse]. Behav Psychol 19:223–236

Garcia-Lopez LJ, Diaz-Castela MM, Muela-Martinez JA, Espinosa-Fernandez L (2014) Can parent training for parents with high levels of expressed emotion have a positive effect on their child's social anxiety improvement? J Anxiety Disord 28:812–822

Gelernter J, Page GP, Stein MB, Woods SW (2004) Genome-wide linkage scan for loci predisposing to social phobia: evidence for a chromosome 16 risk locus. Am J Psychiatry 161:59–66. doi:10.1176/appi.ajp.161.1.59

Gentili C, Ricciardi E, Gobbini MI, Santarelli MF, Haxby JV, Pietrini P, Guazzelli M (2009) Beyond amygdala: default mode network activity differs between patients with social phobia and healthy controls. Brain Res Bull 79:409–413. doi:10.1016/j.brainresbull.2009.02.002

Gilboa-Schechtman E, Franklin ME, Foa EB (2000) Anticipated reactions to social events: differences among individuals with generalized social phobia, obsessive compulsive disorder, and nonanxious controls. Cogn Ther Res 24:731–746. doi:10.1023/A:1005595513315

Gómez-Ariza, C.J., Iglesias-Parro, S., Garcia-Lopez, L.J., Díaz-Castela, M.M., Espinosa-Fernández, L., Muela, J.A., 2013. Selective intentional forgetting in adolescents with social anxiety disorder. Psychiatry Research 208, 151–155.

Grant BF, Hasin DS, Blanco C, Stinson FS, Chou P, Goldstein RB, Dawson DA, Smith S, Saha TD, Huang B (2005) The epidemiology of social anxiety disorder in the United States: results from the national epidemiologic survey on alcohol and related conditions. J Clin Psychiatry 66:1351–1361. doi:10.4088/JCP.v66n1102

Greco LA, Morris TL (2002) Paternal child-rearing style and child social anxiety: investigation of child perceptions and actual father behaviour. J Psychopathol Behav Assess 24:259–267. doi:10.1023/A:1020779000183

Greco LA, Morris TL (2005) Factors influencing the link between social anxiety and peer acceptance: contributions of social skills and close friendships during middle childhood. Behav Ther 36:197–205. doi:10.1016/S0005-7894(05)80068-1

Gros DF, Sarver NW (2014) An investigation of the psychometric properties of the Social Thoughts and Beliefs Scale (STABS) and structure of cognitive symptoms in participants with social anxiety disorder and healthy controls. J Anxiety Disord 28:283–290. doi:10.1016/j.janxdis.2014.01.004

Hattingh CJ, Ipser J, Tromp SA, Syal S, Locher C, Brooks SJ, Stein DJ (2013) Functional magnetic resonance imaging during emotion recognition in social anxiety disorder: an activation likelihood meta-analysis. Front Hum Neurosci 6:1–7. doi:10.3389/fnhum.2012.00347

Hayward C, Killen JD, Kraemer HC, Taylor CB (1998) Linking self-reported childhood behavioural inhibition to adolescent social phobia. J Am Acad Child Adolesc Psychiatry 37:1308–1316. doi:10.1097/00004583-199812000-00015

Hermann C, Ziegler S, Birbaumer N, Flor H (2002) Psychophysiological and subjective indicators of aversive Pavlovian conditioning in generalized social phobia. Biol Psychiatry 52:328–337. doi:10.1016/S0006-3223(02)01385-9

Hettema JM, An SS, Neale MC, Bukszar J, van den Oord EJCG, Kendler KS, Chen X (2006a) Association between glutamic acid decarboxylase genes and anxiety disorders, major depression, and neuroticism. Mol Psychiatry 11:752–762. doi:10.1038/sj.mp.4001845

Hettema JM, Neale MC, Myers JM, Prescott CA, Kendler KS (2006b) A population-based twin study of the relationship between neuroticism and internalizing disorders. Am J Psychiatry 163:857–864. Retrieved from http://ajp.psychiatryonline.org/

Higa-McMillan CK, Ebesutani C (2011) The aetiology of social anxiety disorder in adolescents and young adults. In: Alfano CA, Beidel DC (eds) Social anxiety in adolescents and young adults: translating developmental science into practice. American Psychological Association, Washington, DC, pp 29–51

Hirshfeld-Becker DR, Biederman J, Henin A, Faraone SV, Davis S, Harrington K, Rosenbaum JF (2007) Behavioral inhibition in preschool children at risk is a specific predictor of middle childhood social anxiety: a five-year follow-up. J Dev Behav Pediatr 28:225–233. doi:10.1097/01.DBP.0000268559.34463.d0

Hodges EVE, Boivin M, Vitaro F, Bukowski WM (1999) The power of friendship: protection against an escalating cycle of peer victimization. Dev Psychol 35:94–101. doi:10.1037/0012-1649.35.1.94

Hofmann SG, Barlow DH (2002) Social phobia (social anxiety disorder). In: Barlow DH (ed) Anxiety and its disorders: the nature and treatment of anxiety and panic, 2nd edn. The Guilford Press, New York, pp 454–476

Hofmann SG, Asnaani A, Hinton DE (2010) Cultural aspects in social anxiety and social anxiety disorder. Depress Anxiety 27:1117–1127. doi:10.1002/da.20759

Hudson JL, Dodd HF, Lyneham HJ, Bovopoulous N (2011) Temperament and family environment in the development of anxiety disorders: two-year follow-up. J Am Acad Child Adolesc Psychiatry 50:1255–1264. doi:10.1016/j.jaac.2011.09.009

Hummel RM, Gross AM (2001) Socially anxious children: an observational study of parent–child interaction. Child Fam Beh Ther 23:19–40. doi:10.1300/J019v23n03_02

Inderbitzen-Nolan HM, Anderson ER, Johnson HS (2007) Subjective versus objective behavioral ratings following two analogue tasks: a comparison of socially phobic and non-anxious adolescents. J Anxiety Disord 21:76–90. doi:10.1016/j.janxdis.2006.03.013

Juster HR, Heimberg RG, Frost RO, Hold CS, Mattia JI, Faccenda K (1996) Social phobia and perfectionism. Pers Indiv Differ 21:403–410. doi:10.1016/0191-8869(96)00075-X

Kagan J (1989) Temperamental contributions to social behavior. Am Psychol 44:668–674. doi:10.1037/0003-066x.44.4.668

Kashdan TB, Herbert JD (2001) Social anxiety disorder in childhood and adolescence: current status and future directions. Clin Child Fam Psychol Rev 4:37–61. doi:10.1023/A:1009576610507

Kearney CA (2005) Social anxiety and social phobia in youth: characteristics, assessment, and psychological treatment. Springer Science, New York

Kendler KS, Neale MC, Kessler RC, Heath AC, Eaves LJ (1992) The genetic epidemiology of phobias in women: the interrelationship of agoraphobia, social phobia, situational phobia, and simple phobia. Arch Gen Psychiatry 49:273–281. doi:10.1001/archpsyc.1992.01820040025003

Kendler KS, Karkowski LM, Prescott CA (1999) Fears and phobias: reliability and heritability. Psychol Med 29:539–553. Retrieved from http://journals.cambridge.org/action/displayJournal?jid=PSM

Kendler KS, Myers J, Prescott CA, Neale MC (2001) The genetic epidemiology of irrational fears and phobias in men. Arch Gen Psychiatry 58:257–265. doi:10.1001/archpsyc.58.3.257

Kennedy JL, Neves-Pereira M, King N, Lizak MV, Basile VS, Chartier MJ, Stein MB (2001) Dopamine system genes not linked to social phobia. Psychiatr Genet 11:213–217. Retrieved from http://journals.lww.com/psychgenetics

Kessler RC, Berglund P, Demler O, Jin R, Merikangas KR, Walters EE (2005) Lifetime prevalence and age-of-onset distributions of DSM-IV disorders in the national comorbidity survey replication. Arch Gen Psychiatry 62:593–602. doi:10.1001/archpsyc.62.6.593

Kiff CJ, Lengua LJ, Zalewski M (2011) Nature and nurturing: parenting in the context of child temperament. Clin Child Fam Psychol Rev 14:251–301. doi:10.1007/s10567-011-0093-4
Kimbrel NA (2008) A model of the development and maintenance of generalized social phobia. Clin Psychol Rev 28:592–612. doi:10.1016/j.cpr.2007.08.003
Kley H, Tuschen-Caffier B, Heinrichs N (2012) Safety behaviors, self-focused attention and negative thinking in children with social anxiety disorder, socially anxious and non-anxious children. J Behav Ther Exp Psychiatry 43:548–555. doi:10.1016/j.jbtep.2011.07.008
Klumpp H, Angstadt M, Phan KL (2012) Insula reactivity and connectivity to anterior cingulate cortex when processing threat in generalized social anxiety disorder. Biol Psychol 89:273–276. doi:10.1016/j.biopsycho.2011.10.010
Klumpp H, Fitzgerald DA, Cook E, Shankman SA, Angstadt M, Phan KL (2014) Serotonin transporter gene alters insula activity to threat in social anxiety disorder. NeuroReport 25:926–931. doi:10.1097/WNR.0000000000000210
Knappe S, Beesdo K, Fehm L, Höfler M, Lieb R, Wittchen HU (2009) Do parental psychopathology and unfavourable family environment predict the persistence of social phobia? J Anxiety Disord 23:986–994. doi:10.1016/j.janxdis.2009.06.010
Knappe S, Beesdo-Baum K, Fehm L, Lieb R, Wittchen HU (2012) Characterizing the association between parenting and adolescent social phobia. J Anxiety Disord 26:608–616. doi:10.1016/j.janxdis.2012.02.014
Kolassa I-T, Miltner WHR (2006) Psychophysiological correlates of face processing in social phobia. Brain Res 1118:130–141. doi:10.1016/j.brainres.2006.08.019
Kolassa I-T, Kolassa S, Musial F, Miltner WHR (2007) Event-related potentials to schematic faces in social phobia. Cogn Emot 21:1721–1744. doi:10.1080/02699930701229189
Kolassa I-T, Kolassa S, Bergmann S, Lauche R, Dilger S, Miltner WHR, Musial F (2009) Interpretive bias in social phobia: an ERP study with morphed emotional schematic faces. Cogn Emot 23:69–95. doi:10.1080/02699930801940461
Krämer M, Seefeldt WL, Heinrichs N, Tuschen-Caffier B, Schmitz J, Wolf OT, Blechert J (2012) Subjective, autonomic, and endocrine reactivity during social stress in children with social phobia. J Abnorm Child Psychol 40:95–104. doi:10.1007/s10802-011-9548-9
Kuo JR, Goldin PR, Werner K, Heimberg RG, Gross JJ (2011) Childhood trauma and current psychological functioning in adults with social anxiety disorder. J Anxiety Disord 25:467–473. doi:10.1016/j.janxdis.2010.11.011
La Greca AM, Harrison HM (2005) Adolescent peer relations, friendships, and romantic relationships: do they predict social anxiety and depression? J Clin Child Adolesc Psychol 34:49–61. doi:10.1207/s15374424jccp3401_5
La Greca AM, Lopez N (1998) Social anxiety among adolescents: linkages with peer relations and friendships. J Abnorm Child Psychol 26:83–94. doi:10.1023/A:1022684520514
Lanzenberger RR, Mitterhauser M, Spindelegger C, Wadsak W, Klein N, Mien LK, Holik A, Attarbaschi T, Mossaheb N, Sacher J, Geiss-Granadia T, Kletter K, Kasper S, Tauscher J (2007) Reduced serotonin-1A receptor binding in social anxiety disorder. Biol Psychiatry 61:1081–1089. doi:10.1016/j.biopsych.2006.05.022
Lee CK, Kwak YS, Yamamoto J, Rhee H, Kim YS, Han JH, Choi JO, Lee YH (1990) Psychiatric epidemiology in Korea: I. Gender and age differences in Seoul. J Nerv Ment Dis 178:242–246. doi:10.1097/00005053-199004000-00004
Lengua LJ, Kovacs EA (2005) Bidirectional associations between temperament and parenting and the prediction of adjustment problems in middle childhood. Appl Dev Psychol 26:21–38. doi:10.1016/j.appdev.2004.10.001
Lenzenweger MF (2013) Thinking clearly about the endophenotype–intermediate phenotype–biomarker distinctions in developmental psychopathology research. Dev Psychopathol 25:1347–1357. doi:10.1017/S0954579413000655
Lewis-Morrarty E, Degnan KA, Chronis-Tuscano A, Rubin KH, Cheah CSL, Pine DS, Henderon HA, Fox NA (2012) Maternal over-control moderates the association between early childhood behavioral inhibition and adolescent social anxiety symptoms. J Abnorm Child Psychol 40:1363–1373. doi:10.1007/s10802-012-9663-2

Lieb R, Wittchen HU, Höfler M, Fuetsch M, Stein MB, Merikangas KR (2000) Parental psychopathology, parenting styles, and the risk of social phobia in offspring: a prospective-longitudinal community study. Arch Gen Psychiatry 57:859–866. doi:10.1001/archpsyc.57.9.859

Lissek S, Levenson J, Biggs AL, Johnson LL, Ameli R, Pine DS, Grillon C (2008) Elevated fear conditioning to socially relevant unconditioned stimuli in social anxiety disorder. Am J Psychiatry 165:124–132. doi:10.1176/appi.ajp.2007.06091513

Lochner C, Hemmings S, Seedat S, Kinnear C, Schoeman R, Annerbrink K, Olsson M, Eriksson E, Moolman-Smook J, Allgulander C, Stein DJ (2007) Genetics and personality traits in patients with social anxiety disorder: a case–control study in South Africa. Eur Neuropsychopharmacol 17:321–327. doi:10.1016/j.euroneuro.2006.06.010

Loukas A, Pasch KE (2013) Does school connectedness buffer the impact of peer victimization on early adolescents' subsequent adjustment problems? J Early Adolesc 33:245–266. doi:10.1177/0272431611435117

Magee WJ (1999) Effects of negative life experiences on phobia onset. Soc Psychiatry Psychiatr Epidemiol 34:343–351. doi:10.1007/s001270050154

Martel FL, Hayward C, Lyons DM, Sanborn K, Varady S, Schatzberg AF (1999) Salivary cortisol levels in socially phobic adolescent girls. Depress Anxiety 10:25–27. doi:10.1002/(SICI)1520-6394(1999)10:1<25::AID-DA4>3.0.CO;2-O

Mick MA, Telch MJ (1998) Social anxiety and history of behavioral inhibition in young adults. J Anxiety Disord 12:1–20. doi:10.1016/S0887-6185(97)00046-7

Miers AC, Blöte AW, Westenberg PM (2011) Negative social cognitions in socially anxious youth: distorted reality or a kernel of truth? J Child Fam Stud 20:214–223. doi:10.1007/s10826-010-9423-2

Miers AC, Blöte AW, de Rooij M, Bokhorst CL, Westenberg PM (2013) Trajectories of social anxiety during adolescence and relations with cognition, social competence, and temperament. J Abnorm Child Psychol 41:97–110. doi:10.1007/s10802-012-9651-6

Mohammadi MR, Ghanizadeh A, Mohammadi M, Mesgarpour B (2006) Prevalence of social phobia and its comorbidity with psychiatric disorders in Iran. Depress Anxiety 23:405–411. doi:10.1002/da.20129

Morris TL (2001) Social phobia. In: Vasey MW, Dadds MR (eds) The developmental psychopathology of anxiety. Oxford University Press, Oxford, pp 435–458

Mueller EM, Hofmann SG, Santesso DL, Meuret AE, Bitran S, Pizzagalli DA (2009) Electrophysiological evidence of attentional biases in social anxiety disorder. Psychol Med 39:1141–1152. doi:10.1017/S0033291708004820

Muris P, van Brakel AML, Arntz A, Schouten E (2011) Behavioral inhibition as a risk factor for the development of childhood anxiety disorders: a longitudinal study. J Child Fam Stud 20:157–170. doi:10.1007/s10826-010-9365-8

Murray L, de Rosnay M, Pearson J, Bergeron C, Schofield E, Royal-Lawson M, Cooper PJ (2008) Intergenerational transmission of social anxiety: the role of social referencing processes in infancy. Child Dev 79:1049–1064. doi:10.1111/j.1467-8624.2008.01175.x

Ollendick TH, Benoit KE (2012) A parent–child interactional model of social anxiety disorder in youth. Clin Child Fam Psychol Rev 15:81–91. doi:10.1007/s10567-011-0108-1

Ollendick TH, Hirshfeld-Becker DR (2002) The developmental psychopathology of social anxiety disorder. Biol Psychiatry 51:44–58. doi:10.1016/S0006-3223(01)01305-1

Pannekoek JN, Veer IM, van Tol MJ, van der Werff SJA, Demenescu LR, Aleman A, Veltman DJ, Zitman FG, Rombouts SA, van der Wee NJA (2013) Resting-state functional connectivity abnormalities in limbic and salience networks in social anxiety disorder without comorbidity. Eur Neuropsychopharmacol 23:186–195. doi:10.1016/j.euroneuro.2012.04.018

Pérez-Edgar K, Bar-Haim Y, McDermott JM, Chronis-Tuscano A, Pine DS, Fox NA (2010) Attention biases to threat and behavioral inhibition in early childhood shape adolescent social withdrawal. Emotion 10:349–357. doi:10.1037/a0018486

Phan KL, Fitzgerald DA, Cortese BM, Seraji-Bozorgzad N, Tancer ME, Moore GJ (2005) Anterior cingulated neurochemistry in social anxiety disorder: 1H-MRS at 4 Tesla. NeuroReport 16:183–186. Retrieved from http://journals.lww.com/neuroreport

Pollack MH, Jensen JE, Simon NM, Kaufman RE, Renshaw PF (2008) High-field MRS study of GABA, glutamate and glutamine in social anxiety disorder: response to treatment with levetiracetam. Prog Neuropsychopharmacol Biol Psychiatry 32:739–743. doi:10.1016/j.pnpbp.2007.11.023
Ranta K, Kaltiala-Heino R, Pelkonen M, Marttunen M (2009) Associations between peer victimization, self-reported depression and social phobia among adolescents: the role of comorbidity. J Adolesc 32:77–93. doi:10.1016/j.adolescence.2007.11.005
Ranta K, Kaltiala-Heino R, Fröjd S, Marttunen M (2013) Peer victimization and social phobia: a follow-up study among adolescents. Soc Psychiatry Psychiatr Epidemiol 48:533–544. doi:10.1007/s00127-012-0583-9
Ranta K, Tuomisto MT, Kaltiala-Heino R, Rantanen P, Marttunen M (2014) Cognition, imagery and coping among adolescents with social anxiety and phobia: testing the Clark and Wells model in the population. Clin Psychol Psychother 21:252–263. doi:10.1002/cpp.1833
Rapee RM (2014) Preschool environment and temperament as predictors of social and nonsocial anxiety disorders in middle adolescence. J Am Acad Child Adolesc Psychiatry 53:320–328. doi:10.1016/j.jaac.2013.11.014
Rapee RM, Coplan RJ (2010) Conceptual relations between anxiety disorder and fearful temperament. New Dir Child Adolesc Dev 127:17–31. doi:10.1002/cd.260
Rapee RM, Heimberg RG (1997) A cognitive-behavioral model of anxiety in social phobia. Behav Res Ther 35:741–756. doi:10.1016/S0005-7967(97)00022-3
Rapee RM, Melville LF (1997) Recall of family factors in social phobia and panic disorder: comparison of mother and offspring reports. Depress Anxiety 5:7–11. doi:10.1002/(SICI)1520-6394(1997)5:1<7::AID-DA2>3.0.CO;2-E
Rapee RM, Spence SH (2004) The aetiology of social phobia: empirical evidence and an initial model. Clin Psychol Rev 24:737–767. doi:10.1016/j.cpr.2004.06.004
Rapee RM, Gaston JE, Abbott MJ (2009) Testing the efficacy of theoretically-derived improvements in the treatment of social phobia. J Consult Clin Psychol 77:317–327. doi:10.1037/a0014800
Rapee RM, Kim J, Wang J, Liu X, Hofmann SG, Chen J, Oh KY, Bögels SM, Arman S, Heinrichs N, Alden LE (2011) Perceived impact of socially anxious behaviours on individuals' lives in Western and East Asian countries. Behav Ther 42:485–492. doi:10.1016/j.beth.2010.11.004
Reinelt E, Stopsack M, Aldinger M, John U, Grabe HJ, Barnow S (2013) Testing the diathesis-stress model: 5- HTTLPR, childhood emotional maltreatment, and vulnerability to social anxiety disorder. Am J Med Genet 162B:253–261. doi:10.1002/ajmg.b.32142
Rheingold AA, Herbert JD, Franklin ME (2003) Cognitive bias in adolescents with social anxiety disorder. Cogn Ther Res 27:639–655. doi:10.1023/A:1026399627766
Rothbart MK, Ahadi SA, Evans DE (2000) Temperament and personality: origins and outcomes. J Pers Soc Psychol 78:122–135. doi:10.1037/0022-3514.78.1.122
Rowe DC, Stever C, Gard JMC, Cleveland HH, Sanders ML, Abramowitz A, Kozol ST, Mohr JH, Sherman SL, Waldman ID (1998) The relation of the dopamine transporter gene (DAT1) to symptoms of internalizing disorders in children. Behav Genet 28:215–225. doi:10.1023/A:1021427314941
Rubin KH, Nelson LJ, Hastings P, Asendorpf J (1999) The transaction between parents' perceptions of their children's shyness and their parenting styles. Int J Behav Dev 23:937–957. doi:10.1080/016502599383612
Sanson A, Hemphill SA, Smart D (2004) Connections between temperament and social development: a review. Soc Dev 13:142–170. doi:10.1046/j.1467-9507.2004.00261.x
Sareen J, Campbell DW, Leslie WD, Malisza KL, Stein MB, Paulus MP, Kravetsky LB, Kjernisted KD, Walker JR, Reiss JP, Reiss JP (2007) Striatal function in generalized social phobia: a functional magnetic resonance imaging study. Biol Psychiatry 61:396–404. doi:10.1016/j.biopsych.2006.05.043
Scaini S, Belotti R, Ogliari A (2014) Genetic and environmental contributions to social anxiety across different ages: a meta-analytic approach to twin data. J Anxiety Disord 28:650–656. doi:10.1016/j.janxdis.2014.07.002

Schmitz TW, Kawahara-Baccus TN, Johnson SC (2004) Metacognitive evaluation, self-relevance, and the right prefrontal cortex. Neuroimage 22:941–947. doi:10.1016/j.neuroimage.2004.02.018

Schmitz J, Krämer M, Blechert J, Tuschen-Caffier B (2010) Post-event processing in children with social phobia. J Abnorm Child Psychol 38:911–919. doi:10.1007/s10802-010-9421-2

Schneider F, Weiss U, Kessler C, Müller-Gärtner HW, Posse S, Salloum JB, Grodd W, Himmelmann F, Gaebel W, Birbaumer N (1999) Subcortical correlates of differential classical conditioning of aversive emotional reactions in social phobia. Biol Psychiatry 45:863–871. doi:10.1016/S0006-3223(98)00269-8

Schneier FR, Liebowitz MR, Abi-Dargham A, Zea-Ponce Y, Lin SH, Laruelle M (2000) Low dopamine D2 receptor binding potential in social phobia. Am J Psychiatry 157:457–459. doi:10.1176/appi.ajp.157.3.457

Schwartz CE, Snidman N, Kagan J (1999) Adolescent social anxiety as an outcome of inhibited temperament in childhood. J Am Acad Child Adolesc Psychiatry 38:1008–1015. doi:10.1097/00004583-199908000-00017

Shin LM, Liberzon I (2010) The neurocircuitry of fear, stress, and anxiety disorders. Neuropsychopharmacology 35:169–191. doi:10.1038/npp.2009.83

Siegel RS, La Greca AM, Harrison HM (2009) Peer victimization and social anxiety in adolescents: prospective and reciprocal relationships. J Youth Adolesc 38:1096–1109. doi:10.1007/s10964-009-9392-1

Sipilä T, Kananen L, Greco D, Donner J, Silander K, Terwilliger JD, Auvinen P, Peltonen L, Lönnqvist J, Pirkola S, Partonen T, Hovatta I (2010) An association analysis of circadian genes in anxiety disorders. Biol Psychiatry 67:1163–1170. doi:10.1016/j.biopsych.2009.12.011

Skre I, Onstad S, Torgersen S, Lygren S, Kringlen E (1993) A twin study of DSM-III-R anxiety disorders. Acta Psychiatr Scand 88:85–92. doi:10.1111/j.1600-0447.1993.tb03419.x

Smoller JW, Rosenbaum JF, Biederman J, Kennedy J, Dai D, Racette SR, Laird NM, Kagan J, Snidman N, Hirshfeld-Becker D, Tsuang MT, Sklar PB, Slaugenhaupt SA (2003) Association of a genetic marker at the corticotropin-releasing hormone locus with behavioral inhibition. Biol Psychiatry 54:1376–1381. doi:10.1016/S0006-3223(03)00598-5

Smoller JW, Yamaki LH, Fagerness JA, Biederman J, Racette S, Laird NM, Kagan J, Snidman N, Faraone SV, Hirshfeld-Becker D, Tsuang MT, Slaugenhaupt SA, Rosenbaum JF, Sklar PB (2005) The corticotropin-releasing hormone gene and behavioral inhibition in children at risk for panic disorder. Biol Psychiatry 57:1485–1492. doi:10.1016/j.biopsych.2005.02.018

Spence SH, Donovan C, Brechman-Toussaint M (1999) Social skills, social outcomes, and cognitive features of childhood social phobia. J Abnorm Psychol 108:211–221. doi:10.1037/0021-843X.108.2.211

Stein MB, Chartier MJ, Kozak MV, King N, Kennedy JL (1998) Genetic linkage to the serotonin transporter protein and 5HT2A receptor genes excluded in generalized social phobia. Psychiatry Res 81:283–291. doi:10.1016/S0165-1781(98)00117-6

Stein MB, Jang KL, Livesley WJ (2002) Heritability of social anxiety-related concerns and personality characteristics: a twin study. J Nerv Ment Dis 190:219–224. doi:10.1097/01.NMD.0000012869.70943.98

Stein MB, Schork NJ, Gelernter J (2004) Polymorphism of the β1-adrenergic receptor is associated with low extraversion. Biol Psychiatry 56:217–224. doi:10.1016/j.biopsych.2004.05.020

Steinberg L (2005) Cognitive and affective development in adolescence. Trends Cogn Sci 9:69–74. doi:10.1016/j.tics.2004.12.005

Steinberg L (2010) Adolescence, 9th edn. McGraw-Hill, New York

Storch EA, Masia-Warner C, Crisp H, Klein RG (2005) Peer victimization and social anxiety in adolescence: a prospective study. Aggress Behav 31:437–452. doi:10.1002/ab.20093

Taylor CT, Alden LE (2006) Parental overprotection and interpersonal behavior in generalized social phobia. Behav Ther 37:14–24. doi:10.1016/j.beth.2005.03.001

Tiet QQ, Bird HR, Hoven CW, Moore R, Wu P, Wicks J, Jensen PS, Goodman S, Cohen P (2001) Relationship between specific adverse life events and psychiatric disorders. J Abnorm Child Psychol 29:153–164. doi:10.1023/A:1005288130494

Tiihonen J, Kuikka J, Bergström K, Lepola U, Koponen H, Leinonen E (1997) Dopamine reuptake site densities in patients with social phobia. Am J Psychiatry 154:239–242. Retrieved from http://ajp.psychiatryonline.org/

Tillfors M, Persson S, Willén M, Burk WJ (2012) Prospective links between social anxiety and adolescent peer relations. J Adolesc 35:1255–1263. doi:10.1016/j.adolescence.2012.04.008

Tinoco-González D, Fullana MA, Torrents-Rodas D, Bonillo A, Vervliet B, Pailhez G, Farré M, Andión O, Perez V, Torrubia R (2014) Conditioned subjective responses to socially relevant stimuli in social anxiety disorder and subclinical social anxiety. Clin Psychol Psychother. doi:10.1002/cpp.1883

Tuschen-Caffier B, Kühl S, Bender C (2011) Cognitive-evaluative features of childhood social anxiety in a performance task. J Behav Ther Exp Psychiatry 42:233–239. doi:10.1016/j.jbtep.2010.12.005

van der Wee NJ, van Veen JF, Stevens H, van Vliet IM, van Rijk PP, Westenberg HG (2008) Increased serotonin and dopamine transporter binding in psychotropic medication-naive patients with generalized social anxiety disorder shown by ^{123}I-β-(4-iodophenyl)-tropane SPECT. J Nucl Med 49:757–763. doi:10.2967/jnumed.107.045518

Van Hecke AV, Mundy PC, Acra CF, Block JJ, Delgado CEF, Parlade MV, Meyer JA, Neal AR, Pomares YB (2007) Infant joint attention, temperament, and social competence in preschool children. Child Dev 78:53–69. doi:10.1111/j.14678624.2007.00985.x

Velting ON, Albano AM (2001) Current trends in the understanding and treatment of social phobia in youth. J Child Psychol Psychiatry 42:127–140. doi:10.1111/1469-7610.00705

Vernberg EM, Abwender DA, Ewell KK, Beery SH (1992) Social anxiety and peer relationships in early adolescence: a prospective analysis. J Clin Child Psychol 21:189–196. doi:10.1207/s15374424jccp2102_11

Voncken MJ, Bögels SM (2008) Social performance deficits in social anxiety disorder: reality during conversation and biased perception during speech. J Anxiety Disord 22:1384–1392. doi:10.1016/j.janxdis.2008.02.001

Voncken MJ, Bögels SM, de Vries K (2003) Interpretation and judgmental biases in social phobia. Behav Res Ther 41:1481–1488. doi:10.1016/S0005-7967(03)00143-8

Warren SL, Schmitz S, Emde RN (1999) Behavioral genetic analyses of self-reported anxiety at 7 years of age. J Am Acad Child Adolesc Psychiatry 38:1403–1408. doi:10.1097/00004583-199911000-00015

Wittchen HU, Stein MB, Kessler RC (1999) Social fears and social phobia in a community sample of adolescents and young adults: prevalence, risk factors and co-morbidity. Psychol Med 29:309–323. Retrieved from http://journals.cambridge.org/action/displayJournal?jid=PSM

Wong QJJ, Moulds ML, Rapee RM (2014) Validation of the self-beliefs related to social anxiety (SBSA) scale: a replication and extension. Assessment 21:300–311. doi:10.1177/1073191113485120

Developmental Epidemiology of Social Anxiety and Social Phobia in Adolescents

3

Susanne Knappe, Satoko Sasagawa, and Cathy Creswell

Prevalence of Social Anxiety Disorder and Social Fears in Western and Non-Western Countries

Social anxiety includes a spectrum of phenomena that may range from shyness to more or less isolated social fears up to the clinically relevant diagnostic prototype of SAD, sometimes also extending to avoidant or anxious personality disorder. Social fears may occur in only one or two situations but may also be more pervasive in a wider range of situations. They include performance fears such as fear of public speaking or speaking in front of others or taking tests and fears of being observed by others while writing in public, reading aloud, or eating and/or drinking in public. Other social fears relate to social interactions such as initiating and/or maintaining a conversation, talking to or dealing with others, using public restrooms, or going to (social) activities or participating in social events (APA 2000, 2013).

Contribution upon request for Ranta, K., La Greca, A. M., Garcia-Lopez, L.-J., Marttunen, M., (eds). *Social Anxiety and Phobia in Adolescents: Development, Manifestation and Intervention Strategies*. Springer.

S. Knappe (✉)
Institute of Clinical Psychology and Psychotherapy,
Technische Universität Dresden, Dresden, Germany
e-mail: susanne.knappe@tu-dresden.de

S. Sasagawa, PhD
Faculty of Human Sciences, Mejiro University, Tokyo, Japan
e-mail: sasagawa@mejiro.ac.jp

C. Creswell, BA (Ox) Hons, D Clin Psy, PhD
School of Psychology and Clinical Language Sciences,
University of Reading, Reading, Berkshire, UK
e-mail: c.creswell@reading.ac.uk

K. Ranta et al. (eds.), *Social Anxiety and Phobia in Adolescents: Development, Manifestation and Intervention Strategies*, DOI 10.1007/978-3-319-16703-9_3

Social Anxiety Disorder (SAD)

Social anxiety disorder (SAD) or social phobia is the most frequent anxiety disorder and the second most common of all DSM-IV disorders (Kessler et al. 2005b). Rates are higher in adults as compared to adolescents and children, but as implicated in the studies shown here, the differences between adults and adolescents are at least in part explained by methodological artifacts and the remaining differences are small.

About 13 % of the population meet the diagnostic criteria for SAD at some point in their life (Beesdo et al. 2007; Kessler et al. 1994), and mean lifetime prevalence is estimated at 6.7 % in European (Fehm et al. 2005) and up to 12.1 % in US samples (NCS-R; Kessler et al. 2005a). Twelve-month prevalence rates for SAD range from 0.4 (Neufeld et al. 1999) to 6.8 % (Chavira et al. 2004). Prevalence estimates generally vary across studies due to sampling and assessment strategies (screening tools or self-report measurements vs. standardized or structured interviews, please see Chap. 6), applied diagnostic criteria (DSM vs. ICD), or culture-bound forms of social anxiety such as taijin kyofusho (Kleinknecht et al. 1997) or hikikomori (Nagata et al. 2013). Lifetime rates range between 15.3 and 32.4 % in clinical samples (Last et al. 1992; Lépine et al. 1993; Zhang et al. 2004) and between 2.5 and 24.0 % in community samples (Fehm et al. 2005).

There is a lack of comparable studies in children and adolescents in non-Western countries, specifically East-Asian regions. However, studies among East-Asian adults have yielded lower SAD estimates ranging between 0.5 and 1.2 % according to DSM or ICD (Hwu et al. 1989; Tsuchiya et al. 2009; Kleinknecht et al. 1997; Lee et al. 2009). Of note, culture-specific forms of social anxiety are typically more frequent in the respective culture than DSM-defined social anxiety (Dinnel et al. 2002; Vriends et al. 2013; Lee et al. 2006). Hence, ethnic differences on self-reported social anxiety are likely attenuated when assessments consider views of the self that are typically associated with Western cultures (Hong and Woody 2007; Heinrichs et al. 2006; Essau et al. 2012) and when culture-specific assessment formats and evaluations of impairment are used (Hsu and Alden 2007). Lifetime prevalence estimates in childhood and adolescence are somewhat lower than for adults in Europe and the United States, where rates are up to 10 % (Merikangas et al. 2011; Beesdo et al. 2007; Feehan et al. 1994). Again, reported rates are higher in adolescents than in children and higher in girls than in boys. For example, the overall rate for SAD was 3.9 % in Turkish children and adolescents; 1.8 and 3.5 % for boys and girls aged 9 to 10 years, respectively; and 3.2 and 6.4 % for boys and girls aged 11–13 years (Demir et al. 2013). In Finnish adolescents aged 12–17 years who were drawn from the general population, the 12-month prevalence was 3.2 % for SAD with a further 4.6 % with subclinical SAD (Ranta et al. 2009b). Finally, the prevalence has been found to be 5.5 % in Spanish adolescents (13–18 years) and 5.8 % (12–18-year-old) who were also drawn from the general population (Garcia-Lopez et al. 2014; Garcia-Lopez 2015b, respectively).

Social Fears

The most common social fear both in adolescents and in adults is fear of public speaking (Stein et al. 1994; Faravelli et al. 2000; Magee et al. 1996; Kessler et al. 1994). However, isolated or pure social fears occur rarely, as the majority report at least one other social fear (Kessler et al. 1998; Wittchen et al. 1999b). For the recently introduced specifier for DSM-5 social anxiety disorder, namely, "performance only," reliable prevalence estimates are still rare (Garcia-Lopez et al. 2015a, 2015b; Kerns et al. 2013). Unreasonably strong social fears were found in 22.3 % of male and in 32.2 % of female adolescents and young adults aged 14–24 years (Wittchen et al. 1999b). Similarly, at least one-fifth of adults reported unreasonable strong social fears (Fehm et al. 2008). In a community sample of adolescents and young adults, 20.0, 11.6, and 11.7 % of respondents reported fear of one, two, three or more social situations, respectively, and among individuals with DSM-IV SAD, rates were 24.2, 18.7, and 57.1 % (Knappe et al. 2011). Among Spanish adolescents, the highest anxiety-provoking social situation was speaking in public (11 %), followed by being observed by others (9.7 %), being in an embarrassing situation (9.3 %), and being rejected (9 %) (Garcia-Lopez et al. 2008).

Further, a substantial proportion of adolescents and young adults reported social fears that may not necessarily meet the criteria for the diagnostic threshold of SAD: 23.1 % reported symptomatic SAD, i.e., positively affirmed a diagnostic stem question for "ever having a persistent, irrational fear of, and compelling desire to avoid a situation in which the respondent attended social affairs, like going to a party or meeting," and another 18.4 % met all but one diagnostic criteria for SAD according to the DSM-IV (Knappe et al. 2009a). Of note, the direct and indirect economic and individual costs associated with SAD are substantial, and those of subthreshold SAD approach those of the full-threshold disorder (Acaturk et al. 2009).

Onset, Natural Course, and Persistence

Onset

Retrospective reports of clinical populations have located the age of SAD onset in late adolescence and adulthood (Keller 2006; Wittchen and Fehm 2001), likely reflecting the point in life at which symptoms have led to severe impairment requiring treatment, after the disorder has been present for a considerable proportion of years. In contrast, prospective-longitudinal studies in youth preponed first onset of SAD toward childhood and adolescence between ages 10 and 16.6 years (Wittchen and Fehm 2001; Magee et al. 1996). Specifically, the core high-risk period spans from 9 years of age to the third decade of life (Beesdo et al. 2007). New onsets after the age of 20 are probably rare, though further peaks of incidence may not be strictly excluded. For clinicians, it is worth knowing that most adults with SAD fail to recall the first onset of SAD symptoms or to remember a time when SAD did not affect their daily life – probably because of the early onset in childhood and adolescence (Wittchen and Fehm 2001) (Figs 3.1 and 3.2).

Duration and Course Patterns

The mean duration of SAD symptoms ranges from 19 to 21 years in clinical studies and from 19 to 25 years in community studies (Fehm et al. 2008; Wittchen and Fehm 2001).

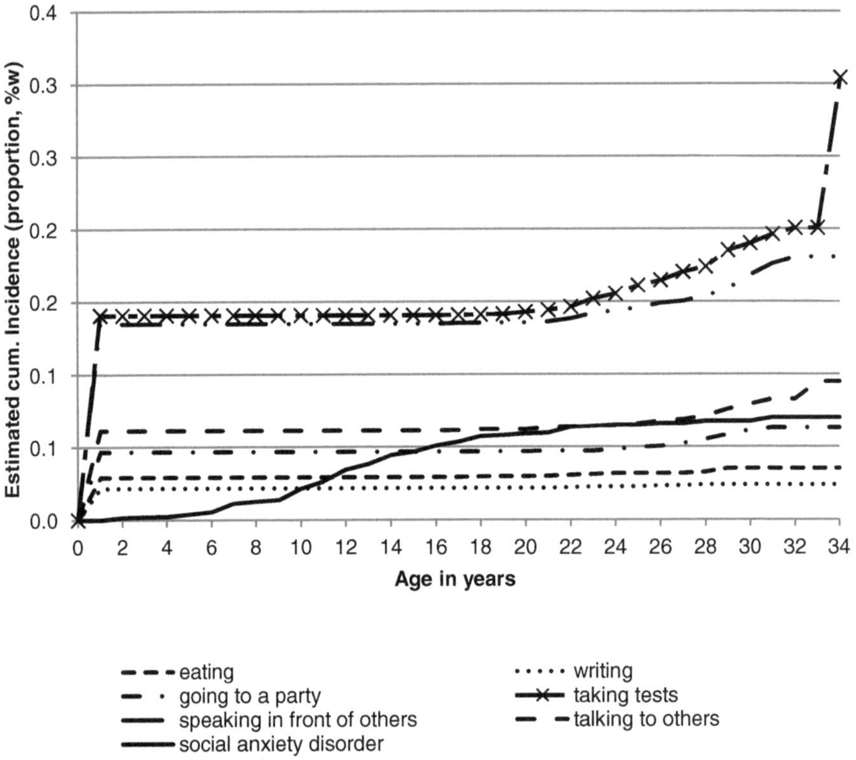

Fig. 3.1 Estimated cumulative incidence of social fears and social anxiety disorder in a sample of adolescents and young adults (T0–T3, last observation carried forward, Source: EDSP 2014)

Little is however known about the natural course of SAD, and the majority of findings are based on adult samples. Studies are needed that cover the high-risk period for SAD onset as well as tracking subsequent chronification vs. alleviation of SAD symptoms. Prospective examinations in adult clinical samples and primary care patients indicate a chronic, i.e., long-lasting, course with enduring symptom load (Chartier et al. 1998; Beard et al. 2010). One small retrospective cross-sectional study of 39 socially anxious adults (Chartier et al. 1998) revealed four patterns of course: "worsening" (8 %), "stability" (33 %), "slight improvement" (21 %), and "remission" (38 %) of symptoms across an average illness duration of 29 years (±2.7 years). Notably, all respondents reported to meet DSM-IV diagnostic criteria of SAD continuously during the course of the disorder, with the exception of the remission pattern, which was associated with a marked improvement of social anxiety, none or a minimal level of distress, lack of avoidance, and interference. Larger, predominantly community studies indicate, however, that meeting the disorder criteria continuously over long time periods is rare. Comparing the ratios of the 12-month to lifetime rate (90.9 %) with 30-day to 12-month prevalence rate of SAD (55.7 %) in the cross-sectional NCS-A, Kessler and colleagues concluded that persistence of SAD is better characterized by recurrences than by constant chronicity (Kessler et al. 2012). In accordance, prospective-longitudinal examinations have revealed

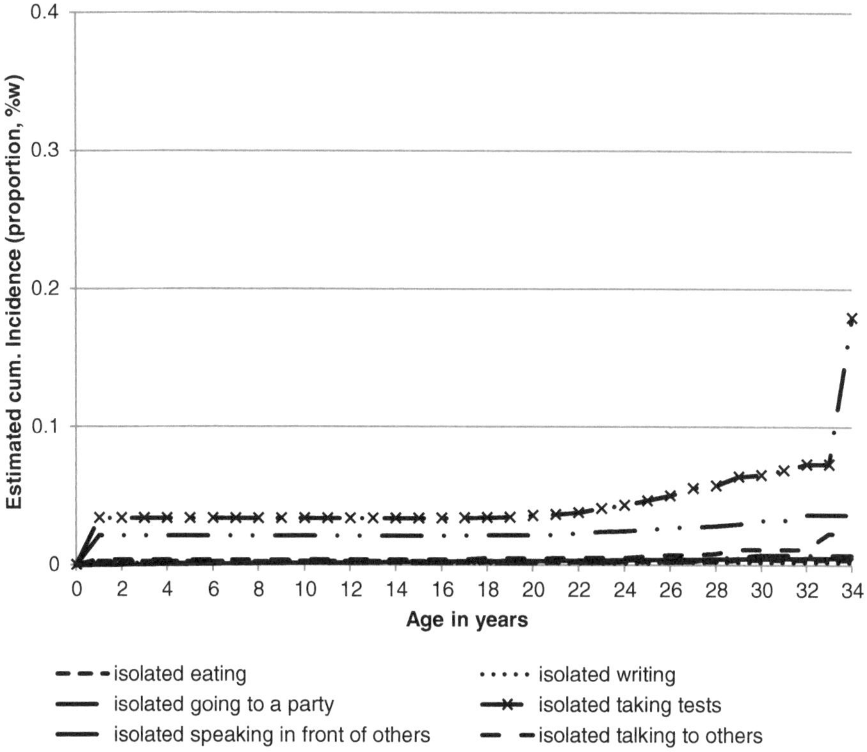

Fig. 3.2 Estimated cumulative incidence of isolated social fears in a sample of adolescents and young adults (T0–T3, last observation carried forward, Source: EDSP 2014)

considerable persistence of SAD, but also substantial fluctuations of symptom severity. In the 15-year prospective multi-wave Zurich Cohort Study (Angst and Vollrath 1991), no individual with SAD was diagnosed continuously at each follow-up assessment after the disorder had manifested (Merikangas et al. 2002). Thus, diagnostic stability of SAD is presumed to be low, consistent with findings that stability rates of threshold SAD (defined as meeting the full DSM-IV criteria again at a subsequent assessment) ranged between 7.1 and 15.1 % in a prospective-longitudinal study (Beesdo-Baum et al. 2012), depending on the assessment times that were considered and the follow-up periods. Rates increase to 56.7 % when also symptomatic and subthreshold SAD is taken into account. These stability rates for SAD may appear rather moderate, but SAD at each time point was associated with a considerably increased risk to also have the disorder or signs and symptoms of the disorder at later points in time, compared to the rates for those without SAD. In fact, a substantial proportion of SAD cases reported at least some significant SAD symptoms (21.5 %) or subthreshold SAD (19.7 %) at subsequent waves (Beesdo-Baum et al. 2012), indicating an oscillating course of SAD (i.e., waxing and waning) around the diagnostic threshold (Wittchen et al. 1999a). Stability of social anxiety symptomatology has been found to be moderate in adolescents after 6 months reassessment (Garcia-Lopez et al. 2008).

Remission, Recovery, and Relapse

Few studies have considered the natural course of SAD among young people, so available findings may lead to misinterpretations and underestimations of disorder severity. We have therefore first drawn on studies with adult populations, where more extensive data is available. Generally, the course of SAD in adults is considered to be less favorable in clinical than in primary care or community samples (27 % vs. 40 % recovery rate after 5 years) (Steinert et al. 2013). Between 45 and 56 % of patients who underwent routine treatment in outpatient care centers experienced at least partial remission from their symptoms over 6–8 years (Alnaes and Torgersen 1999; Keller 2003), while in the community this rate was 77 % after 3 years (Steinert et al. 2013). In a female community sample, 64 % of SAD cases were at least partially recovered, and 36 % showed full recovery 1.5 years later, i.e., no longer experienced any of the DSM-IV criteria of social phobia (Vriends et al. 2007). Roughly estimated, less than half of affected adults experience spontaneous remissions or full recovery (Sibrava et al. 2013; Keller 2006; Bruce et al. 2005; Alnaes and Torgersen 1999).

As noted, few studies have examined natural remission among children, adolescents, and young people with SAD. However, one study with a clinical population (many of whom received treatment) reported remission of SAD and other anxiety disorders in 80 % of children aged 5–18 years (Last et al. 1996), but 30 % of the cases reported another anxiety disorder 3–4 years later. In a community sample of adolescents and young adults, the rate of full remission of SAD was 15.1 % (Beesdo-Baum et al. 2012), that is, they revealed neither SAD symptoms nor other disorders across a time period of up to 10 years. Hence, even though the frequency or intensity of SAD symptoms may decrease over time, the risk for other mental problems (disorders) increases (Essau et al. 2002).

Mental and Physical Comorbidity

Comorbidity with Other Mental Disorders

Co-occurrence of other anxiety and mental disorders with SAD is frequent in adolescence and adulthood and is the rule rather than the exception (Wittchen and Fehm 2001). In general, comorbidity rates range from between about 69 and 99 % (Steinert et al. 2013; Schneier et al. 1992) depending on the study sample, setting, and assessments. The most frequent comorbid mental conditions in adolescents and adults are other anxiety disorders, depressive disorders, substance use, and somatoform disorders (Coles et al. 2006; Fu et al. 2007; Rogers et al. 1996; Beesdo-Baum and Knappe 2012), as well as personality disorders in adults (Massion et al. 2002; Lampe et al. 2003; Cox et al. 2009). Compared to non-SAD cases, an increased risk for suicidal ideation but not for suicide attempts was reported in both cross-sectional and longitudinal analyses of NEMESIS data drawn from adults (Sareen et al. 2005a).

Among the anxiety disorders, SAD most commonly co-occurs with specific phobias, agoraphobia, panic disorder, and generalized anxiety disorder (e.g.,

Alonso et al. 2004; Kessler et al. 2005b; Lampe et al. 2003; Merikangas et al. 2002). Prospective epidemiological studies indicate that children and adolescents meeting the criteria for SAD or any other anxiety disorder are at high risk for meeting the criteria for the same or comorbid disorders also in adulthood (Costello et al. 2003), and vice versa, adults with SAD or other anxiety disorders reported that the same or comorbid disorder was already present in childhood and adolescence (Gregory et al. 2007; Kim-Cohen et al. 2003; Rutter et al. 2006). Compared to unaffected individuals, higher rates of SAD have also been observed in adult patients with obsessive-compulsive disorders (e.g., Assuncao et al. 2012). Among individuals with anorexia nervosa, elevated rates for SAD were observed relative to those without anorexia, though findings are yet inconclusive (Godart et al. 2002; Swinbourne and Touyz 2007); lifetime and current prevalence rates for SAD in threshold or subsyndromal bulimia nervosa are significantly higher than in nonclinical controls (Godart et al. 2002).

Comorbidity with Physical Disorders

Elevated rates of SAD have also been found to be associated with physical problems, specifically sleep problems and insomnia (Stein et al. 1993; Johnson et al. 2006), diabetes, thyroid disease, lupus, or other autoimmune disease (Sareen et al. 2005b). Findings are however limited to adults. For adolescents, a history of early language impairment was associated with a greater likelihood to meet diagnostic criteria for DSM-IV SAD by the age of 19 years (Voci et al. 2006) (Table 3.1).

SAD as a Risk Factor for Incident Conditions

While acknowledging the variability in definitions and applied assessment methods, analyses of comorbidity can inform understanding of shared and non-shared risk factors for SAD and can help delineate hypotheses about underlying pathogenic mechanisms. The most basic assumptions about the co-occurrence (comorbidity) of mental and/or physical conditions are probably that co-occurrence is either at random or that two or more conditions overlap or even represent the same underlying clinical phenomenon. Comorbidity may also be due to the fact that one condition temporally precedes the other, potentially as a (causal) risk factor for the other condition. In this regard, SAD is presumed to serve as a risk factor for a cascade of secondary psychopathology. Because longitudinal data (starting in childhood or adolescence and with sufficient follow-up periods) are needed to resolve these questions, findings from studies in adolescents and young adults up to the third decade of life are presented. Therein, longitudinal studies have provided evidence for the role of SAD as a putative causal risk factor for depressive disorders (Beesdo et al. 2007; Stein et al. 2001b; Pine et al. 1998), substance use disorders (Buckner et al. 2006, 2008; Sonntag et al. 2000; Sareen et al. 2006; Zimmerman et al. 2004), and, in some studies, psychosis (Schutters et al. 2011; Rietdijk et al. 2013).

Table 3.1 Selected community studies reporting comorbidity rates of social anxiety disorder with mental and physical conditions

Condition	Study	*N*	Age (in years)	% rate in SAD cases	OR (95 %CI)	Time frame	Reference
Anxiety disorders							
Generalized anxiety disorder	NCS	9,098	15–54	13.3	3.8 (2.8–5.03)	Lifetime	Magee et al. (1996)
	NSMHWB	10,641	18+	33.9	3.0 (1.9–4.6)	12 months	Lampe et al. (2003)
	ESEMeD	21,425	18+	nr	13.5 (7.7–23.5)	12 months	Alonso et al. (2004)
	NEMESIS	7,076	18–64	16.7	8.9 (6.3–12.6)	12 months	Acarturk et al. (2008)
	ECA (Baltimore)	320	18+	nr	3.9 (1.5–9.7)	Lifetime	Bienvenue et al. (2001)
	BJS	1,035	12–17	0	ns	Lifetime	Essau et al. (1998)
	Zurich Study	591	19–35	nr	3.1 (1.5–5.7)	12 months	Merikangas et al. (2002)
Agoraphobia	NEMESIS	7,076	18–64	12.4	12.7 (8.5–19.1)	Lifetime	Acarturk et al. (2008)
	BJS	1,035	12–17	9.5	nr	Lifetime	Essau et al. (1998)
Agoraphobia with or without panic disorder	EDSP	3,021	14–24	8.8	5.5 (2.9–10.3)	Lifetime	Wittchen et al. (1999b)
Specific phobias	NCS	9,098	15–54	37.6	7.75 (6.4–9.5)	Lifetime	Magee et al. (1996)
	Zurich Study	591	19–35	nr	5.9 (3.2–11.1)	12 months	Merikangas et al. (2002)
	NEMESIS	7,076	18–64	37.0	8.6 (6.7–11.1)	12 months	Acarturk et al. (2008)
	BJS	1,035	12–17	2.7	nr	Lifetime	Essau et al. (1998)
Panic disorder	NCS	9,098	15–54	10.9	4.83 (3.5–6.6)	Lifetime	Magee et al. (1996)
	ECA	18,571	18+	4.7	3.24 (1.9–5.4)	Lifetime	Schneier et al. (1992)
	NSMHWB	10,641	18+	20.6	4.9 (2.4–9.9)	12 months	Lampe et al. (2003)
	BJS	1,035	12–17	0	ns	Lifetime	Essau et al. (1998)
Panic attacks	NCS	9,098	15–54	20.7	4.67 (3.7–5.9)	Lifetime	Magee et al. (1996)
	EDSP	3,021	14–24	20.1	3.1 (1.8–5.3)	Lifetime	Goodwin et al. (2004)

Affective disorders							
Major depressive episode	NCS	9,098	15–54	26.5	2.9 (2.3–3.6)	Lifetime	Kessler et al. (1999)
	NSMHWB	10,641	18+	40.5	2.4 (1.3–4.5)	12 months	Lampe et al. (2003)
	ESEMeD	21,425	18+	nr	10.2 (6.1–15.1)	12 months	Alonso et al. (2004)
Dysthymia	NCS	9,098	15–54	28.5	2.7 (1.9–3.8)	Lifetime	Kessler et al. (1999)
	NEMESIS	7,076	18–64	20.3	9.1 (6.6–12.5)	12 months	Acarturk et al. (2008)
	ESEMeD	21,425	18+	nr	5.4 (2.6–11.5)	12 months	Alonso et al. (2004)
Any depressive disorder	EDSP	3,021	14–24	31.1	3.04 (2.1–4.4)	Lifetime	Wittchen et al. (1999b)
Mania	NCS	9,098	15–54	5.1	4.6 (2.6–8.3)	Lifetime	Magee et al. (1996)
Bipolar disorder	NCS	9,098	15–54	41.7	5,9 (1.8–19.6)	Lifetime	Kessler et al. (1999)
	NEMESIS	7,076	18–64	11.0	13.1 (8.5–19.9)	12 months	Acarturk et al. (2008)
Suicidality							
Suicidal ideation	NEMESIS	7,076	18–64	25.0	1.6 (1.2–2.1)	Lifetime	Sareen et al. (2005a)
Suicide attempts	NEMESIS	7,076	18–64	27.7	0.7 (0.5–1.2)	Lifetime	Sareen et al. (2005a)
Alcohol use disorder (abuse, dependence)							
	Zurich Study	591	19–35	nr	1.9 (1.0–3.8)	12 months	Merikangas et al. (2002)
	EDSP	3,021	14–24	nr	15 (0.9–2.4)	Lifetime	Zimmermann et al. (2003)
Physical conditions							
Insomnia	HMO	1,014	13–16	32.4	4.4 (2.1–9.2)	Lifetime	Johnson et al. (2006)

nr not reported, *ns* not significant, *BJS* Bremer Jugendstudie (Bremen Adolescents Study), *ECA* Epidemiological Catchment Area, *EDSP* Early Developmental Stages of Psychopathology (-study), *ESEMeD* European Study of the Epidemiology of Mental Disorders, *HMO* Health Maintenance Organization, *NCS* National Comorbidity Survey, *NEMESIS* Netherlands Mental Health Survey and Incidence Study, *NSMHWB* National Survey on Mental Health and Well-Being

References available upon request from the first author

SAD as a Risk Factor for Substance Use

While depressive disorders may be considered a consequence of SAD, it is widely assumed that the consumption of alcohol or other substances as a form of coping or safety behavior bears the risk for alcohol-related problems (Schry and White 2013) and/or other substance use disorders. Consumption of alcohol or other substances prior or during social situations is expected to reduce self-perceived social anxiety but also to affect attentional processes such as preferential processing of external stimuli and physical symptoms such as facial blushing (Stevens et al. 2014). In addition, findings in college student samples point to the role of different drinking motives; that is, alcohol may be consumed in order to reduce social anxiety in situations where intake of alcohol is deemed socially acceptable but fear of cognitive performance deficits may also reduce the motivation for alcohol intake, particularly in performance-related situations (Cludius et al. 2013). Similar observations were made in relation to smoking and nicotine dependence and social anxiety; that is, socially anxious individuals, in particular females, who use cigarettes to cope with feelings of loneliness or social rejection may be particularly vulnerable to more severe nicotine dependence (Buckner and Vinci 2013). Here, the potential mediating role of depression also needs to be considered.

SAD as a Risk Factor for Psychosis

Research on early signs and prodromal states of psychosis in adolescents and young adults has pointed to SAD (Schutters et al. 2011) and social anxiety (Rietdijk et al. 2013) as a useful screener for paranoid symptoms in help-seeking individuals at high risk for psychosis. Again, the associations between SAD and psychosis may relate to shared and non-shared risk factors and to the temporal sequence of these two conditions.

Risk Factors for SAD Onset and Course

A range of correlates and putative risk factors for SAD conditions have been examined. The findings are sometimes unclear as studies focus on selected factors and use cross-sectional designs with diverging assessment strategies and outcome criteria. For descriptive purposes, we will consider factors relevant for SAD onset and SAD course.

Female Gender

Community samples have identified that females across all ages are about twice as often affected by SAD as males (Demir et al. 2013; DeWit et al. 2005; De Graaf et al. 2002; Merikangas et al. 2011; Ruscio et al. 2008; Wittchen et al. 1999b).

In contrast, an equal gender distribution has been observed in clinical samples or even slightly higher rates for men (Fehm et al. 2005). This may be due to the difference in social expectations between genders that is still influential in many societies. Of note, though some studies on convenience samples have suggested differences in the prevalence of social fears between males and females, effect sizes were low (Garcia-Lopez et al. 2008) but appear to increase with advanced puberty (Deardoff et al. 2007).

In relation to the course of SAD, females report higher rates of comorbid anxiety and depressive disorders (MacKenzie and Fowler 2013), whereas males more often report comorbid externalizing disorders and substance use (Xu et al. 2012).

Peer Status and Social Skills

Mixed results have been found regarding the causal relationship of peer status and social skills on SAD. There is ample evidence that negative peer status during childhood and adolescence is linked with higher levels of social anxiety (Erath et al. 2008; La Greca et al. 1988; La Greca and Stone 1993; Ranta et al. 2009a; Rao et al. 2007; Siegel et al. 2009; Storch et al. 2005; Tillfors et al. 2012; Vernberg et al. 1992), and both adolescents and adults with SAD are more likely to report a history of peer victimization than their healthy counterparts or patients with other anxiety disorders (Gren-Landell et al. 2011; McCabe et al. 2003; Roth et al. 2002; Garcia-Lopez et al. 2011; Ranta et al. 2009a, 2013). However, some studies show that the variable with the largest impact in predicting prospective anxiety symptoms is the self-report of victimization and the reaction to these negative experiences (i.e., personal perceptions of the incident) (Bouman et al. 2012; Levinson et al. 2013). Since many existing studies rely on retrospective accounts and lack objective peer ratings, measurement issues need to be considered when comparing specific results.

The relationship between peer rejection and heightened social anxiety is likely to be bidirectional (Tillfors et al. 2012). Thus, children and adolescents with elevated social anxiety behave in a reserved way toward their peers, and their peers tend to evaluate these children negatively. Negative evaluation from others may then reinforce children's fear of social situations, making the child more reluctant to interact with his or her peers (Rapee and Spence 2004).

Whether the reserved social behaviors shown by children with social anxiety reflect a lack of social skills is a matter of ongoing debate. Early studies by Spence and colleagues (Spence et al. 2000) and Beidel et al. (1999) showed that SAD is associated with not only lower subjective ratings of social skills but also lower observer ratings on behavioral measures. Many subsequent studies have replicated these findings in both clinical and nonclinical samples (Alfano et al. 2006; Beidel et al. 2014; Inderbitzen-Nolan et al. 2007; Morgan and Banerjee 2006) and thus have provided the basis for the application of social skills training in child and adolescent social anxiety intervention programs (e.g., Beidel et al. 2000; Spence et al. 2000). However, evaluating social skills in situations where children are anxious makes it difficult to ascertain whether group differences reflect social communication skill deficits or a lack of social confidence. For example, Cartwright-Hatton and colleagues (Cartwright-Hatton et al. 2003; Cartwright-Hatton et al. 2005) recruited a group of non-referred school children and assessed their performance in a speech/conversation task and found that, although more anxious children had more negative perceptions of their performance, micro-behaviors and global impression of the performance did not differ significantly between anxious and non-anxious children. The authors concluded that socially anxious children may benefit from cognitive interventions that focus on maladaptive beliefs about how they appear to others during social encounters.

One approach to teasing apart social skills deficits and a lack of social confidence is to consider the social communication difficulties that may underlie restricted social behaviors. For example, Banerjee and Henderson (2001) reported that community children with high levels of social anxiety were rated by teachers as being less skilled in social tasks that involved insight into others' mental states, compared to their low-anxious peers. Consistent with this finding are recent reports that clinically referred children with anxiety disorders have inflated levels of traits of autistic spectrum disorders (van Steensel et al. 2013) and that this is particularly the case among children with SAD (Halls et al. 2014). Whether similar patterns are found among adolescents with social anxiety requires investigation given findings that adolescents show less impairment in behavioral measures of social skills than younger children (Rao et al. 2007).

Clearly, more research is needed to clarify the causal relationship between peer status, social skills, and SAD. However, existing evidence strongly suggests that interpersonal relationships during the adolescent years shape subjective image of the social self, and this image has a lasting impact which persists into adulthood. Social skills training on the part of the individual as well as classwide prevention and early intervention programs to change the environmental factors within the school may have a synergistic effect for both anxious and non-anxious adolescents. For example, reactions from classmates moderate anxious adolescents' performance level in social tasks (Blöte et al. 2007), and children's risk for peer difficulties is moderated by classroom emotional climate (Gazelle 2006; Avant et al. 2011).

Familial Load and Parental Psychopathology

Family and high-risk studies strongly indicate that SAD aggregates in families, that is, offspring are at increased risk for SAD when parents are affected themselves (Knappe et al. 2009c; Lieb et al. 2000; Bandelow et al. 2004; Elizabeth et al. 2006; Merikangas et al. 2003; Stein et al. 2001a). Associative family studies however do not provide information on the mechanisms of intergenerational transmission, i.e., whether, when, and to which degree genetic factors, environmental factors, or a combination thereof contribute to offspring SAD. The vast majority of literature has demonstrated that both gene and environmental influences and their interaction contribute to SAD.

Findings are mixed with regard to specificity of the parent-to-offspring transmission. The Reading longitudinal study recruited mothers during pregnancy on the basis of their meeting diagnostic criteria for SAD (n=96), generalized anxiety disorder (n=58), or having no history of an anxiety disorder (n=94). At the most recent assessment (age 4–5 years), inflated levels of internalizing difficulties and SAD (15 %), specifically, were already apparent among the offspring of mothers with SAD compared to those with generalized anxiety disorder (2 %) and those with no history of anxiety disorder (0 %) (Murray et al. 2014). These findings are consistent with early diagnostic specificity in transmission, at least in the case of SAD.

However, epidemiological data with adolescent or adult populations indicate parental SAD, but also other parental anxiety, depressive, and alcohol use disorders confer risk to offspring SAD above and below the diagnostic threshold and to other offspring disorders as well (Knappe et al. 2009a, b; Lieb et al. 2000). Interestingly, SAD cases with isolated performance-related fears had substantially lower rates of parents with SAD or alcohol use disorders than SAD cases who reported fears in interaction or both interaction or performance-related social situations (Knappe et al. 2011). In addition, different risks for the development of social anxiety disorder may be associated with different developmental phases. For example, increased social fears have been documented among infant and toddler offspring of parents with social anxiety disorder (Murray et al. 2007, 2008; Akatr et al. 2014), indicating that infancy and early childhood are sensitive time windows for learning social fears through observation of parental behaviors.

Heritability and Candidate Genes

Heritability estimates specifically for SAD based on twin samples are modest, range from 0.20 to 0.50 across studies (Knappe et al. 2010), and are generally comparable across ages (McGrath et al. 2012). However, it has been suggested that men and women differ in the extent to which genetic and environmental factors contribute to SAD. Specifically, twin resemblance was best explained by (non-shared) family-environment factors in females and by (shared) genetic factors in males (Kendler et al. 2002). It is likely that there are common genetic risk factors underlying many of the childhood anxiety disorders and traits, although the magnitude of overlap differs depending on the age of the sample, measures used, and disorders or traits considered (for reviews cf. Gregory and Eley 2007; McGrath et al. 2012). For example, overlap in familial and non-shared environmental factors was observed between specific phobia and SAD (Eley et al. 2008). Particularly for SAD, there is some evidence for developmental dynamics; that is, genetic contributions to SAD in childhood are different from those in adolescence and adulthood, indicating only a limited degree of genetic continuity across time. Compared to other phobias, the genetic effects on SAD were observed to dramatically change in adolescence and young adulthood, when new and substantial genetic influences contributed to the course of SAD and the development of comorbid conditions (Kendler et al. 2008).

With regard to potential candidate genes, the focus has been on specific genes encoding components of serotonergic (5-HT) and dopaminergic pathways

(Domschke et al. 2009; Gelernter et al. 2004) without notable results for SAD. Progress in this field is slow and limited given that multiple genes of small effect size are likely to contribute to SAD as well as to other anxiety-related conditions (Gregory and Eley 2007) and because of a range of methodological issues such as small or heterogeneous samples with broad age ranges, diverse comorbidity profiles, false-positive results that do not hold up for replication, and vague thresholds to differentiate between normative and pathological (social) anxiety conditions (McGrath et al. 2012). Similarly, genome-wide association studies (GWAS), including both linkage and association designs, have mostly focused on anxiety-related traits, the broader category of anxiety disorders in general, or predominantly panic disorder (for an overview, cf. McGrath et al. 2012; Domschke and Deckert 2012). Genetic polymorphisms are of further interest in understanding and predicting outcomes related to SAD treatment, though findings are not yet convincing (Andersson et al. 2013). For more details on genetics and heritability in SAD, refer to Tillfors et al. (2012), and Chap. 4 of this book.

Behavioral Inhibition and Other Temperamental and Personality Factors

A further potential mechanism underlying the familial and genetic factors that are associated with SAD is behavioral inhibition (BI). BI is a temperamental trait that has been consistently associated with an increased risk for SAD. Originally derived from laboratory-based direct observation, BI is defined as a chronic tendency to "show an initial avoidance of or behavioral restraint to novelty" (Kagan et al. 1988a). Behavioral signs of BI in children include "long latencies to interact with unfamiliar adults, retreat from unfamiliar objects, cessation of play and vocalization, and long periods remaining proximal to the mother" (Kagan et al. 1988b). In recent years, it has been shown that BI is a heritable trait that has a strong neurophysiological basis (DiLalla et al. 1994; Kagan et al. 1987; Matheny 1989; Robinson et al. 1992).

Early studies by Kagan et al. (1988a, b) found that children with extreme BI tendencies at age 2 showed stable social avoidance and withdrawal behavior at ages 4, 5.5, and 7.5. In diagnostic terms, a follow-up study of this same cohort at age 13 showed higher rates of SAD for children with BI (Schwartz et al. 1999). Similar results have been obtained using retrospective self-reports in SAD patients (Van Ameringen et al. 1998) and adolescents (Hayward et al. 1998). Results from a recent meta-analysis (Clauss and Blackford 2012) indicate that BI is associated with a greater than sevenfold increase in risk for developing SAD. This association remained significant after considering study differences in temperament assessment, control group, parental risk, age at temperament assessment, and age at anxiety diagnosis. Collectively, it is well established that BI has the strongest relationship with SAD above all other mental disorders.

There is an ongoing controversy regarding whether BI is a distinct construct from SAD. Some researchers regard BI on a quantitative continuum from shyness to SAD (e.g., McNeil 2001). However, for the most part, BI is conceptualized as a temperamental vulnerability that is linked to the later development of anxiety disorders. Cultural differences in the manifestation of BI (Chen et al. 1998) and interactions with parenting variables (e.g., Natsuaki et al. 2013) are some areas of future research that may clarify such distinctions.

Biological Factors

Central to adolescent development are hormonal changes associated with growth and puberty. As part of normative functional changes, morphological and neural maturations significantly impact on cognition and information processing (Haller et al. 2014; Blakemore 2008). The rapid increase of studies using structural and functional imaging procedures with special interest in limbic and prefrontal brain areas has contributed tremendously to our understanding of social anxiety and SAD, though most findings are based on young adult samples between ages 20 and 35. Structural data indicate enlarged amygdala and left hippocampal regions (Machado-de-Sousa et al. 2014), increased thickness of the left inferior temporal cortex, and reduced thickness of the right rostral anterior cingulate cortex (Frick et al. 2013) in socially anxious young adults relative to controls. Some of these brain areas are associated with dysfunctional regulation and processing of emotions in SAD which is further supported by functional imaging studies.

Functional imaging studies in SAD focus on face perception, social cue processing, and processing and inhibition of social threat stimuli as neural correlates for SAD-relevant cognitive distortions and bias (Anderson et al. 2013; Pejic et al. 2013; Gentili et al. 2009), as well as emotional hyperreactivity and ineffective emotion regulation. For example, Goldin and colleagues (Goldin et al. 2009) examined neural correlates of emotional reactivity and cognitive regulation during processing of harsh facial expressions (i.e., social threat) and violent scenes (physical threat) in 15 adults with SAD and matched unaffected controls. As a result, viewing social threat resulted in greater emotion-related neural responses and reduced cognitive and attention regulation-related neural activation in patients than controls, with social anxiety symptom severity related to activity in a network of emotion- and attention-processing regions only in patients (Goldin et al. 2009). For more details on the neurobiological factors, regions, and processes in SAD (see Chap. 4).

Family Environment

Given the early onset of SAD in childhood and adolescence, the strong familial aggregation, and the importance of the family for the social, emotional, and cognitive development of an individual, diverse family processes have been hypothesized to promote the onset or persistence or to affect the treatment of SAD (for a comprehensive overview, see Knappe et al. 2010), such as insecure attachment (Stevenson-Hinde and Shouldice 1990; Eng et al. 2001; van Brakel et al. 2006), higher levels of expressed emotion (Suveg et al. 2005; Garcia-Lopez et al. 2009, 2014), excessive family cohesion (Peleg-Popko and Dar 2001), and disturbed family functioning (Ballash et al. 2006; Bögels and Brechmann-Toussaint 2006; Tamplin and Goodyer 2001). It should be noted though that some of these concepts have been linked with anxiety disorders, but their specific association with social anxiety disorder has rarely been examined. An exception is Garcia-Lopez et al.'s (2009) study revealing that parental psychopathology (parents with high expressed emotion, EE) should be taken into consideration to prevent poor treatment outcomes for socially anxious adolescent. More recently, Garcia-Lopez et al. (2014) have found that the inclusion of parent training to reduce EE in a treatment program designed to address social anxiety in adolescents had a positive effect on their improvement, particularly when the parents' EE status changed from high to low expressed emotion after treatment. In addition, different roles for maternal and paternal behavior in the development of child anxiety have been suggested (Bögels et al. 2011; Bögels and Perotti 2011; Teetsel et al. 2014), for example, that fathers' parenting behavior may have a particularly important role in encouraging the child to playfully test limits, approach new situations, and actively cope with fears (Majdandzic et al. 2014), whereas maternal parenting behavior may be particularly critical for teaching social wariness (Bögels et al. 2011). Few studies to date have distinguished between maternal and paternal behaviors; however, this is clearly a priority for future research. In fact, awareness and investigations of the father's role for SAD and other anxiety disorders in offspring are increasing (i.e., Majdandzic et al. 2014; Aktar et al. 2014; Bögels and Perotti 2011; Bögels and Phares 2008).

"Anxiogenic" Parenting

It is likely that parents who are anxious, depressed, or stressed display potentially anxiogenic parenting behaviors and that offspring with SAD elicit adverse parenting. Prospective evaluations are limited, but findings so far point to independent as well as accumulated contributions of parental psychopathology and parental rearing to offspring SAD.

Parenting styles and behaviors characterized by expressed anxiety, overcontrol, and low warmth have been implicated in the development and maintenance of childhood anxiety disorders (e.g., Murray et al. 2009), with most consistent support from both questionnaire and observational assessments of overcontrol (McLeod et al. 2007; Wood et al. 2003). It has been suggested that negative parenting behaviors may be particularly pertinent to the development of SAD, where sensitivity to negative evaluation from others is a core feature (Gulley et al. 2014). Results of a recent prospective study using observational methods have implicated parental overcontrol in the development of social anxiety symptoms and disorder, particularly among children with a stable history of high levels of behavioral inhibition (Lewis-Morrarty et al. 2012). However, few studies have examined associations between parental behaviors and SAD specifically (i.e., in contrast to other anxiety disorders). A notable exception is a prospective-longitudinal study in adolescents and young adults, in which offspring-reported dysfunctional parental rearing (rejection, overprotection, and lack of emotional warmth) was associated with offspring threshold SAD and, albeit less strong and less consistently, also with subthreshold SAD (Knappe et al. 2009a). Here, the constellation of higher paternal rejection and lower paternal (but not maternal) emotional warmth and higher maternal (but not paternal) overprotection was observed in offspring SAD but not in other offspring anxiety disorders, suggesting that there may be specificity in parenting factors associated with offspring SAD and that particular patterns of behaviors of mothers and fathers may have distinct functions (Knappe et al. 2012).

Whether parenting behaviors account for the intergenerational transmission of SAD has also received little empirical investigation. Notably, in the prospective-longitudinal study described above, associations between offspring-reported parenting behaviors and offspring SAD did not change after controlling for parental psychopathology and vice versa, suggesting that both risk factors may contribute independently to offspring SAD (Knappe et al. 2009a, c). However, offspring-reported parenting on questionnaire measures may be subject to biases and may not pick up on situationally specific parenting responses. Murray et al. (2012), for example, found that differences in parenting behaviors (specifically increased passivity and reduced encouragement and warmth) between mothers with SAD or GAD and non-anxious mothers were principally evident in the context of disorder-specific challenge. In line with these findings, parents with SAD have demonstrated less warmth and more criticism and doubts of child competency than parents with other anxiety disorders when observed with their child conducting two performance tasks, although notably no differences were found in parental overcontrol or autonomy granting (Budinger et al. 2013).

In addition to particular parental responses being more likely to occur in the context of parental anxiety, depression, or stress, child experiences and characteristics are likely to elicit particular parental responses. For example, natal complications have been found to relate to later overprotection and low emotional warmth, with a trend toward serious health problems predicting unfavorable parenting (Knappe et al. 2012). Furthermore, adverse experiences or particular child characteristics may provoke particular parenting styles more readily among more anxious parents. Consistent with this suggestion, Hirshfeld et al. (1997) found that maternal criticism of the child was a function of a significant interaction between child behavioral inhibition and maternal anxiety disorder status: Within the group of anxious mothers, 65 % of those with inhibited children were critical compared to 18 % of those with non-inhibited children. Similarly Murray et al. (2008) reported that mothers with SAD showed low levels of encouragement to their infants to engage with a stranger *only* when the infant was behaviorally inhibited. Together these findings highlight the likely complex reciprocal and interacting relationships between child and parent characteristics and behaviors.

Information Processing Biases

Biases in information processing have been emphasized in theories of the development and maintenance of anxiety disorders in both adults (Beck et al. 1985) and children (Kendall 1985) and in models of social anxiety disorder specifically (Clark and Wells 1995; Rapee and Heimberg 1997). Central to these theories are the hypotheses that anxiety is reinforced by a tendency to (1) selectively or preferentially respond to threat and (2) to interpret ambiguous information in a negative or threatening manner. However, Spence et al. (1999) suggested that negative expectancies about social situations may not be a key factor in the development of social anxiety in children, but may initially be a response to a lack of social success, which then later maintains anxiety by promoting avoidance of social situations. Findings to date have not yet been able to fully evaluate this possibility, although, in contrast, there is some evidence that infants at risk of SAD (by virtue of having a parent with SAD) differ from low-risk infants (with non-socially anxious parents) in their looking responses to emotional faces (Creswell et al. 2008) and that this is associated with later anxiety symptoms (Creswell et al. 2011). In a similar vein, compared to children of non-anxious mothers, 4 to 5-year-old children of mothers with SAD were significantly more likely to give negative responses to school-based scenarios presented in a doll-play format prior to the child starting school (Pass et al. 2012). Furthermore, negative doll play predicted teacher reported anxious-depressed and social worry problems at the end of the child's first term at school. Despite these intriguing findings which might suggest a developmental role of information processing biases, cross-sectional studies that have examined associations between information processing biases and SAD in children have failed to deliver a clear pattern of results in relation to the maintenance of SAD.

Associations between attention biases and anxiety in children and adolescents have varied across studies, with some finding that anxiety is associated with attention toward threat (e.g., Roy et al. 2008) but others finding attention away from (or avoidance of) threat (e.g., Monk et al. 2006). Differences in findings may be explained by methodological and sample characteristics, for example, the specific anxiety disorder subtypes that make up the sample (Waters et al. 2014). Specific associations between social anxiety and attention bias in children and adolescents have received little attention; however, Stirling, Eley, and Clark (2006) reported that social anxiety symptoms (and not general anxiety symptoms) in a community population of 8–11-year-olds were significantly associated with a bias *away* from negative facial expressions. In contrast, Gulley, Oppenheim, and Hankin (2014) recently reported a bias *toward* angry faces among children (9–15 years) with higher symptoms of social anxiety in both a community and a psychiatrically enriched sample. Of particular note, the association between observed authoritarian and negative parenting and child social anxiety was mediated by attention to angry faces in the community sample. These cross-sectional findings provide preliminary support for the hypothesis that environmental factors (such as parenting) may present a risk for SAD by virtue of their influence on emerging information processing styles. These findings are fascinating, but the lack of consistency in reported results to date emphasizes the need for caution and further examination of the role of attentional biases in the development and maintenance of SAD in childhood and adolescence.

Although a number of studies have demonstrated that children with anxiety disorders interpret ambiguous situations in a more negative manner than non-anxious children (e.g., Barrett et al. 1996; Creswell et al. 2005), there has been little examination of disorder-specific associations. The studies that have considered this have provided inconsistent findings, with some finding no SAD-specific associations when compared to children with other anxiety disorders (Barrett et al. 1996) or non-anxious controls (Creswell et al. 2014), but with one recent study reporting higher fear and threat ratings in response to ambiguous situations in children with SAD compared to both other anxious and non-anxious children (Alkozei et al. 2014). These discrepancies may be accounted for by methodological and sample characteristics, and further clarification is required. In addition, little is known about the role of interpretation biases in SAD in adolescence. On the basis of Spence et al.'s (1999) proposal, prospective studies are clearly required that follow children into adolescence to examine the potentially changing association between interpretation biases, social functioning, and social anxiety over time.

Although studies with children and adolescents have focused predominantly on attention and interpretation biases, adult models of the maintenance of SAD emphasize other information processing biases, such as recall biases, self-focused attention, and the tendency to view anxiety symptoms as having negative consequences (e.g., Clark and Wells 1995; Rapee and Heimberg 1997). Accordingly, consideration of broader indices of information processing in relation to SAD is required with adolescent populations. One such recent example reported that adolescents with SAD were more likely to recall information that they had been instructed to forget than non-anxious children (Gómez-Ariza et al. 2013). These findings are consistent with the hypothesis that young people with SAD may be particularly likely to hold on to negative or unhelpful memories (e.g., relating to social failure), and that this may underlie negative expectancies when entering novel social situations.

Given the limited available evidence and lack of consistency found in relation to information processing biases and SAD in adolescents, replication of positive findings is required, as are prospective and experimental methods to establish the directional nature of associations at different stages in development.

Predictors for SAD Course and Persistence

In contrast to the substantial literature reporting on correlates and (risk) factors for SAD or SAD onset, data on risk factors for the (natural) course of SAD, (i.e., with regard to remission or persistence of SAD symptoms), are limited. Again, findings vary between retrospective and clinical studies and prospective samples with varying follow-up periods and whether SAD or anxiety disorders in general are examined as outcomes. Most studies are based on adult samples. Among distal factors, in a study of adolescents and young adults, presence of parental psychopathology was unrelated to persistence of offspring SAD, but higher levels of parental overprotection were associated with higher persistence of offspring SAD (Knappe et al. 2009c). Also cumulative effects were suggested; that is, lack of emotional warmth and disturbed family functioning predicted higher SAD persistence, particularly when parents were affected by a mental disorder themselves (Knappe et al. 2009c). Distal vulnerability characteristics such as parental SAD and depression, behavioral inhibition, and harm avoidance predicted SAD persistence and also, but less consistently, diagnostic stability of SAD (Beesdo-Baum et al. 2012).

Among proximal factors, clinical characteristics of onset patterns and early course are of interest (Noyes et al. 2005), with early age of onset (de Menezes et al. 2005; Lim et al. 2013; but see Crippa et al. 2007), degree of impairment (Davidson et al. 1994), or symptom severity (DeWit et al. 1999), as well as comorbid conditions (Yonkers et al. 2003; Massion et al. 2002), being associated with an unfavorable outcome. One study in young women did not find that SAD symptom severity or duration predicted recovery 1.5 years later (Vriends et al. 2007), while other studies with longer follow-up periods and including both genders reported that baseline severity (van Beljouw et al. 2010), a longer duration of SAD, comorbid panic disorder with agoraphobia, and lower psychosocial functioning predicted lower rates of recovery from SAD (Beard et al. 2010). Blanco et al. (2011) recorded treatment seeking in the past 12 months to predict an unfavorable course. In contrast, being employed, no lifetime depression, fewer than three lifetime psychiatric disorders, less anxiety sensitivity, and fewer daily hassles were associated with recovery from SAD (Vriends et al. 2007). In adolescents and young adults, predominantly clinical features in terms of early onset, generalized subtype, more anxiety cognitions, severe avoidance and impairment, and co-occurring panic attacks were associated with SAD persistence (Beesdo-Baum et al. 2012).

A Heuristic Framework for the Epidemiology of SAD

In parallel to a number of psychological models for SAD (Hughes et al. 2006; Clark and Wells 1995; Hoffman 2002; Christensen et al. 2003; Morrison and Heimberg 2013), clinical-epidemiological research focusing on natural course patterns as well as identification of correlates and risk factors and their interplay has stimulated a diathesis-stress model (vulnerability stress model) linking societal, biological, and psychological vulnerabilities with environmental stressors. This heuristic approach may help to delineate hypotheses about multiple factors relevant for the onset and course of SAD, as well as putative mechanisms and processes and their occurrence within sensitive developmental periods. In the past decade, a range of studies have provided findings in line with this approach (for a review, cf. Brook and Schmidt 2008). Childhood and adolescence have emerged as a sensitive time window for first SAD onset, though indicators and early signs for SAD may already be observed in infancy. The observed familial aggregation of SAD and the importance of the family and environment (in addition or combination with genetics) for the societal, emotional, and cognitive development of the offspring may denote a more family-oriented approach for targeted prevention and early intervention (Knappe et al. 2010; Elizabeth et al. 2006). However, dissection of the complex interplay of risk factors, correlates, and consequences is warranted to also understand underlying mechanisms and, more specifically, to identify moderators and mediators for SAD onset and course.

Summary and Conclusions

SAD is a debilitating condition that affects a large number of children and adolescents in both Western and non-Western countries. Most patients report an onset age of 20 years or younger, and symptoms tend to be persistent, although considerable fluctuations are seen over time. High co-occurrence is found with other mental problems, such as other anxiety disorders, depressive disorders, bulimia nervosa, substance use and somatoform disorders, and even psychosis. In addition, individuals with SAD are at increased risk for physical disorders, including insomnia, diabetes, and autoimmune diseases. In light of these facts, early intervention and prevention of SAD are a research imperative.

A wide range of risk factors have been identified to heighten incidence rates of SAD. Demographic variables include female gender and parental history of psychopathology. Low peer status and social skills and maladaptive familial environment and parenting are some typical psychological risk factors. Biological and physiological factors as represented by behavioral inhibition also play an important role in the manifestation and maintenance of symptoms. In recent years, cognitive factors such as information processing bias have received increased attention in relation to the etiology of SAD. These risk factors do not function independently, but rather constitute a complex interplay underpinning multiple trajectories to the onset of the disorder.

Current literature has come a long way since SAD was described as a "neglected anxiety disorder" (Liebowitz et al. 1985). However, information regarding temporal alteration and the longitudinal course of the disorder is very limited. Future studies may benefit from a family-oriented perspective to depict the divergent developmental sequence, to provide a comprehensive model in promoting epidemiological understanding of SAD, and to delineate targeted prevention and early interventions.

References

Acaturk C, Smit F, De Graaf R, van Straten A, Ten Have M, Cuijpers P (2009) Economic costs of social phobia: a population-based study. J Affect Disord 115:421–429

Aktar M, Majdandzic M, De Vente W, Bogels SM (2014) Parental social anxiety disorder prospectively predicts toddlers' fear/avoidance in a social referencing paradigm. J Child Psychol Psychiatry 55:77–87

Alfano CA, Beidel DC, Turner SM (2006) Cognitive correlates of social phobia among children and adolescents. J Abnorm Child Psychol 34:189–201

Alkozei A, Cooper P, Creswell C (2014) Emotional reasoning and anxiety sensitivity: associations with social anxiety disorder in childhood. J Affect Disord 152–154:219–228
Alnaes R, Torgersen S (1999) A 6-year follow-up study of anxiety disorders in psychiatric outpatients: development and continuity with personality disorders and personality traits as predictors. Nord J Psychiatry 53:409–416
Alonso J, Angermeyer C, Bernert S (2004) 12-month comorbidity patterns and associated factors in Europe: results from the European Study of the Epidemiology of Mental Disorders (ESEMeD) project. Acta Psychiatr Scand 109:28–37
American Psychiatric Association (2000) DSM-IV-TR. Diagnostic and statistical manual of mental disorders (Text revision). Author, Washington, DC
American Psychiatric Association (2013) DSM-5. Diagnostic and statistical manual of mental disorders, 5th edn. American Psychiatric Publishing, Arlington
Anderson EC, Dryman MT, Worthington J, Hoge EA, Fischer LE, Pollack MH, Barrett LF, Simon NM (2013) Smiles may go unseen in generalized social anxiety disorder: evidence from binocular rivalry for reduced visual consciousness of positive facial expressions. J Anxiety Disord 27:619–626
Andersson E, Ruck C, Lavebratt C, Hedman E, Schalling M, Lindefors N, Eriksson E, Carlbring P, Andersson G, Furmark T (2013) Genetic polymorphisms in monoamine systems and outcome of cognitive behavior therapy for social anxiety disorder. PLoS One 8
Angst J, Vollrath M (1991) The natural history of anxiety disorders. Acta Psychiatr Scand 84:446–452
Assuncao MC, Costa DLD, De Mathis MA, Shavitt RG, Ferrao YA, Do Rorsario MC, Miguel EC, Torres AR (2012) Social phobia in obsessive-compulsive disorder: prevalence and correlates. J Affect Disord 143:138–147
Avant TS, Gazelle H, Faldowski R (2011) Classroom emotional climate as a moderator of anxious solitary children's longitudinal risk for peer exclusion: a child x environment model. Dev Psychol 6:1711–1727
Ballash NG, Pemble MK, Usui WM, Buckley AF, Woodruff-Borden J (2006) Family functioning, perceived control, and anxiety: a mediational model. J Anxiety Disord 20:486
Bandelow B, Torrente AC, Wedekind D, Broocks A, Hajak G, Rüther E (2004) Early traumatic life events, parental rearing styles, family history of mental disorders, and birth risk factors in patients with social anxiety disorder. Eur Arch Psychiatr Clin Neurosci 254:397–405
Banerjee R, Henderson L (2001) Social-cognitive factors in childhood social anxiety: a preliminary investigation. Social Develop 10:558–572
Barrett PM, Rapee RM, Dadds MR, Ryan ND (1996) Family enhancement of cognitive style in anxious and aggressive children. J Abnorm Child Psychol 24:187–203
Beard C, Moitra E, Weisberg RB, Keller MB (2010) Characteristics and predictors of social phobia course in a longitudinal study of primary care patients. Depress Anxiety 27:839–845
Beck AT, Emery G, Greenberg RL (1985) Anxiety disorders and phobias: a cognitive perspective. Basic Books, New York
Beesdo K, Bittner A, Pine DS, Stein MB, Höfler M, Lieb R, Wittchen H-U (2007) Incidence of social anxiety disorder and the consistent risk for secondary depression in the first three decades of life. Arch Gen Psychiatry 64:903–912
Beesdo-Baum K, Knappe S (2012) Developmental epidemiology of anxiety disorders. Child Adolesc Psychiatr Clin N Am 21:457–478
Beesdo-Baum K, Knappe S, Fehm L, Höfler M, Lieb R, Hofmann SG, Wittchen H-U (2012) The natural course of social anxiety disorder among adolescents and young adults. Acta Psychiatr Scand 126:411–425
Beidel DC, Turner SM, Morris TL (1999) Psychopathology of childhood social phobia. J Am Acad Child Adolesc Psychiatry 38:643–650
Beidel DC, Turner SM, Morris TL (2000) Behavioral treatment of childhood social phobia. J Consult Clin Psychol 68:1072–1080
Beidel DC, Alfano CA, Kofler MJ, Rao, PA, Scharfstein L, Sarver, NW (2014). The impact of social skills training for social anxiety disorder: A randomized controlled trial. 28:908–918

Blakemore S-J (2008) The social brain in adolescence. Nat Rev Neurosci 9:267–277
Blanco C, Xu Y, Schneier FR, Okuda M, Liu SM, Heimberg GRG (2011) Predictors of persistence of social anxiety disorder: a national study. J Psychiatr Res 45:1557–1563
Blöte AW, Kint MJW, Westenberg PM (2007) Peer behavior towards socially anxious adolescents: classroom observations. Behav Res Ther 45:2773–2779
Bögels SM, Brechmann-Toussaint ML (2006) Family issues in child anxiety: attachment, family functioning, parental rearing and beliefs. Clin Psychol Rev 26:834–856
Bögels SM, Perotti EC (2011) Does father know best? A formal model of the paternal influence on childhood social anxiety. J Child Fam Stud 20:171–181
Bögels SM, Phares V (2008) Fathers' role in the etiology, prevention and treatment of child anxiety: a review and new model. Clin Psychol Rev 28:539–558
Bögels S, Stevens J, Majdandzic M (2011) Parenting and social anxiety: fathers' versus mothers' influence on their children's anxiety in ambiguous social situations. J Child Psychol Psychiatry 52:599–606
Bouman T, van der Meulen M, Goossens FA, Olthof T, Vermande MM, Aleva EA (2012) Peer and self-reports of victimization and bullying: their differential association with internalizing problems and social adjustment. J Sch Psychol 50:759–774
Brook CA, Schmidt LA (2008) Social anxiety disorder: a review of environmental risk factors. Neuropsychiatr Dis Treat 4:123–143
Bruce SE, Yonkers KA, Otto MW, Eisen JL, Weisberg RB, Pagano ME, Shea MT, Keller MB (2005) Influence of psychiatric comorbidity on recovery and recurrence in generalized anxiety disorder, social phobia, and panic disorder: a 12-year prospective study. Am J Psychiatry 162:1179–1187
Buckner JD, Vinci C (2013) Smoking and social anxiety: the roles of gender and smoking motives. Addict Behav 38:2388–2391
Buckner JD, Schmidt NB, Bobadilla L, Taylor J (2006) Social anxiety and problematic cannabis use: evaluating the moderating role of stress reactivity and perceived coping. Behav Res Ther 44:1007–1015
Buckner JD, Schmidt NB, Lang AR, Small JW, Schlauch RC, Lewinsohn PM (2008) Specificity of social anxiety disorder as a risk factor for alcohol and cannabis dependence. J Psychiatr Res 42:230–239
Budinger MC, Drazdowski TK, Ginsburg GS (2013) Anxiety-promoting parenting behaviors: a comparison of anxious parents with and without social anxiety disorder. Child Psychiatr Human Developt 44:412–418
Cartwright-Hatton S, Hodges L, Porter J (2003) Social anxiety in childhood: the relationship with self and observer rated social skills. J Clin Psychol Psychiatry 44:737–742
Cartwright-Hatton S, Tschernitz N, Gomersall H (2005) Social anxiety in children: social skills deficit, or cognitive distortion? Behavr Res Ther 43(1):131–141
Chartier MJ, Hazen AL, Stein MB (1998) Lifetime patterns of social phobia: a retrospective study of the course of social phobia in a nonclinical population. Depress Anxiety 7:113–121
Chavira DA, Stein MB, Bailey K, Stein MT (2004) Child anxiety in primary care: prevalent but untreated. Depress Anxiety 20:155–164
Chen X, Hastings PD, Rubin KH, Chen H, Cen G, Stewart SL (1998) Child-rearing attitudes and behavioral inhibition in Chinese and Canadian toddlers: a cross-cultural study. Dev Psychol 34:677–686
Christensen PN, Stein MB, Means-Christensen A (2003) Social anxiety and interpersonal perception: a social relations model analysis. Behav Res Ther 41:1355–1371
Clark DM, Wells A (1995) A cognitive model of social phobia. In: Heimberg RG, Liebowitz M, Hope DA, Schneier FR (eds) Social phobia: diagnosis, assessment, and treatment. Guilford, New York
Clauss JA, Blackford JU (2012) Behavioral inhibition and risk for developing social anxiety disorder: A meta-analytic study. J Am Acad Child Adolesc Psychiatry 51:1066–1075
Cludius B, Stevens S, Bantin T, Gerlach AL, Hermann C (2013) The motive to drink due to social anxiety and its relation to hazardous alcohol use. Psychol Addict Behav 27:806–813

Coles ME, Philipps BM, Menard W, Pagano ME, Fay C, Weisberg RB, Stout RL (2006) Body dysmorphic disorder and social phobia: cross-sectional and prospective data. Depress Anxiety 23:26–33

Costello EJ, Mustillo S, Erkanli A, Keeler G, Angold A (2003) Prevalence and development of psychiatric disorders in childhood and adolescence. Arch Gen Psychiatry 60:837–844

Cox BJ, Pagura J, Stein MB, Sareen J (2009) The relationship between generalized social phobia and avoidant personality disorder in a national mental health survey. Depress Anxiety 26:354–362

Creswell C, Schniering CA, Rapee RM (2005) Threat interpretation in anxious children and their mothers: comparison with nonclinical children and the effects of treatment. Behav Res Ther 43:1375–1381

Creswell C, Woolgar M, Cooper P, Giannakakis A, Schofield E, Young AW, Murray L (2008) Processing of faces and emotional expressions in infants at risk of social phobia. Cogn Emot 22:437–458

Creswell C, Cooper P, Giannakakis A, Schofield E, Woolgar M, Murray L (2011) Emotion processing in infancy: specificity in risk for social anxiety and associations with two year outcomes. J Exp Psychopathol 2:490–508

Creswell C, Murray G, Cooper P (2014) Interpretation and expectation in childhood anxiety disorders: age effects and social specificity. J Abnorm Child Psychol 42:453–465

Crippa JAS, Loureiro SR, Bapista CA, Osorio F (2007) Are there differences between early- and late-onset social anxiety disorder? Revista Brasileira De Psiquiatria 29:195–196

Davidson JRT, Hughes DC, George LK, Blazer DG (1994) The boundary of social phobia: exploring the threshold. Arch Gen Psychiatry 51:975–983

De Graaf R, Bijl RV, Smit F, Vollebergh WAM, Spijker J (2002) Risk factors for 12-month comorbidity of mood, anxiety, and substance use disorders: findings from the Netherlands Mental Health Survey and Incidence Study. Am J Psychiatry 159(4):620–629

De Menezes GB, Fontenelle LF, Versiani MR (2005) Early-onset social anxiety disorder in adults: Clinical and therapeutic features. Rev Bras Psiquiatr 27:32–36

Deardorff J, Hayward C, Wilson KA, Bryson S, Hammer LD, Agras S (2007) Puberty and gender interact to predict social anxiety symptoms in early adolescence. J Adolesc Health 41(1):102–124

Demir T, Karacetin G, Demir DE, Uysal O (2013) Prevalence and some psychosocial characteristics of social anxiety disorder in an urban population of Turkish children and adolescents. Eur Psychiatry 28:64–69

Dewit DJ, Ogborne A, Offord DR, MacDonald K (1999) Antecedents of the risk of recovery from DSM-III-R social phobia. Psychol Med 29:569–582

Dewit DJ, Chandler-Coutts M, Offord DR, King G, McDougall J, Specht J, Stewart S (2005) Gender differences in the effects of family adversity on the risk of onset on DSM III-R social phobia. J Anxiety Disord 19:479–502

DiLalla LF, Kagan J, Reznick JS (1994) Genetic etiology of behavioral inhibition among 2-year-old children. Infant Behav Dev 17:405–412

Dinnel DL, Kleinknecht RA, Tanaka-Matsumi J (2002) A cross-cultural comparison of social phobia symptoms. J Psychopathol Behavl Assess 24:75–84

Domschke K, Deckert J (2012) Genetics of anxiety disorders – status Quo and quo vadis. Curr Pharm Des 18:5691–5698

Domschke K, Stevens S, Beck B, Baffa A, Hohoff C, Deckert J, Gerlach AL (2009) Blushing propensity in social anxiety disorder: influence of serotonin transporter gene variation. J Neural Transm 116:663–666

Eley TC, Rijsdijk FV, Perrin S, O'Connor TG, Bolton D (2008) A multivariate genetic analysis of specific phobia, separation anxiety and social phobia in early childhood. J Abnorm Child Psychol 36:839–848

Elizabeth J, King N, Ollendick TH, Gullone E, Tonge B, Watson S, Macdermott S (2006) Social anxiety disorder in children and youth: a research update on aetiological factors. Couns Psychol Q 19:151–163

Eng W, Heimberg RG, Hart TA, Schneier FR, Liebowitz MR (2001) Attachment in individuals with social anxiety disorder: the relationship among adult attachment styles, social anxiety, and depression. Emotion 1
Erath SA, Flanagan KS, Biedermann KL (2008) Early adolescent school-adjustment: associations with friendship and peer victimization. Soc Devel 17:853–870
Essau CA, Conradt J, Petermann F (2002) Course and outcome of anxiety disorders in adolescents. J Anxiety Disord 16:67–81
Essau CA, Sasagawa S, Ishikawa S, Okajima I, O'Callaghan J, Bray D (2012) A Japanese form of social anxiety (taijin kyofusho): frequency and correlates in two generations of the same family. Int J Soc Psychiatry 58:635–642
Faravelli C, Zucchi T, Viviani B, Salmoria R, Perone A, Paionni A, Scarpato A, Vigliaturo D, Rosi S, D'Adamo D, Bartolozzi D, Cecchi C, Abrardi L (2000) Epidemiology of social phobia: a clinical approach. Eur Psychiatry 15:17–24
Feehan M, McGee R, Raha SN, Williams SM (1994) DSM-III-R disorders in New Zealand 18-year-olds. Aust N Z J Psychiatry 28:87–99
Fehm L, Pelissolo A, Furmark T, Wittchen H-U (2005) Size and burden of social phobia in Europe. Eur Neuropsychopharmacol 15:453–462
Fehm L, Beesdo K, Jacobi F, Fiedler A (2008) Social anxiety disorder above and below the diagnostic threshold: prevalence, comorbidity and impairment in the general population. Soc Psychiatry Psychiatr Epidemiol 43:257–265
Frick A, Howner K, Fischer H, Eskildsen SF, Kristiansson M, Furmark T (2013) Cortical thickness alterations in social anxiety disorder. Neurosci Lett 536:52–55
Fu C-W, Tan AW, Sheng F, Luan R-S, Zhan S-Y, Chen W-Q et al (2007) The prevalence of anxiety symptoms and depressive symptoms in patients with somatic disorders in urban China: a multi-center cross-sectional study. Int J Psychiatry Med 37:185–199
Garcia-Lopez LJ, Ingles C, Garcia-Fernandez JM (2008) Exploring the relevance of gender and age differences in the assessment of social fears in adolescence. Soc Behav Personal 36:385–390
Garcia-Lopez LJ, Beidel DC, Hidalgo MD, Olivares J, Turner S (2008a) Brief form of the Social Phobia and Anxiety Inventory (SPAI-B) for adolescents. Eur J Psychol Assess 24:150–156
Garcia-Lopez LJ, Muela JA, Espinosa-Fernández L, Diaz-Castela MM (2009) Exploring the relevance of expressed emotion to the treatment of social anxiety disorder in adolescence. J Adolesc 32:1371–1376
Garcia-Lopez LJ, Irurtia MJ, Caballo VE, Díaz-Castela MM (2011) Ansiedad social y abuso psicológico [Social anxiety and psychological abuse]. Behav Psycholy 19:223–236
Garcia-Lopez LJ, Diaz-Castela MM, Muela-Martinez JA, Espinosa-Fernandez L (2014) Can parent training for parents with high levels of expressed emotion have a positive effect on their child's social anxiety improvement? J Anxiety Disord 28:812–822
Garcia-Lopez LJ, Moore H (2015a) The Mini-Social Phobia Inventory: psychometric properties in an adolescent general and clinical population. PLOS One (in press)
Garcia-Lopez LJ, Saez-Castillo A, Beidel DC, La Greca AM (2015b) Brief measures to screen for social anxiety in adolescents. Manucript submitted for publication
Gazelle H (2006) Class climate moderates peer relations and emotional adjustment in children with an early history of anxious solitude: a child x environment model. Dev Psychol 42:1179–1192
Gelernter J, Page GP, Stein MB, Woods SW (2004) Genome-wide linkage scan for loci predisposing to social phobia: evidence for a chromosome 16 risk locus. Am J Psychiatry 161:59–66
Gentili C, Ricciardi E, Gobbini MI, Santarelli MF, Haxby JV, Pietrini P, Guazzelli M (2009) Beyond amygdala: default Mode Network activity differs between patients with social phobia and healthy controls. Brain Res Bull 79:409–413
Godart N, Flament M, Perereau F, Jeammet P (2002) Co-morbidity between eating disorders and anxiety disorders: a review. Int J Eat Diosrd 32:253–270
Goldin PR, Manber T, Hakimi S, Canli T, Gross JJ (2009) Neural bases of social anxiety disorder. Emotional reactivity and cognitive regulation during social and physical threat. Arch Gen Psychiatry 66:170–180

Gómez-Ariza CJ, Iglesias-Parro S, Garcia-Lopez LJ, Díaz-Castela MM, Espinosa-Fernández L, Muela JA (2013) Selective intentional forgetting in adolescents with social anxiety disorder. Psychiatry Res 208:151–155
Gregory AM, Eley TC (2007) Genetic Influences on anxiety in children: what we've learned and where we're heading. Clin Child Fam Psychol 10:199–212
Gregory AM, Caspi A, Moffitt TE, Koenen K, Eley TC, Poulton R (2007) Juvenile mental health histories of adults with anxiety disorders. Am J Psychiatry 164:301–308
Gren-Landell M, Aho N, Andersson G, Svedin CG (2011) Social anxiety disorder and victimization in a community sample of adolescents. J Adolesc 34:569–577
Gulley LD, Oppenheimer CW, Hankin BL (2014) Associations among negative parenting, attention bias to anger, and social anxiety among youth. Dev Psychol 50(2):577–585
Haller SPW, Kadosh KC, Lau JYF (2014) A developmental angle to understanding the mechanisms of biased cognitions in social anxiety. Front Hum Neurosci 7:846
Halls G, Cooper PJ, Creswell C (2015) Social communication deficits: specific associations with Social Anxiety Disorder. J Affect Disord 172:38–42
Hayward C, Killen JD, Kraemer HC, Taylor CB (1998) Linking self-reported behavioral inhibition to adolescent social phobia. J Am Acad Child Adolesc Psychiatry 27:1308–1316
Heinrichs N, Rapee RM, Alden LA, Bögels S, Hofmann SG, Ja Oh K, Sakano Y (2006) Cultural differences in perceived social norms and social anxiety. Behav Res Ther 44:1187–1197
Hirshfeld DR, Biederman J, Brody L, Faraone SV, Rosenbaum JF (1997) Expressed emotion toward children with behavioral inhibition: associations with maternal anxiety disorder. J Am Acad Child Adolesc Psychiatry 36:910–917
Hoffman SO (2002) Die Psychodynamik der Sozialen Phobien (The psychodynamics of social anxiety disorder). Forum der Psychoanalyse 18:51–71
Hong JJ, Woody SR (2007) Cultural mediators of self-reported social anxiety. Behav Res Ther 45:1779–1789
Hsu L, Alden L (2007) Social anxiety in Chinese- and European-heritage students: the effect of assessment format and judgments of impairment. Behav Ther 38:120–131
Hughes AA, Heimberg RG, Coles ME, Gibb BE, Liebowitz MR, Schneier FR (2006) Relations of the factors of the tripartite model of anxiety and depression to types of social anxiety. Behav Res Ther 44:1629–1641
Hwu HG, Yeh EK, Chang LY (1989) Prevalence of psychiatric disorders in Taiwan defined by the Chinese Diagnostic Interview Schedule. Acta Psychiatr Scand 79:136–147
Inderbitzen-Nolan HM, Anderson ER, Johnson HS (2007) Subjective versus objective behavioral ratings following two analogue tasks: a comparison of socially phobic and non-anxious adolescents. J Anxiety Disord 21:76–90
Johnson EO, Roth T, Breslau N (2006) The association of insomnia with anxiety disorders and depression: exploration of the direction of risk. J Psychiatr Res 40(8):700–708
Kagan J, Reznick JS, Snidman N (1987) The physiology and psychology of behavioral inhibition in children. Child Dev 58:1459–1473
Kagan J, Reznick JS, Snidman N (1988a) Biological bases of childhood shyness. Science 240:167–171
Kagan J, Reznick JS, Snidman N, Gibbons J, Johnson MO (1988b) Childhood derivates of inhibition and lack of inhibition to the unfamiliar. Child Dev 59:1580–1589
Keller MB (2003) The lifelong course of social anxiety disorder: a clinical perspective. Acta Psychiatr Scand 108:85–94
Keller MB (2006) Social anxiety disorder clinical course and outcome: Review of Harvard/Brown Anxiety Research Project (HARP) findings. J Clin Psychiatry 67:14–19
Kendall PC (1985) Toward a cognitive-behavioral model of child psychopathology and a critique of related interventions. J Abnorm Child Psychol 13:357–372
Kendler KS, Prescott CA, Jacobson K, Myers J, Neale MC (2002) The joint analysis of personal interview and family history diagnoses: evidence for validity of diagnosis and increased heritability estimates. Psychol Med 32:829–845

Kendler KS, Gardner CO, Annas P, Lichtenstein P (2008) The development of fears from early adolescence to young adulthood: a multivariate study. Psychol Med 38:1759–1769

Kerns CE, Comer JS, Pincus DB, Hofmann SG (2013) Evaluation of the proposed social anxiety disorder specifier change for DSM-5 in a treatment-seeking sample of anxious youth. Depress Anxiety 30:709–715.

Kessler RC, McGonagle KA, Zhao S, Nelson CB, Hughes M, Eshleman S, Wittchen H-U, Kendler KS (1994) Lifetime and 12-month prevalence of DSM-III-R psychiatric disorders in the United States: results from the National Comorbidity Study. Arch Gen Psychiatry 51:8–19

Kessler RC, Stein MB, Berglund P (1998) Social phobia subtypes in the national comorbidity survey. Am J Psychiatry 155:613–619

Kessler RC, Berglund P, Demler O, Jin R, Merikangas KR, Walters EE (2005a) Lifetime prevalence and age-of-onset distributions of DSM-IV disorders in the National Comorbidity Survey Replication. Arch Gen Psychiatry 62:593–602

Kessler RC, Chui WT, Demler O, Merikangas KR, Walters EE (2005b) Prevalence, severity, and comorbidity of 12-month DSM-IV disorders in the National Comorbidity Survey Replication. Arch Gen Psychiatry 62:617–627

Kessler RC, Avenevoli S, Costello EJ, Georgiades K, Green JG, Gruber MJ, He JP, Koretz D, McLaughlin KA, Petukhova M, Samspon NA, Zaslavsky AM, Merikangas KR (2012) Prevalence, persistence, and sociodemographic correlates of DSM-IV disorders in the National Comorbidity Survey Replication Adolescent Supplement. Arch Gen Psychiatry 69:372–380

Kim-Cohen J, Caspi A, Moffitt TE, Harrington HL, Milne BJ, Poulton R (2003) Prior juvenile diagnosis in adults with mental disorders: developmental follow-back of a prospective-longitudinal cohort. Arch Gen Psychiatry 60:709–717

Kleinknecht RA, Dinnel DL, Kleinknecht EE, Hiruma N (1997) Cultural factors in social anxiety: a comparison of social phobia symptoms and Taijin Kyofusho. J Anxiety Disord 11:157–177

Knappe S, Beesdo K, Fehm L, Lieb R, Wittchen H-U (2009a) Associations of familial risk factors with social fears and social phobia: evidence for the continuum hypothesis in social anxiety disorder ? J Neural Transm 116:639–648

Knappe S, Lieb R, Beesdo K, Fehm L, Low NCP, Gloster AT, Wittchen H-U (2009b) The role of parental psychopathology and family environment for social phobia in the first three decades of life. Depress Anxiety 26:363–370

Knappe S, Beesdo K, Fehm L, Höfler M, Lieb R, Wittchen H-U (2009c) Do parental psychopathology and unfavorable family environment predict the persistence of social phobia? J Anxiety Disord 23:986–994

Knappe S, Beesdo-Baum K, Wittchen H-U (2010) Familial risk factors in social anxiety disorder: calling for a family-oriented approach for targeted prevention and early intervention. Eur Child Adolesc Psychiatry 19:857–871

Knappe S, Beesdo K, Fehm L, Stein MB, Lieb R, Wittchen HU (2011) Social fear and social phobia types among community youth: differential clinical features and vulnerability factors. J Psychiatr Res 45:111–120

Knappe S, Beesdo-Baum K, Fehm L, Lieb R, Wittchen H-U (2012) Characterizing the association between parental rearing and adolescent social phobia. J Anxiety Disord 26:608–616

La Greca AM, Stone WL (1993) Social anxiety scale for children-revised: factor structure and concurrent validity. J Clin Child Psychol 22:17–27

La Greca AM, Dandes SK, Wick P, Shaw K (1988) Development of the social anxiety scale for children: reliability and concurrent validity. J Clin Child Psychol 17:84–91

Lampe L, Slade T, Issakidis C, Andrews G (2003) Social phobia in the Australian National Survey of Mental Health and Well-Being (NSMHWB). Psychol Med 33:637–646

Last CG, Perrin S, Hersen M, Kazdin AE (1992) DSM-III-R anxiety disorders in children: sociodemographic and clinical characteristics. J Am Acad Child Adolesc Psychiatry 31:1070–1076

Last CG, Perrin S, Hersen M, Kazdin AE (1996) A prospective study of childhood anxiety disorders. J Am Acad Child Adolesc Psychiatry 35:1502–1510

Lee MR, Okazaki S, Yoo HC (2006) Frequency and intensity of social anxiety in Asian Americans and European Americans. Cultu Divers Ethnic Minor Psychol 12:291–305
Lee S, Ng KL, Kwok KPS, Tsang A (2009) Prevalence and correlates of social fears in Hong Kong. J Anxiety Disord 23:327–332
Lépine J-P, Wittchen H-U, Essau CA (1993) Lifetime and current comorbidity of anxiety and depressive disorders: results from the International WHO/ADAMHA CIDI Field Trials. Int J Methods Psychiatr Res 3:67–78
Levinson CA, Langer JK, Rodebaugh TL (2013) Reactivity to social exclusion prospectively predicts social anxiety symptoms in young adults. Behav Ther 44
Lewis-Morrarty E, Degnan KA, Chronis-Tuscano A, Rubin KH, Cheah CS, Pine DS, Henderon HA, Fox NA (2012) Maternal over-control moderates the association between early childhood behavioral inhibition and adolescent social anxiety symptoms. J Abnorm Child Psychol 40(8):1363–1373
Lieb R, Wittchen H-U, Höfler M, Fuetsch M, Stein MB, Merikangas KR (2000) Parental psychopathology, parenting styles and the risk of social phobia in offspring: a prospective-longitudinal community study. Arch Gen Psychiatry 57:859–866
Liebowitz MR, Gorman JM, Fyer AJ, Klein DF (1985) Social phobia: review of a neglected anxiety disorder. Arch Gen Psychiatry 42:729
Lim SW, Ha J, Shin YC, Shin DW, Bae SM, Oh KS (2013) Clinical differences between early- and late-onset social anxiety disorders. Early Interv Psychiatry 7:44–50
Machado-de-Sousa JP, Osorio FD, Jackowski AP, Bressan RA, Chagas MHN, Torro-Alves N, Depaula ALD, Crippa JAS, Hallak JEC (2014) Increased amygdalar and hippocampal volumes in young adults with social anxiety. PLoS One 9(2):e88523
MacKenzie MB, Fowler KF (2013) Social anxiety disorder in the Canadian population: exploring gender differences in sociodemographic profile. J Anxiety Disord 27:427–434
Magee WJ, Eaton WW, Wittchen HU, McGonagle KA, Kessler RC (1996) Agoraphobia, simple phobia, and social phobia in the National Comorbidity Survey. Arch Gen Psychiatry 53:159–168
Majdandzic M, Moller EL, de Vente W, Bogels SM, van den Boom DC (2014) Fathers' challenging parenting behavior prevents social anxiety development in their 4-year-old children: a longitudinal observational study. J Abnorm Child Psychol 42:301–310
Massion AO, Dyck IR, Shea MT, Phillips KA, Warshaw MG, Keller MB (2002) Personality disorders and time to remission in generalized anxiety disorder, social phobia, and panic disorder. Arch Gen Psychiatry 59:434–440
Matheny AP (1989) Children's behavioral inhibition over age and across situations: genetic similarity for a trait during change. J Pers 57:215–235
McCabe RE, Antony MM, Summerfeldt LJ, Liss A, Swinson RP (2003) Preliminary examination of the relationship between anxiety disorders in adults and self-reported history of teasing. Cogn Behav Ther 32:187–193
McGrath LM, Weill S, Robinson EB, MacRae R, Smoller JW (2012) Bringing a developmental perspective to anxiety genetics. Dev Psychopathol 24:1179–1193
McLeod BD, Wood JJ, Weisz JR (2007) Examining the association between parenting and childhood anxiety: a meta-analysis. Clin Psychol Rev 27:155–172
McNeil DW (2001) Terminology and evolution of constructs in social anxiety and social phobia. In: Hofmann SG, Dibartolo PM (eds) From social anxiety to social phobia. Allyn & Bacon, Needham Heights
Merikangas KR, Avenevoli S, Acharyya S, Zhang H, Angst J (2002) The spectrum of social phobia in the Zurich cohort study of young adults. Biol Psychiatry 51:81–91
Merikangas KR, Lieb R, Wittchen H-U, Aveneoli S (2003) Family and high-risk studies of social anxiety disorder. Acta Psychiatr Scand 108:28–37
Merikangas KR, He JP, Burstein M, Swanson SA, Avenevoli S, Cui LH, Benjet C, Georgiades K, Swendsen J (2011) Lifetime prevalence of mental disorders in US adolescents: results from the National Comorbidity Survey Replication-Adolescent Supplement (NCS-A). J Am Acad Child Adolesc Psychiatry 49:980–989

Monk CS, Nelson EE, McClure EB, Mogg K, Bradley BP, Leibenluft E, Blair RJ, Chen G, Charney DS, Ernst M, Pine DS (2006) Ventrolateral prefrontal cortex activation and attentional bias in response to angry faces in adolescents with generalized anxiety disorder. Am J Psychiatry 163:1091–1097

Morgan J, Banerjee M (2006) Social anxiety and self-evaluation of social performance in a nonclinical sample of children. J Clin Child Adolesc Psychol 35:292–301

Morrison AS, Heimberg RG (2013) Social anxiety and Social anxiety disorder. Annu Rev Clin Psychol 9(9):249–274

Murray L, Cooper P, Creswell C, Schofield E, Sack C (2007) The effects of maternal social phobia on mother-infant interactions and infant social responsiveness. J Child Psychol Psychiatry 48:45–52

Murray L, de Rosney M, Pearson J, Bergeron C, Schofield E, Royal-Lawson M, Cooper PJ (2008) Intergenerational transmission of social anxiety: the role of social referencing processes in infancy. Child Dev 79:1049–1064

Murray L, Creswell C, Cooper PJ (2009) The development of anxiety disorders in childhood: an integrative review. Psychol Med 39:1413–1423

Murray L, Lau PY, Arteche A, Creswell C, Russ S, Zoppa LD, Muggeo M, Stein A, Cooper P (2012) Parenting by anxious mothers: effects of disorder subtype, context and child characteristics. J Child Psychol Psychiatry 53:188–196

Murray L, Pella J, De Pascalis L, Arteche A, Pass L, Percy R, Creswell C, Cooper P (2014) Socially anxious mothers' narratives to their children, and their relation to child representations and adjustment. Dev Psychopathol 26(4 Pt 2):1531–1546

Nagata T, Yamada H, Teo AR, Yoshimura C, Nakajima T, van Vliet I (2013) Comorbid social withdrawal (hikikomori) in outpatients with social anxiety disorder: clinical characteristics and treatment response in a case series. Int J Soc Psychiatry 59:73–78

Natsuaki MN, Leve LD, Neiderhiser JM, Shaw DS, Scaramella LV, Ge X, Reiss D (2013) Intergenerational transmission of risk for social inhibition: the interplay between parental responsiveness and genetic influences. Dev Psychopathol 25:261–274

Neufeld KJ, Swartz KL, Bienvenu OJ, Eaton WW, Cai G (1999) Incidence of DIS/DSM-IV social phobia in adults. Acta Psychiatr Scand 100:186–192

Noyes R, Holt CS, Woodman CL (2005) Natural course of anxiety disorders. In: Mavissakalian MR, Prien RF (eds) Long-term treatment of anxiety disorders. American Psychiatric Press, Inc, Washington, DC

Pass L, Arteche A, Cooper P, Creswell C, Murray L (2012) Doll Play narratives about starting school in children of socially anxious mothers, and their relation to subsequent child school-based anxiety. J Abnormal Child Psychol 40(8):1375–1384

Pejic T, Hermann A, Vaitl D, Stark R (2013) Social anxiety modulates amygdala activation during social conditioning. Soc Cogn Affect Neurosci 8:267–276

Peleg-Popko O, Dar R (2001) Marital quality, family patterns, and children's fears and social anxiety. Contemp Fam Ther: Int Jl 23:465–487

Pine DS, Cohen P, Gurley D, Brook J, Ma Y (1998) The risk for early adulthood anxiety and depressive disorders in adolescents with anxiety and depressive disorders. Arch Gen Psychiatry 55:56–64

Ranta K, Kaltiala-Heino R, Pelkonen M, Marttunen M (2009a) Associations between peer-victimization, self-reported depression and social phobia among adolescents: the role of comorbidity. J Adolesc 32:77–93

Ranta K, Kaltiala-Heino R, Rantanen P, Marttunen M (2009b) Social phobia in Finnish general adolescent population: Prevalence, comorbidity, individual and family correlates, and service use. Depress Anxiety 26:528–236

Ranta K, Kaltiala-Heino R, Fröjd S, Marttunen M (2013) Peer victimization and social phobia: a follow-up study among adolescents. Soc Psychiatry Psychiatr Epidemiol 48:533–544

Rao PA, Beidel DC, Turner SM, Ammerman RT, Crosby LE, Sallee FR (2007) Social anxiety disorder in childhood and adolescence: descriptive psychopathology. Behav Res Ther 45:1181–1191

Rapee RM, Heimberg RG (1997) A cognitive-behavioral model of anxiety in social phobia. Behav Res Ther 35:741–756
Rapee RM, Spence SH (2004) The etiology of social phobia: empirical evidence and an initial model. Clin Psychol Rev 24:737–767
Rietdijk J, Ising HK, Dragt S, Klaassen R, Nieman D, Wunderink L, Cuijpers P, Linszen D, van der Gaag M (2013) Depression and social anxiety in help-seeking patients with an ultra-high risk for developing psychosis. Psychiatry Res 209:309–313
Robinson JL, Kagan J, Reznick JS, Corley R (1992) The heritability of inhibited and uninhibited behavior: a twin study. Dev Psychol 28:1030–1037
Rogers MP, Weinshenker NJ, Warshaw MG, Goisman RM, Rodriguez-Villa FJ, Fierman EJ, Keller MB (1996) Prevalence of somatoform disorders in a large sample of patients with anxiety disorders. Psychosomatics: J Consult Liaison Psychiatry 37:17
Roth DA, Coles ME, Heimberg RG (2002) The relationship between memories for childhood teasing and anxiety and depression in adulthood. J Anxiety Disord 16(2):149–164
Roy AK, Vasa RA, Bruck M, Mogg K, Bradley BP, Sweeney M, Bergman RL, McClure-Tone EB, Pine DS (2008) Attention bias toward threat in pediatric anxiety disorders. J Am Acad Child Adolesc Psychiatry 47:1189–1196
Ruscio AM, Brown TA, Chiu WT, Sareen J, Stein MB, Kessler RC (2008) Social fears and social phobia in the USA: results from the National Comorbidity Survey Replication. Psychol Med 38:15–28
Rutter M, Kim-Cohen J, Maughan B (2006) Continuities and discontinuities in psychopathology between childhood and adult life. J Child Psychol Psychiatry 47:276–295
Sareen J, Cox BJ, Afifi TO, de Graaf R, Asmundson GJG, ten Have M, Stein MB (2005a) Anxiety disorders and risk for suicidal ideation and suicide attempts: a population-based longitudinal study of adults. Arch Gen Psychiatry 62:1249–1257
Sareen J, Cox BJ, Clara I, Asmundson GJG (2005b) The relationship between anxiety disorders and physical disorders in the U.S. National Comorbidity Survey. Depress Anxiety 21: 193–202
Sareen J, Chartier MJ, Paulus MP, Stein MB (2006) Illicit drug use and anxiety disorders: findings from two community surveys. Psychiatry Res 142:11–17
Schneier FR, Johnson J, Hornig CD, Liebowitz MR, Weissman MM (1992) Social phobia: comorbidity and morbidity in an epidemiologic sample. Arch Gen Psychiatry 49:282–288
Schry AR, White SW (2013) Understanding the relationship between social anxiety and alcohol use in college students: a meta-analysis. Addict Behav 38:2690–2706
Schutters SIJ, Dominguez MD, Knappe S, Lieb R, van Os J, Schruers KRJ, Wittchen HU (2011) The association between social phobia, social anxiety cognitions and paranoid symptoms. Acta Psychiatr Scand 125:213–227
Schwartz CE, Snidman N, Kagan J (1999) Adolescent social anxiety as an outcome of inhibited temperament in childhood. J Am Acad Child Adolesc Psychiatry 38:1008–1015
Sibrava NJ, Beard C, Bjornsson AS, Moitra E, Weisberg RB, Keller MB (2013) Two-year course of generalized anxiety disorder, social anxiety disorder, and panic disorder in a longitudinal sample of African American adults. J Consult Clin Psychol 81:1052–1062
Siegel RS, La Greca AM, Harrison HM (2009) Peer victimization and social anxiety in adolescents: prospective and reciprocal relationships. J Youth Adolesc 38
Sonntag H, Wittchen HU, Höfler M, Kessler RC, Stein MB (2000) Are social fears and DSM IV social anxiety disorder associated with smoking and nicotine dependence in adolescents and young adults? Eur Psychiatry 15:67–74
Spence SH, Donovan C, Brechman-Toussaint M (1999) Social skills, social outcomes, and cognitive features of childhood social phobia. J Abnorm Psychol 108:211–221
Spence SH, Donovan C, Brechman-Toussaint M (2000) The treatment of childhood social phobia: the effectiveness of a social skills training-based, cognitive-behavioural intervention, with and without parental involvement. J Child Psychol Psychiatry 41:713–726
Stein MB, Kroft CDL, Walker JR (1993) Sleep impairment in patients with social phobia. Psychiatry Res 49:251–256

Stein MB, Walker JR, Forde DR (1994) Setting diagnostic thresholds for social phobia. Considerations from a community survey of social anxiety. Am J Psychiatry 151:408–412
Stein MB, Chavira DA, Jang KL (2001a) Bringing up a bashful baby: developmental pathways to social phobia. Psychiatr Clin North Am 24:661–675
Stein MB, Fuetsch M, Müller N, Höfler M, Lieb R, Wittchen H-U (2001b) Social anxiety disorder and the risk of depression: a prospective community study of adolescents and young adults. Arch Gen Psychiatry 58:251–256
Steinert C, Hofmann M, Leichsenring F, Kruse J (2013) What do we know today about the prospective long-term course of social anxiety disorder? A systematic literature review. J Anxiety Disord 27:692–702
Stevens S, Cludius B, Bantin T, Hermann C, Gerlach AL (2014) Influence of alcohol on social anxiety: an investigation of attentional, physiological and behavioral effects. Biol Psychol 96:126–133
Stevenson-Hinde J, Shouldice A (1990) Fear and attachment in 2,5 year olds. Br J Dev Psychol 8:319–333
Stirling LJ, Eley TC, Clark DM (2006) Preliminary evidence for an association between social anxiety symptoms and avoidance of negative faces in school-age children. J Clin Child Adolesc Psychol 35:431–439
Storch EA, Masia-Warner C, Crisp H, Klein RG (2005) Peer victimization and social anxiety in adolescence: a prospective study. Aggress Behav 31:437–452
Suveg C, Zeman J, Flannery-Schroeder E, Cassano M (2005) Emotion socialization in families of children with an anxiety disorder. J Abnorm Child Psychol 33:145
Swinbourne JM, Touyz SW (2007) The co-morbidity of eating disorders and anxiety disorders: a review. Eur Eat Disord Rev 15:253–274
Tamplin A, Goodyer IM (2001) Family functioning in adolescents at high and low risk for major depressive disorder. Eur Child Adolesc Psychiatry 10:170–179
Teetsel RN, Ginsburg GS, Drake KL (2014) Anxiety-promoting parenting behaviors: a comparison of anxious mothers and fathers. Child Psychiatry Hum Dev 45:133–142
Tillfors M, Persson S, Willen M, Burk WJ (2012) Prospective links between social anxiety and adolescent peer relations. J Adolesc 35:1255–1263
Tsuchiya M, Kawakami N, Ono Y, Nakane Y, Nakamura Y, Tachimori H, Wata N, Uda H, Nakane H, Watanabe M, Naganuma Y, Furukawa TA, Hata Y, Kobayashi M, Miyake Y, Takeshima T, Kikkawa T, Kessler RC (2009) Lifetime comorbidities between phobic disorders and major depression in Japan. Results from the World Mental Health Japan 2002-2004 Survey. Depress Anxiety 26:949–955
Van Ameringen M, Mancini C, Oakman JM (1998) The relationship of behavioral inhibition and shyness to anxiety disorder. J Nerv Mental Dis 186:425–431
van Beljouw IMJ, Verhaak PFM, Cuijpers P, van Marwijk HWJ, Penninx B (2010) The course of untreated anxiety and depression, and determinants of poor one-year outcome: a one-year cohort study. BMC Psychiatry 10:86
van Brakel AML, Muris P, Bögels SM, Thomassen C (2006) A multifactorial model for the etiology of anxiety in non-clinical adolescents: main and interactive effects of behavioral inhibition, attachment and parental rearing. J Child Fam Stud 15:569–579
Van Steensel FJ, Bögels SM, Wood JJ (2013) Autism spectrum traits in children with anxiety disorders. J Autism Dev Disord 43:361–370
Vernberg EM, Abwender DA, Ewell KK, Beery SH (1992) Social anxiety and peer relationships in early adolescence: a prospective analysis. J Clin Child Psychol 21:189–196
Voci SC, Beitchman JH, Brownlie EB, Wilson B (2006) Social anxiety in late adolescence: the importance of early childhood language impairment. J Anxiety Disord 20:915–930
Vriends N, Becker ES, Meyer A, Williams SL, Lutz R, Margraf J (2007) Recovery from social phobia in the community and its predictors: data from a longitudinal epidemiological study. J Anxiety Disord 21:320–337
Vriends N, Pfaltz MC, Novianti P, Hadiyono J (2013) Taijin kyofusho and social anxiety and their clinical relevance in Indonesia and Switzerland. FrontPsychol 4:3

Waters AM, Bradley BP, Mogg K (2014) Biased attention to threat in paediatric anxiety disorders (generalized anxiety disorder, social phobia, specific phobia, separation anxiety disorder) as a function of 'distress' versus 'fear' diagnostic categorization. Psychol Med 44:607–616

Wittchen H-U, Fehm L (2001) Epidemiology, patterns of comorbidity and associated disabilities of social phobia. Psychiatr Clin North Am 24:617–641

Wittchen H-U, Lieb R, Schuster P, Oldehinkel AJ (1999a) When is onset? Investigations into early developmental stages of anxiety and depressive disorders. In: Rapoport JL (ed) Childhood onset of "adult" psychopathology, clinical and research advances. American Psychiatric Press, Washington

Wittchen HU, Stein MB, Kessler RC (1999b) Social fears and social phobia in a community sample of adolescents and young adults: prevalence, risk factors and comorbidity. Psychol Med 29:309–323

Wood JJ, McLeod BD, Sigman M, Hwang W-C, Chu BC (2003) Parenting and childhood anxiety: theory, empirical findings, and future directions. J Child Psychol Psychiatry 44:134–151

Xu Y, Schneier F, Heimberg RG, Princisvalle K, Liebowitz MR, Wang S, Blanco C (2012) Gender differences in social anxiety disorder: results from the national epidemiologic sample on alcohol and related conditions. J Anxiety Disord 26:12–19

Yonkers KA, Bruce SE, Dyck IR, Keller MB (2003) Chronicity, relapse, and illness – course of manic disorder, social phobia, and generalized anxiety disorder: findings in men and women from 8 years of follow-up. Depress Anxiety 17:173–179

Zhang W, Ross J, Davidson JRT (2004) Social anxiety disorder in callers to the Anxiety Disorders Association of America. Depress Anxiety 20:101–106

Zimmerman G, Pin MA, Krenz S, Bouchat A, Favrat B, Besson J, Zullino DF (2004) Prevalence of social phobia in a clinical sample of drug dependent patients. J Affect Disord 83:83–87

4 Easier to Accelerate Than to Slow Down: Contributions of Developmental Neurobiology for the Understanding of Adolescent Social Anxiety

Maria Tillfors and Nejra Van Zalk

Introduction

Social anxiety tends to increase in early adolescence, and age 13 is considered the typical age of onset for social anxiety disorder (SAD) or social phobia (see Rapee and Spence 2004 for a review, as well as Chap. 3). Social anxiety is characterized by social fears, excessive discomfort, anticipatory worry, rumination, and somatic symptoms such as trembling, blushing, and sweating before, during, and/or after social situations (Heiser et al. 2009). High levels of social anxiety are associated with lower peer acceptance (Erath et al. 2010; Flanagan et al. 2008; La Greca and Lopez 1998; La Greca and Harrison 2005) as well as increased peer victimization (Garcia-Lopez et al. 2011; Siegel et al. 2009; Ranta el al. 2009, 2013; Storch et al. 2003; see also Chap. 5), impairment in romantic relationships (Hebert et al. 2013; see also Chap. 8 of this book), high levels of loneliness (Stoeckli 2010), and poor relationships with parents (Van Zalk and Kerr 2011; see also Chap. 2). As such then, social anxiety can become a huge problem for young people's social development.

Anxiety is a negative emotion, and when people experience negative emotions, they tend to try to reduce them by regulating their feelings. *Emotion regulation* refers to a number of automatic or controlled processes that people use to influence their feelings (Gross 1998). It also involves attempting to influence when to have these emotions and how to express them—both consciously and unconsciously (Gross 1998). Commonly used emotion regulation strategies are escape and avoidance. When people are afraid of external stimuli such as social situations or internal stimuli such as frightening, intrusive thoughts, unpleasant bodily sensations, or

M. Tillfors, PhD (✉) • N. Van Zalk, PhD
Department of Law, Psychology and Social Work,
Örebro University, Örebro, Sweden
e-mail: maria.tillfors@oru.se

K. Ranta et al. (eds.), *Social Anxiety and Phobia in Adolescents: Development, Manifestation and Intervention Strategies*, DOI 10.1007/978-3-319-16703-9_4

intense emotions, it is natural to want to escape from these threatening situations and unpleasant inner experiences and avoid them in the future. These common transdiagnostic (or across-disorder) emotion regulation strategies have been shown to play a central role in maintaining a range of different forms of psychological ill–health, including SAD. In addition to helping maintain problems, these strategies are believed to play important roles in the development of psychological ill–health and are thus counterproductive. Nonetheless, compared to the maintenance of ill–health, there is far less research focused on the development of ill–health (Harvey et al. 2004).

During adolescence, major neurobiological changes take place in several regions in the prefrontal cortex. These changes pertain to the neurobiological *brake system*, which is believed to have the function of regulating emotions, among other things. During this developmental period, the neurobiological brake system is rather immature in relation to the brain's more matured *gas system*. This gas or alarm system is located in the subcortical areas of the amygdala/hippocampus. Interestingly, this gap between the brain's brake system and its ability to accelerate, or gas, is larger in adolescence than during both childhood and adulthood (for a review of a neurobiological model of adolescent behavior, see Sommerville et al. 2010). The amygdala is the area in the limbic system that is believed to play an important role regarding many aspects of emotional information processing and behaviors, such as processing of facial expressions of fear, and associative aversive learning (Davis and Whalen 2001; Tillfors 2004). The frontal part of the brain, or the prefrontal cortex, which is important for emotional regulation, is assumed to inhibit amygdala activity much like the brakes in a car (Davidson et al. 2000). Hence, the combination of neurobiological changes during adolescence, and the fact that young people are faced with an array of other changes in the social, cognitive, and behavioral domains, is likely to have important implications for how they perceive and experience emotions, how they learn to regulate them, and whether their regulation—or lack thereof—leads to the development of psychological ill–health.

Adolescence: A Critical Time

Despite much debate about whether adolescence is a period characterized by *sturm und drang* or is far less dramatic than previously believed, one thing is for certain—young people are faced with various changes on neurobiological, social, cognitive, and behavioral levels. Adolescents must learn to juggle the majority of these changes fairly successfully, while changing physically and emotionally and learning to adapt to their social environments. Whether dramatic or not, therefore, these changes are likely to have an impact on early adolescent development.

Vulnerability for Developing Social Anxiety: The Genetic, Neurobiological, Cognitive, Behavioral, and Social Level

The Genetic Level

Twin and family studies jointly suggest that rather than inheriting the risk for developing a specific anxiety disorder such as SAD, people inherit a general vulnerability to fearfulness (Fyer et al. 1995; Hettema et al. 2005; Rapee and Spence 2004; Tillfors et al. 2001). This general vulnerability, which could be manifested through the body's reactive alarm system via the amygdala/hippocampus, might be expressed through the personality trait *negative affect*. Evidence suggests that negative affect underlying different anxiety disorders could explain the high comorbidity between them (Hudson and Rapee 2000). Additionally, indications exist that as opposed to other anxiety disorders, SAD and depression also share a specific vulnerability noticeable in the personality trait *positive affect* (Brown et al. 1998). This so-called double vulnerability with high levels of negative affect in combination with low levels of positive affect could help explain the high level of comorbidity observed between SAD and depression (Brown et al. 1998).

Another genetic risk factor which has been linked specifically to SAD is *behavioral inhibition* (Kagan et al. 1993; Robinson et al. 1992). Behavioral inhibition is a temperamental dimension found very early on and is marked by subdued affect and distressed and avoidant behaviors in toddlers and small children (Kagan 1999; Kagan et al. 1988). Conceptual similarities between childhood behavioral inhibition and social anxiety in adulthood, including avoidance behavior and reticence in contact with unfamiliar people, have received focus in the literature. However, previous studies have found only a weak to moderate association between childhood behavioral inhibition and later developed SAD (e.g., Rapee and Spence 2004). One possible explanation for this moderate correlation could be that the relationship between behavioral inhibition and later developed social anxiety is moderated and/or mediated by dysfunctional emotion regulation strategies, such as avoidance. This explanation still awaits testing, nonetheless.

The Neurobiological Level

Common underlying *neurobiological correlates* for the general genetic vulnerability in anxiety disorders that have been observed in both emotional information processing and emotion regulation are several subcortical areas such as the *amygdala/hippocampus*, which is the body's alarm system and is involved in external stimulus-driven attention and appraisal, among other things. These types of processes are referred to as bottom-up processes, because they are effortless and preconscious. Top-down processes, on the other hand, are viewed as effortful and reflective. Another area is *insula*, which is the so-called limbic integration cortex involved in internal stimulus-driven attention. The subcortical areas and insula work in interaction with several regions of the *prefrontal cortex*, which is involved in goal-directed top-down processes like emotional regulation, and the *anterior cingulate cortex*, which is involved in both bottom-up and top-down processes (e.g., Clark and Beck 2010; Gorman et al. 2000; Tillfors 2004). These areas are also involved in the abovementioned neurobiological gap or imbalance between emotional reactivity and control, which is large during adolescence (Sommerville et al. 2010), and has been studied in research about self-regulation (see, e.g., Heatherton and Wagner 2011 for a review).

Another hypothesis concerning anxiety disorders relates to dysfunctions in the brain's serotonin system (see, e.g., Bell et al. 1999). Some evidence for the latter is found in the fact that selective serotonin reuptake inhibitors (SSRIs) are effective in the treatment of SAD. That is, an increased concentration of serotonin in the brain appears to provide an anxiolytic effect (Van Ameringen et al. 1999). There is also evidence that increased levels of serotonin may inhibit activity in the amygdala (or the brain's gas system), which in turn might result in a higher amygdala threshold regarding when emotional stimuli trigger neural activity (Faria et al. 2014). Additionally, it is not only successful medical treatment with SSRI that is linked to inhibited activity of the amygdala, but the same is also true for successful psychological treatment using cognitive–behavioral therapy (e.g., Furmark et al. 2002). Interestingly, in addition to inhibiting the activity in the amygdala after successful medical treatment, the coupling between prefrontal cortex and the amygdala also changes, indicating that the interaction between the brain's gas system (the amygdala) and its brake system (the prefrontal cortex) is central (e.g., Faria et al. 2014; Phan et al. 2013).

There are further indications that the interactions between prefrontal regions and subcortical regions can be both unidirectional, as regions in the prefrontal cortex appear to inhibit the subcortical regions, and bidirectional (Davidson et al. 2000). One way to explain this bidirectionality may be through the activity in the amygdala, via respondent learning earlier in life, which has been associated with increased reactivity to certain external as well as internal stimuli. These stimuli have thus become emotionally colored, and the processes in the prefrontal cortex may this way be controlled by emotions through bottom-up processes (Thompson and Goodman 2010). Some support for this notion is provided by findings showing that appraisal of both external and internal negative stimuli involves regions of the prefrontal as well the anterior cingulate cortex via elevated activity in the amygdala and the insula, respectively (Etkin et al. 2011). Hence, for those persons with a genetic and/or a psychological vulnerability, a bidirectional influence between prefrontal and subcortical regions may pose a double risk during adolescence, via the imbalance between prefrontal cortex and amygdala with its immature brake system and the more matured gas system, as well as the suggested bidirectional effects on each other. To summarize, there are indications in the literature that the prefrontal cortex and the anterior cingulate cortex work in a dysfunctional way in concert with the subcortical areas of the brain, which may be of importance for the development of psychological ill–health in general and social anxiety in particular.

The Behavioral and Cognitive Level

The core problem in social anxiety is a fear of being negatively evaluated by others. For socially anxious individuals, this fear could be described as a struggle characterized by wanting to take part in social interactions, but simultaneously wanting to avoid the anxiety-provoking social situations (i.e., avoidance on an overt level) as well as the unpleasant inner experiences such as negative emotions and thoughts associated with approaching others (i.e., avoidance on a covert level; Garcia-Lopez 2013; Kimbrel et al. 2010). Hence, people who suffer from SAD show high levels of avoidance when faced with anxiety-provoking social situations, despite their wishes to take part in the social interactions. Avoidance on an overt behavioral level is a further strategy to regulate emotions, which is likely learned early in childhood through, for example, respondent learning or modeling, and which, when paired with an individual variation in genetic vulnerability such as behavioral inhibition or the body's alarm system, may constitute a risk factor for later development of social anxiety (Tillfors 2004).

Nevertheless, people with SAD are characterized by intense anxiety not only in the anxiety-provoking social situations but also in the anticipation of such situations (characterized by anticipatory anxiety or worry) as well as afterwards (characterized by postmortem processing, or rumination). In addition, socially anxious people are quick in attending to potential threats. That is, they show high levels of *selective attention* toward both external stimuli and internal stimuli (i.e., self-focused attention) (Harvey et al. 2004). Furthermore, selective attention plays a central role in well-known cognitive theoretical models (e.g., Clark and Wells' cognitive model, Clark et al. 1995, 2003) as well as in cognitive–behavioral theoretical models (e.g., Rapee and Heimberg 1997). Excessive self-focused attention has especially been highlighted during the last decades as one main candidate for explaining the maintenance of SAD (cognitive model, Clark et al. 1995, 2003). This theoretical model assumes that the fear and/or the anxiety a person experiences when attending a social situation brings with it an elevated level of selective attention toward internal stimuli (i.e., self-focused attention) as well as increase in the risk of using control strategies (e.g., safety behavior, catastrophic thinking, worry, and rumination), thus resulting in an increase in overt and covert avoidance and disability. Hence, on a *cognitive* level, selective attention directed in the form of external attention toward the surrounding environment and inward in the form of internal self-focused attention appears to be one of the key concepts in central theories about how and why social anxiety emerges and is maintained. In line with this, selective attention also has been found to be a maintaining factor for SAD (Harvey et al. 2004).

This notion may be supported and mirrored on a neurobiological level via both bottom-up processes by the amygdala (attention of external stimuli) and the insula (attention of internal stimuli) exhibiting increased neuronal activity in relation to appraisal of threatening stimuli. It could also be mirrored in top-down processes by prefrontal regions activating attention to emotional colored memories of past events, which in turn could generate negative emotions and increased neural activity in the amygdala (Oschner and Gross 2007). Interestingly, recurrent memories and imagery have been shown to be a maintaining factor not only for posttraumatic stress disorder but also for SAD and may function as a warning signal for avoiding future danger (Harvey et al. 2004). Hence, social anxiety could be maintained via selective attention both via neurobiological bottom-up and top-down processes. Additionally, the recurrent intrusive memories activated before a threatening social situation also can lead to an increased risk for completely avoiding the feared situation in the future (i.e., overt avoidance).

One question comes to mind regarding Clark and Wells' cognitive model of SAD (1995). Namely, is it just the high level of internal, self-focused attention in itself that may act as a mediator between selective attention to external social threats and the development of SAD? Interestingly, thought processes such as worry and rumination (i.e., repetitive negative thinking) that characterize socially anxious people refer to a conceptual–evaluative mode of self-focused processing and have also been associated with maintenance of ill–health in general and SAD specifically (Ehring and Watkins 2008; Harvey et al. 2004). Consequently, these control strategies might set in motion a negative vicious cycle that could explain both the development and continuance of ill–health.

Indeed, repetitive negative thinking is believed to constitute a cognitive risk. Repetitive negative thinking is a generic term comprising thought processes such as worry and rumination, which are both characterized by the repetitive, abstract, and passive focus on topics of a negative nature that are perceived difficult to control (Ehring and Watkins 2008). Furthermore, worry and rumination are believed to fulfill emotional regulatory purposes for unpleasant inner experiences. By their abstract and predominantly verbal styles, worry and rumination are thought to reduce both aversive imagery and unpleasant physical anxiety reactions related to potential problems and threats. The consequences are assumed to be an increased level of covert avoidance and thus a decline in emotional processing. This indicates a close link between selective attention and worry/rumination, as, for example, the prefrontal regions may direct attention selectively to emotionally colored memories or imagery through top-down processes. Without external inputs, these processes may generate negative emotions and further increase the risk to make use of worry and rumination to minimize discomfort. The latter may also partly contribute to explaining a paradoxical observation. That is, when asked to upregulate negative emotions, trait ruminators show a correlation with greater activity in the amygdala (Ray et al. 2005). Even though cautiousness should be applied to inferences of causality, it does seem that the use of repetitive negative thinking has short-term functional gains in potential reduction of negative emotions. Nevertheless, this could have dysfunctional consequences in the long run, such as impaired emotional processing and a higher reactivity to negative emotions. This in turn increases the probability of using repetitive negative thinking as an emotion regulation strategy and thus, the vicious cycle spins on.

In adolescence, rumination appears to be used as an emotion regulation strategy more often by early adolescent females than males in relation to stress and depression. Compared to boys, girls start to use rumination as an emotion regulation strategy as early as 12 years of age, which may partly explain why depression is twice as common in girls. Boys seem to start using rumination as a strategy later on, at 15 years of age (e.g., Jose and Brown 2008). It would therefore be interesting to examine if rumination and worry predict an increase in social anxiety, whether rumination and worry mediate the relationship between social anxiety and depression, and if there are gender differences regarding using rumination and worry in relation to social anxiety and depression over time.

Another important note is that high levels of worry and rumination are associated with impaired and less flexible problem-solving abilities. According to the reduced concreteness theory of worry (Stöber and Borkovec 2002), this may be explained by the fact that an abstract thinking style is less detailed and specific and therefore performs more poorly in generating alternatives. The latter process is serious and may have implications for adolescents, especially in Western society where flexible solutions are of utmost importance both at school and in social situations. In conclusion, avoidance on a behavioral overt level as well as avoidance on a covert level are likely dysfunctional ways to regulate emotions and both are strategies used by socially anxious individuals.

The Social Level

Furthermore, covert avoidance, like worry and rumination has been shown to interfere with curiosity and positive experiences in a social situation. This is likely due to an increased level of internal self-focused attention, which could be both a risk factor by itself and an assumed consequence of frequent use of other dysfunctional emotion regulation strategies (Kashdan 2007). For example, being highly self-focused could give off a lack of presence in social situations, which may be interpreted by others as a lack of interest. An increased level of self-focused attention could therefore have implications for developing and maintaining interpersonal relations. From a developmental perspective, this may pose a serious issue on a social level, because peer relationships play a significant role in adolescence (e.g., Bukowski et al. 1991). In addition, well-functioning social relationships are a general protective factor against developing ill–health (Alden and Taylor 2004; Rubin et al. 2009). Taken together, selective attention as well as the functional aspect of repetitive negative thinking are probably important contributing factors to the development of social anxiety.

In conclusion, a number of common, cognitive transdiagnostic factors, such as external and internal attention as well as repetitive negative thinking, are represented in the common underlying neurobiological areas mentioned above and believed to be involved in the development of SAD. More specifically, adolescents with an underlying vulnerability who experience social fears are at specific risk, as it is likely easier for them to attend to and learn to fear both internal stimuli (such as negative intrusive thoughts and memories, intense feelings, and unpleasant bodily sensations) and external stimuli (such as feared social situations) through a more reactive amygdala (the brain's gas system). This in turn may increase the risk of recognizing these unpleasant internal stimuli as threats that must be controlled. To compensate for an immature neurobiological brake system in relation to the more matured gas system, adolescents with an underlying vulnerability may feel a quicker need to compensate for this imbalance by using dysfunctional emotion regulation strategies to reduce their internal unpleasant experiences, as compared to those without the underlying vulnerability. This may start a vicious circle, which could lead to developing clinical levels of social anxiety in the long run.

The Development of the Social Brain and Its Links to Social Anxiety and Problem Behavior: When Peers Take Center Stage

In addition to a larger *gap* or an imbalance between the brain's brake and gas systems in adolescence compared to anytime in childhood or after adolescence, the *social brain* also develops. The social brain is defined as those areas of the brain involved in social cognition. Broadly speaking, social cognition is defined as becoming aware of one's own intentions, thoughts, and desires and the fact that other people have them as well. By developing this so-called theory of mind, adolescents begin to understand what impact other people's intentions, thoughts, and desires have in relation to oneself (Sebastian et al. 2010). Another part of the concept of social cognition is a greater degree of *self-awareness*, which also develops during adolescence. One personality trait, self-consciousness, refers to people's individual differences in the degree of self-awareness or self-focused attention (Fenigstein et al. 1975). Self-consciousness has been shown to consist of two separate aspects. One is a private aspect that directs a person's attention inward toward thoughts and feelings, and the other is a public aspect that directs a person's attention toward the self as a social object. Examples of private and public self-consciousness, respectively, are "I reflect about myself a lot" and "I usually worry about making a good impression." As previously mentioned, the core problem with SAD is a fear of being negatively evaluated by others. This implies a high degree of public self-consciousness, in that an individual cares very much about how he or she appears in the eyes of others. To reflect upon oneself as a social object is something that is both necessary for and precedes the development of social anxiety, according to Fenigstein and colleagues (1975). Nevertheless, this in itself is not enough for developing social anxiety, which could explain why there is only a weak to moderate correlation between the concepts of public self-consciousness and social anxiety in the general population (Fenigstein et al. 1975). In addition, private self-consciousness seems to interact with the personality traits of *negative affect* and *positive affect*. That is, if a person has high levels of private self-consciousness paired with high levels of negative affect, the feelings of anxiety, sadness, and fear appear to be intensified and vice versa. Interestingly, high levels of negative affect and low levels of positive affect are both believed to be underlying traits for developing SAD as well as depression (Brown et al. 1998).

The areas of the brain involved in the development of the social brain are basically the same as those supposedly underlying anxiety disorders in general and SAD in particular. These regions are also involved in the neurobiological gap or imbalance between prefrontal regions and subcortical regions, which is greatest during adolescence. Additionally, the development of the social brain is thought to parallel the development of the dopamine system and manifests itself by adolescents' becoming more reward seeking in general (Sebastian et al. 2010). Specifically, social rewards in the form of spending more and more time with peers become more important during this period (see Steinberg and Morris 2001 for a review). The *striatum* (consisting of the *caudate* and the *putamen*), which is a subcortical brain region with many dopamine receptors, is involved in reward seeking. This region is also connected to the prefrontal cortex. If the knowledge about the striatum with its reward-seeking function is added to the knowledge about the function of the regions that are involved in the neurobiological gap or imbalance in adolescence and its bidirectional coupling, this could implicate that both reward incentives and emotions can drive decisions for adolescents to a greater degree than in adult life, which could explain several behaviors that are associated with teens. Indeed, reward seeking has in turn been linked to increases in problem behaviors such as alcohol use and delinquency, and there is a general increase in problem behaviors specifically during the early adolescent period (Sebastian et al. 2010). Furthermore, problem behaviors are associated with poor impulse control. People with lesions in the orbitofrontal cortex, a region in the prefrontal cortex, have been characterized by emotional instability and poor impulse control. The phenomenon has been termed *acquired psychopathy* (see e.g., Davidson et al. 2000) and may partly be analogous to adolescents' exhibition of an immature neurological brake system manifested in, for example, poor impulse control.

In a prominent conceptual model about delinquent behavior, Moffitt (1993) has proposed two developing paths for delinquent behavior reflecting two different subgroups. One subgroup is small by size and is characterized by a life-course-persistent behavioral pattern that has an early onset in childhood. This subgroup comprises about 10 % of males and 1 % of females in the general population. A hallmark feature of this life-course-persistent subgroup is physical aggression that appears to persist into midlife (Moffitt and Caspi 2001). The other larger subgroup has been described as adolescence limited, shows a gender ratio of 1.5 boys to 1 girl, and is expected to reflect normative rather than pathological behavior in adolescence as well as a more temporary involvement in delinquent behavior. In addition, according to Moffitt's theory (1993), adolescents in the different subgroups tend to engage in different patterns of delinquent behavior. On the one hand, adolescents in the life-course-persistent group tend to get involved in victim-oriented crimes such as violence to a higher degree and also show a stronger association with psychopathic personality traits, such as lack of empathy, anxiety, and guilt (Moffitt and Caspi 2001). This link may mirror an observed negative correlation in children with psychopathic traits and trait anxiety (Vermeiren et al. 2002). It may also refer to the new specifier "*with limited prosocial emotions, such as limited empathy and guilt*," which has recently been added to the symptomatology of conduct disorder in the

DSM-5 (APA 2013). On the other hand, adolescents in the adolescence-limited subtype tend to engage primarily in nonviolent acts that demonstrate autonomy from parental control. Moffitt's abovementioned theoretical model has received ample support in empirical studies (e.g., Moffitt and Caspi 2001).

When thinking of a socially fearful person, one does not immediately think of externalizing problem behaviors such as delinquency or alcohol misuse. Nevertheless, there are reasons to believe that social fears might put early adolescents at risk for these problems. First, socially fearful adolescents tend to have low self-esteem, which is a strong predictor of susceptibility to peer influence (Brown 1989). In adolescence, it becomes more rewarding to be with peers, and at the same time, the imbalance between the brake and the gas system is large, which may result in socially negative experiences such as peer exclusion being experienced more intensely. Hence, in the context of problem behaviors, socially fearful adolescents might go along with peers' suggestions of deviant behavior rather than speak up against it (Cheek and Krasnoperova 1999). In addition, adolescents might start using alcohol as a way to relieve their social anxiety, and this could be a gateway to problem behaviors through associations with socially deviant peers. Thus, although it is not an intuitive way of thinking about socially anxious adolescents, social anxiety might serve a gateway for involvement in problem behaviors.

Empirical investigations of social anxiety and problem behaviors show mixed results, however. A number of studies have shown protective effects for early adolescents concerning delinquency, alcohol use, and risky sexual behavior (Fröjd et al. 2011; Kerr et al. 1997; Van Zalk et al. 2011a), but social anxiety has also been linked to alcohol misuse in late adolescence and adulthood (Zimmerman et al. 2003). Furthermore, social anxiety has been associated with antisocial behaviors in adults (e.g., Sareen et al. 2004) and adolescent boys (Tillfors et al. 2009). The reason for these contradictory findings might lie in a subgroup of individuals with social anxiety who also show impulsive, risk-prone behavioral tendencies. Even if such behaviors seem to be complete opposites of socially fearful behaviors, they could have the same underlying purpose—avoiding negative evaluation. The latter is exactly what we have shown in one study where we investigated what consequences social anxiety has for adolescents' external adjustment (Tillfors et al. 2013b). We identified different subgroups of socially anxious adolescents—those who were behaviorally inhibited, which is how we typically think about socially anxious individuals, and those who were impulsive, which is an atypical combination recently identified among adults (Kashdan et al. 2009). Our study was the first to identify a socially anxious–impulsive subgroup of adolescents and to show that boys in this subgroup had high levels of both intoxication frequency and delinquency (Tillfors et al. 2013b). In another study, we also identified a socially anxious–impulsive subgroup of young adults and showed that young women who were anxious–inhibited or anxious–impulsive had high levels of depressive symptoms and low levels of life satisfaction (Tillfors et al. 2013a). Jointly, these results indicate that there may be more to social anxiety than first meets the eye and that an anxious–impulsive subgroup of socially anxious adolescent boys may fit in well with Moffitt's adolescence-limited subgroup mentioned above.

Another point worth mentioning in more detail is that adolescents are hypersensitive to social exclusion compared to adults, which may be linked to the abovementioned neurobiological gap or imbalance between emotional reactivity and control. This may be of particular significance specifically in relation to the development of social anxiety, as using avoidance to downregulate negative emotions may become problematic because early adolescents perceive socially avoidant behaviors negatively (Rubin et al. 2006). The more avoidance strategies are used, the more peers might find such behaviors unattractive during this period of time. Indeed, it has been shown that low acceptance by peers can increase social anxiety over time and social anxiety, in turn, is linked to decreased relationship support for boys and increased peer victimization for girls (Tillfors et al. 2012). One important contribution of this study was prospectively identifying the unique impact of social anxiety on multiple aspects of peer relations (peer acceptance, peer victimization, and relationship quality) simultaneously and vice versa. From a neurobiological perspective, the same area of the brain activated for social pain, such as social exclusion, is also activated during physical pain (MacDonald and Leary 2005), interestingly enough. In line with this, observations show that the sensitivity to physical pain and sensitivity to social rejection are mutually reinforcing each other (Eisenberger et al. 2006). These findings could in part explain the comorbidity between social anxiety and chronic pain that has been observed in both general and clinical populations (see, e.g., Asmundson and Katz 2009 for a review).

The abovementioned findings about social anxiety and peer relations go hand in hand with other findings showing that social anxiety could be partly socialized by peers. In one study, adolescents who were socially anxious were found to be less popular and chose fewer friends in their peer social network (Van Zalk et al. 2011b). They also tended to choose friends who were socially anxious, and over time they influenced each other into becoming more socially anxious—over and above other effects (Van Zalk et al. 2011b). Interestingly, girls' social anxiety was more influenced than boys' by their friends' social anxiety levels (Van Zalk et al. 2011b). In another study, peer crowd affiliation was shown to be an important factor for socializing social anxiety (Van Zalk et al. 2011c). The results showed that being a member of a peer crowd in itself did not predict socialization of social anxiety, but adolescents in Radical crowds, such as Punks or Goths, were more influenced by their peers' social anxiety, compared to adolescents who did not affiliate with the Radical crowd group (Van Zalk et al. 2011c). These results suggest that adolescents who affiliate with certain types of peer crowds may narrow their peer relationship ties over time and in turn socialize each other's social anxiety through a bidirectional process (Van Zalk et al. 2011c). Jointly, these studies expand the current knowledge about direct and indirect peer influences on social anxiety and help to identify how social anxiety, in turn, interferes with the quality of peer relationships.

In conclusion, changes that occur in adolescence create social novelty as well as the need to face new people and assume new roles, which is problematic for adolescents with social anxiety. Social novelty increases as adolescents move into larger, less familiar school environments and develop romantic and sexual interests. In addition, adolescence is also a period of time with a larger imbalance between the brain's brake and gas system compared to adulthood, which is likely to lead to difficulties for some adolescents. Indeed, adolescents often react more intensely than adults to social stimuli, such as social exclusion or ostracism, and some adolescents are more sensitive to peer influence than others. Entering teenage years often entails a changing lifestyle, such as a new school environment, new peers, more homework, and less sleep. During this period, adolescents start turning to peers instead of parents for emotional support, and peers become more important than ever before. At the same time, cognitive changes make adolescents aware of being social objects, which can bring about self-consciousness regarding social situations more so than during childhood (see Rubin et al. 2009 for a review). Despite all of these marked changes that adolescence poses, some individuals manage to cope with their social fears fairly well. Others struggle, however, which might lead to even more problems in the future. Knowledge about what strategies adolescents use to deal with social novelty and elevated social fears is, therefore, of significance. As we have mentioned before, these strategies are often referred to as emotion regulation.

The Role of Emotion Regulation

Emotion regulation has been defined as consisting of "*extrinsic and intrinsic processes responsible for monitoring, evaluating, and modifying emotional reactions, especially their intensive and temporal features, to accomplish one's goals*" (Thompson and Goodman 2010, pp. 39–40). From a developmental perspective, extrinsic processes usually appear first, as parents or other caregivers teach young children to manage their emotions through extrinsic influence. With increasing age, however, children learn to regulate their emotions more and more by their own efforts, or via intrinsic processes. Extrinsic processes still take place during adolescence, nonetheless, and it is not only parents who exert extrinsic influence but also peers. Concerning socially anxious adolescents, extrinsic processes could mean talking at length with friends about one's negative social experiences and failures, a process known as *co-rumination*. Indeed, this construct has been shown to explain why high levels of self-disclosure, which is usually related to good psychological health, can lead to increased anxiety and depression for adolescent girls (Rose 2002; Rose et al. 2007). Nonetheless, results from a preliminary study indicate that co-rumination could be beneficial for adolescents with high social anxiety in terms of being less likely to develop depressive symptoms over time (Van Zalk and Tillfors 2014). Indeed, our preliminary results show no direct but rather moderating effects of co-rumination on the link between social anxiety and depressive symptoms. For girls, however, co-rumination predicted a decrease in social anxiety over time, whereas the reverse was true for boys (Van Zalk and Tillfors 2014). These results indicate that boys and girls may co-ruminate in different ways, but not much research has been focused on how and for what purposes they co-ruminate. Further research is needed to test in which way co-rumination is relevant for the development of social anxiety.

Intrinsic processes could mean avoiding anxiety-provoking situations or unpleasant inner experiences, such as suppressing intense negative thoughts, or by aforementioned excessive worry and rumination. Both extrinsic and intrinsic strategies remove the unpleasant inner experiences in the short term, thus providing negative reinforcement and increasing the likelihood that they will be repeated. These are dysfunctional ways of regulating emotions, however, which have been shown to maintain instead of alleviate problems in the long run (Harvey et al. 2004). As the factors that maintain a problem are not necessarily the same as those involved in its development, however, more research is needed about which role emotion regulation strategies play in the development of social anxiety, specifically.

In sum, the consequences of all the changes taking place during adolescence are likely to lead to more intense emotions, which could be mirrored in the more reactive neurobiological gas pedal in the amygdala/hippocampus, and an increased difficulty in controlling or managing these emotions. If the negative emotions are highly intense, a further consequence could be that they are more readily interpreted as real threats and indications of something bad happening. These inner experiences may thus become construed as a true description of reality, or a high degree of cognitive fusion, a concept used in acceptance and commitment therapy and believed to mediate ill–health (Herbert and Cardaciotto 2005). One outcome may thus be an increased risk of wanting to get rid of these unpleasant internal experiences more quickly. For some adolescents, thus, it may become easier to use various emotion regulation strategies when trying to compensate for the immature neurobiological brake system in interaction with an accelerating gas system, in order to get rid of the unpleasant emotions. This strategy is bound to become dysfunctional in the long term, nevertheless, and SAD often makes its debut during this critical phase.

The Role of Peers and Parents in Emotion Regulation During Adolescence: A Proposed Model

Theoretically, experiences with parents and peers could play important roles in emotion regulation processes. Parental behaviors such as negative control and unpredictability, for instance, could set adolescents up for using dysfunctional emotion regulation strategies. These parenting behaviors have been linked to the development of low levels of control, which is believed to increase children's risk of learning dysfunctional strategies such as escape and avoidance behaviors to regulate their emotions, especially during stressful and negative experiences (e.g., Allen et al. 2008). These same parental behaviors have been linked to the development of internalizing problems such as social anxiety later in life (e.g., Rubin et al. 2010), but these links are relatively weak, which could indicate that factors such as emotion regulation strategies might mediate the links between parenting and the development of internalizing problems. Thus, parental behaviors might have an impact on how children and adolescents learn to regulate their emotions.

In addition, due to the amount of time spent with peers in combination with the fact that adolescents are hypersensitive to social exclusion, peers could play at least two different roles in the development of social anxiety, emotion regulation strategies, or both. First, mistreatment by peers could contribute to the negative emotions that adolescents attempt to regulate. Second, co-rumination with close peers about socially anxious feelings could be an extrinsic emotion regulation strategy. In both of these cases, peers could affect the levels of emotion regulation strategies, which in turn might affect social anxiety. In addition, certain emotion regulation strategies might make peer relationships worse. For instance, early adolescents perceive socially avoidant behaviors by their peers in an undesirable way, which may become an issue for those adolescents who use avoidance to downregulate their emotions (Rubin et al. 2006). By using avoidance, socially anxious individuals decrease their levels of unpleasantness and anxiety. Their peers may not approve these behaviors, which may make it difficult for socially anxious adolescents to initiate social interactions, become accepted within a larger peer group, and develop close intimate friendships. Indeed, previous research has found that peers seem to play a significant role for socially anxious adolescents' mental health (e.g., Siegel et al. 2009; Tillfors et al. 2012), whereas social anxiety, in turn, seems to interfere with healthy peer relationships (e.g., Flanagan et al. 2008; Tillfors et al. 2012). Hence, emotion regulation might also be an important mediator in the links between peer relationships and social anxiety.

Current studies on parent and peer relationships and social anxiety in childhood and adolescence have reported mixed findings. Some of these differences may be due to differences in design, however, as most of these studies are cross sectional. Nevertheless, there could be at least two additional explanations. First, as mentioned above, emotion regulation strategies that socially anxious adolescents apply might work as *mediators* in the links between peer relationships and the development of social anxiety, as well as vice versa. Second, the quality of the parent–child relationships might *moderate* these effects, thus explaining the mixed findings. As an example of the latter process, if socially anxious adolescents have experienced warm and supportive relationships with their parents, this could protect them from increasing in social anxiety over time due to poor peer relationships. This should be particularly important during early adolescence specifically, when intense emotions are brought to life more easily, but are unfortunately harder to resist by adolescents' immature neurobiological brake systems. However, the joint roles that peers and parents play during adolescence in the development of social anxiety are relatively unexplored in the literature. Indeed, scholars have emphasized the need to "*examine parent–child and friendship relationships in concert*" for socially withdrawn children and adolescents (Rubin et al. 2010, p. 90). In a study of early adolescents, we found that care and connectedness with mothers, fathers, and friends jointly predicted decreases in social anxiety (Van Zalk and Van Zalk in press). Based on this reasoning, then, we propose a theoretical model as a broad framework for the development of social anxiety, which is

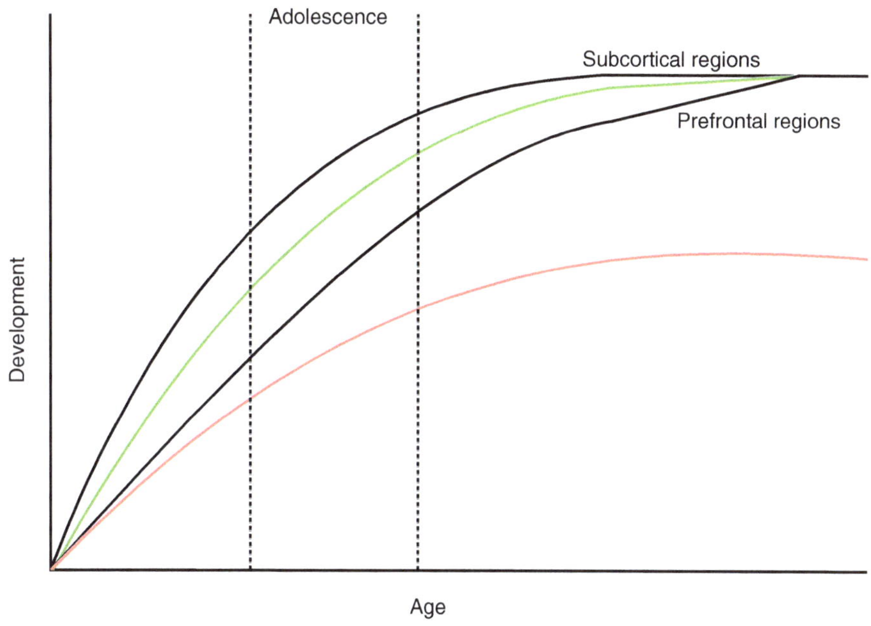

Fig. 4.1 Proposed model for the development of social anxiety. According to Sommerville et al. (2010), early development of the subcortical regions (e.g., amygdala), as illustrated by the *top black line*, in combination with late development of the prefrontal cortical regions, as illustrated by the *bottom black line*, predicts a boost in emotionally driven behavior as well as difficulties to control them during adolescence. The *red line* represents adolescents with poor peer and parent relationships, who show a larger developmental gap, compared to adolescents with supportive peer and parent relationships (as illustrated by the *green line*)

paired with an empirically driven model proposed by Sommerville and colleagues (2010) and is shown in Fig. 4.1.

As both peer and parent relationships are likely to contribute to the development of social anxiety, both should be considered as predictors, controlling for initial levels of social anxiety in order to address change over time. The associations between peer relationships and social anxiety in this model could be different for adolescents who experience different types of parenting, however, which would imply moderating effects. Traditionally, the causal direction has been assumed from parents' behaviors to their children's social anxiety, but recent empirical evidence suggests that adolescents' social anxiety might likewise influence how their parents and peers behave toward them, which in turn influences the levels of social anxiety (Van Zalk and Kerr 2011). These links can therefore be assumed to be bidirectional, where emotional regulation could act as a mediator in both directions. Hence, by using this broad model in longitudinal designs, specific hypotheses across different contexts can be generated in order to obtain more detailed information about the mechanisms underlying the development of social anxiety.

The Role of Sleep Habits and Consequences for Emotion Regulation in Relation to Social Anxiety

As mentioned before, entering teenage years often entails a changing lifestyle, such as a new school environment, new peers, more homework, and less sleep. For some adolescents, getting less sleep could turn into developing sleep problems. Sleep problems are in turn related to many different psychological problems such as depression and SAD (Ohayon and Roth 2003). Traditionally, sleep problems have been viewed as consequences of psychological problems, rather than vice versa. Nonetheless, recent research indicates that these links are likely bidirectional, as sleep problems have been found to precede as well as follow psychological problems. For example, insomnia has been shown to predict later developed depression episodes both in adolescents and in adults (for a meta-analysis, see Baglioni et al. 2011). Social anxiety has, in turn, been shown to precede depressive symptoms in a number of longitudinal studies (Stein and Gorman 2001; Wittchen et al. 2003). Due to these links, some scholars propose that sleep problems may be an underlying transdiagnostic factor for later psychological problems (Harvey 2002). It is therefore of interest to take a closer look at what underlying mechanisms may link sleep problems to the development of ill–health and particularly social anxiety.

Two neurobiological hypotheses regarding the role of sleep in relation to emotional regulation have been highlighted in the current literature (Van der Helm and Walker 2010). The first hypothesis states that sleep deprivation can lead to an increased risk of using dysfunctional emotion regulation strategies. Support for this notion comes partly from the knowledge that after being sleep deprived, people show an elevated emotional reactivity through a higher level of activity in the brain's gas system or amygdala. That is, people who have been sleep deprived tend to react more easily and more frequently to emotional stimuli compared to people who had not been subjected to sleep deprivation. In addition, sleep-deprived individuals have shown a decreased functional connectivity with the prefrontal cortex, or the brain's brake system. For certain people with an underlying vulnerability, this might entail difficulties to resist emotion-driven behaviors that are associated with the specific emotions, such as an impulse to flee driven by fear or an impulse to attack either verbally or physically driven by anger. Other people might instead do the opposite of their impulses and conclude nothing dangerous is happening even if the emotion is unpleasant (Allen et al. 2008).

The second hypothesis states that sleep deprivation seems to further contribute to negatively charged memories having priority over positive and neutrally charged memories (Van der Helm and Walker 2010). That is, the negative emotional memories during sleep, mainly during REM (rapid eye movement) sleep, are assumed to be processed and stored in the long-term memory at the expense of the positive and neutral ones. Interestingly, people who are sleep deprived during the REM phase have shown an occurrence of increased neuronal activity of the limbic areas of the brain, while the connectivity with the prefrontal cortex appears to be impaired.

Thus, it may be easier to hold on to the negative emotional memories at the expense of the positive ones. Furthermore, due to lack of sleep, people do not appear to get rid of this negative "emotional coloration" in their memory over time, as people with normal sleep patterns manage to do more readily. In other words, the negatively charged memories still evoke as much negative emotions as when they were encoded for sleep-deprived people. If people's autobiographical memories are largely made up of memories of a negative nature, they may run the risk of using worry and rumination to a greater degree as a way to solve their problems related to these negative memories and/or get rid of the unpleasantness related to it. On a related note, worry also interferes with sleep by increased sleep-onset latency (Harvey 2002), thus setting the stage for a vicious cycle.

In order to achieve an understanding about the physiology of emotions, and as an interesting analogue to the two abovementioned neurobiological hypotheses regarding the role of sleep in emotion regulation, current research has mainly been focused on the amygdala and its interaction with the prefrontal parts of the brain and the hippocampus (Davidson et al. 2000; Gorman et al. 2000; LeDoux 1996). Much like braking while driving a car, the prefrontal cortex inhibits the amygdala activity (Davidson et al. 2000). Support for this notion has been found in animal studies, as results imply that animals with lesions in these cortical areas appear to be resistant to extinction of aversive stimuli (LeDoux 1996). In a similar vein, lack of sleep could have analogous consequences to those seen in animals with lesions in prefrontal brain areas. One may speculate that people with prolonged sleep problems might have difficulties in taking advantage of some central components in cognitive–behavioral treatments, such as exposure techniques that are built upon learning theories. Hence, if socially anxious people have comorbid sleep problems, it might be important to start treating the sleep problem before starting exposure. Indeed, some support for the latter was found in a study showing that poor sleep quality is a predictor of cognitive–behavioral therapy outcomes in people with SAD (Zalta et al. 2013).

The two abovementioned hypotheses provide no specific explanation for the development of social anxiety, however, but offer a general explanation regarding the development of various forms of psychiatric disorders such as anxiety disorders. So what could be behind the development of social anxiety, specifically? One hypothetical scenario may be found in the way that young people live their lives in today's society. Most teenagers use computers and their phones for texting, chatting, and other forms of communication, which can interfere with their sleep (Cain and Gradisar 2010). Furthermore, it is more common for young people than adults to shift their circadian rhythms (Wolfson and Carskadon 1998). In addition, for adolescents who experience higher levels of social fears, it is extra difficult to withhold from behaving in the same way as their peers (Brown 1989). As it is particularly rewarding to spend time with peers during this period, adolescents in general are sensitive to peer influence. Given all of these factors, some socially anxious adolescents might therefore run an extra risk of developing sleep problems, which could be linked to the development of SAD later on.

Conclusions and Implications

As we have attempted to show in this chapter, adolescence is a highly critical time for the onset of SAD for many various reasons. Adolescents are vulnerable on a wide array of levels—genetically, neurobiologically, cognitively, behaviorally, and socially. On a genetic level, research indicates that people inherit a general vulnerability for fearfulness, rather than inheriting a direct risk for developing SAD (Fyer et al. 1995; Hettema et al. 2005; Rapee and Spence 2004; Tillfors et al. 2001). This genetic susceptibility may be apparent very early in the form of behavioral inhibition, which is another genetic risk factor specifically associated with SAD (Kagan et al. 1993; Robinson et al. 1992). Thus, for some people, social fear may be present from birth. On a neurobiological level, several correlates for the genetic vulnerability in anxiety disorders regarding how emotional information is processed, and how emotions are regulated, are to be found in the amygdala/hippocampus, the insula, and the prefrontal areas of the brain. The amygdala/hippocampus represents the body's alarm system, which is involved in external stimulus-driven attention and appraisal. On a neurobiological level, then, some individuals might be primed for later development of SAD. On cognitive and behavioral levels, an important problem in social anxiety is fear of negative evaluation by other people. This is often present in the form of an internal struggle, where people want to partake in social interactions, but also want to avoid anxiety-provoking situations and unpleasant inner emotions at the same time (Kimbrel et al. 2010). On a social level, covert avoidance, such as excessive worry and rumination, appears to interfere with positive experiences in social situations, which is likely due to increased levels of internal self-focused attention that socially anxious individuals exhibit (Kashdan 2007). In sum then, several factors may contribute to the development of social anxiety. Nonetheless, the knowledge about which of these factors are necessary in order for SAD to develop, and whether other processes may interfere or mediate these links, has not been thoroughly investigated in the literature.

Another point we have brought up in this chapter which is worth noting is that adolescent girls, as opposed to boys, start using rumination as an emotion regulation strategy already at age 12. In a sense, then, their risk of developing SAD might be higher compared to boys, because they are more vulnerable. An interesting follow-up question is therefore why girls ruminate more than boys. One part of the answer may be linked to sleep disturbances. People who do not sleep regularly have intense reactions to slightly stressful situations, such as during social encounters. This may lead to dysfunctional emotion regulation strategies such as rumination in order to get rid of the discomfort or anxiety, which in turn may impact a person's sleeping patterns in terms of the amount of times waking up at night, which then further disrupts sleep. These processes may affect how emotional memories are coded and may thus result in a more negative emotional coloration over time, which is likely to help maintain a vicious cycle. Thus, for adolescent girls with an underlying vulnerability, a disturbed circadian rhythm paired with using dysfunctional emotion regulation strategies might help explain the onset of SAD and could be one of the reasons why SAD is more common among adolescent girls than boys.

To make matters more complex, young people face an array of other changes during adolescence that may contribute to the development of SAD. Adolescents tend to shift schools during early adolescence, which often implies a new social network of peers, paired with the fact that peers take center stage during adolescence and are crucial for the development of the social brain, as well as new challenges that may be faced with parents. As we have also attempted to illustrate in this chapter, the role of emotion regulation for the development of SAD is a very important one, and parents and peers may contribute to this development in numerous ways. We have proposed a theoretical model for how SAD may develop throughout adolescence (shown in Fig. 4.1). Based on a model by Somerville and colleagues (2010), this model assumes that early development of the subcortical regions such as the amygdala, in combination with late development of the prefrontal cortical regions, predicts an increase in emotionally driven behavior during adolescence. In our addition to the proposed model, we suggest that for adolescents with poor peer and parent relationships, however, the developmental gap is expected to be larger, compared to adolescents with supportive peer and parent relationships. As both peer and parent relationships affect the development of social anxiety in adolescence, we believe that both should be considered as predictors of SAD. Nonetheless, as the links between peer relationships and social anxiety in our model may differ for adolescents who experience different types of parenting, parental behavior may be a moderator between these links instead. Also, as recent empirical evidence suggests bidirectional links between adolescents' social anxiety and how parents and peers behave toward them (Van Zalk and Kerr 2011), these links can therefore be assumed to be bidirectional with emotion regulation acting as a mediator in both directions. We believe that the model we have proposed allows for generating specific hypotheses about the development of SAD and should be tested using longitudinal and/or experimental designs.

There are many gaps in the current literature that need answering before a clear picture of the *processes* behind the development of SAD can be understood more fully. This entails understanding both the *how* and the *why* some adolescents end up as adults with SAD. In order to understand these processes on a broad level, nonetheless, certain microprocesses deserve more research attention in future studies. For instance, regarding emotion regulation, the concept of co-rumination has been largely overlooked in the literature, and our own preliminary results indicate that boys and girls may co-ruminate in different ways. Further research is needed to test the way in which co-rumination is relevant for the development of social anxiety. Also of interest would be to longitudinally examine multiple aspects of emotion regulation strategies (e.g., the extrinsic process of co-rumination in relation to the intrinsic processes of rumination and worry) simultaneously, with the purpose to identify their impact on social anxiety. In addition, interactions with mothers compared to fathers may affect the development of social anxiety differently, and especially for boys and girls, but this research area has been largely overlooked. Indeed, the connection between parents and peers may be such that it affects how adolescent social anxiety develops, as our own findings indicate that supportive relationships with peers *and* parents help decrease social anxiety over time (Van Zalk and Van Zalk in press). Additionally, as adolescents in general and socially anxious adolescents in particular are sensitive to peer influence, peers' sleeping behavior could be a gateway for developing sleep disturbances for some adolescents, which could be further linked to dysfunctional emotion regulation strategies and developing SAD later on. Indeed, social anxiety and emotion regulation in relation to sleep problems is another research area that has also been largely unnoticed. It would be of significance to examine sleep deprivation in relation to emotional reactivity and emotion regulation in different age groups. Because adolescents have a relatively immature neurobiological brake system in relation to a more matured gas system compared to adults, this may make adolescents more sensitive to sleep deprivation compared to adults. Thus, incorporating mothers, fathers, and peers in the study of social anxiety and taking into account both emotion regulation and sleep patterns may be a further important stepping stone in helping to paint a broader picture of who may be at risk for developing social anxiety and why. Consequently, mothers, fathers, and peers may make a difference when it comes to learning to slow down rather than accelerating the "socially anxious car" during the adolescent years.

References

Alden LE, Taylor CT (2004) Interpersonal processes in social phobia. Clin Psychol Rev 24(7): 857–882, http://dx.doi.org/10.1016/j.cpr.2004.07.006

Allen LB, McHugh K, Barlow DH (2008) Emotional disorders: a unified protocol. In: Barlow DH (ed) Clinical handbook of psychological disorders: a step-by-step treatment manual. Guilford Press, New York, pp 216–249

APA (2013) Diagnostic and statistical manual of mental disorders, 5th edn, American Psychiatric Association. American Psychiatric Association, Washington, DC

Asmundson GJG, Katz J (2009) Understanding the co-occurrence of anxiety disorders and chronic pain: state-of-the-art. Depress Anxiety 26(10):888–901, http://dx.doi.org/10.1002/da.20600

Baglioni C, Battagliese G, Feige B, Spiegelhalder K, Nissen C, Voderholzer U et al (2011) Insomnia as predictor of depression: a metaanalytic evaluation of longitudinal epidemiological studies. J Affect Disord 135(1–3):10–19. doi:10.1016/j.jad.2011.01.011

Bell CJ, Malizia AL, Nutt DJ (1999) The neurobiology of social phobia. Eur Arch Psychiatry Clin Neurosci 249(S1):S11–S18, http://dx.doi.org/10.1007/PL00014162

Brown BB (1989) The role of peer groups in adolescents' adjustment to secondary school. In: Berndt TJ, Ladd GW (eds) Peer relationships in child development. Wiley, New York, pp 188–215

Brown TA, Chorpita BF, Barlow DH (1998) Structural relationships among dimensions of the DSM-IV anxiety and mood disorders and dimensions of negative affect, positive affect, and autonomic arousal. J Abnorm Psychol 107(2):179–192, http://dx.doi.org/10.1037/0021-843X.107.2.179

Bukowski WM, Gauze C, Hoza B, Newcomb AF (1991) Differences and consistency between same-sex and other-sex peer relationships during early adolescence. Dev Psychol 29(2): 255–263. doi:10.1037//0012-1649.29.2.255

Cain N, Gradisar M (2010) Electronic media use and sleep in school-aged children and adolescents: a review. Sleep Med 11(8):735–742, http://dx.doi.org/10.1016/j.sleep.2010.02.006

Cheek JM, Krasnoperova EN (1999) Varieties of shyness in adolescence and adulthood. In: Schmidt LA, Schulkin J (eds) Extreme fear, shyness, and social phobia: origins, biological mechanisms, and clinical outcomes. Oxford University Press, Inc., New York, pp 224–250

Clark DA, Beck AT (2010) Cognitive theory and therapy of anxiety and depression: convergence with neurobiological findings. Trends Cogn Sci 14(9):418–424, http://dx.doi.org/10.1016/j.tics.2010.06.007

Clark DM, Wells A (1995) A cognitive model of social phobia. In: Heimberg RG, Liebowitz MR, Hope DA, Schneier FR (eds) Social phobia: diagnosis, assessment and treatment. Guilford Press, New York, pp 69–93

Clark DM, Ehlers A, McManus F, Hackmann A, Fennell M, Campbell H et al (2003) Cognitive therapy versus fluoxetine in generalized social phobia: a randomized placebo-controlled trial. J Consult Clin Psychol 71(6):1058–1067, http://dx.doi.org/10.1037/0022-006X.71.6.1058

Davidson RJ, Jackson DC, Kalin NH (2000) Emotion, plasticity, context, and regulation: perspectives from affective neuroscience. Psychol Bull 126(6):890–909, http://dx.doi.org/10.1037//0033-2909.126.6.890

Davis M, Whalen PJ (2001) The amygdala: vigilance and emotion. Mol Psychiatry 6(1):13–34, http://dx.doi.org/10.1038/sj.mp.4000812

Ehring T, Watkins ER (2008) Repetitive negative thinking as a transdiagnostic process. Int J Cogn Ther 1(3):192–205, http://dx.doi.org/10.1680/ijct.2008.1.3.192

Eisenberger NI, Jarcho JM, Lieberman MD, Naliboff BD (2006) An experimental study of shared sensitivity to physical pain and social rejection. Pain 126(1–3):132–138, http://dx.doi.org/10.1016/j.pain.2006.06.024

Erath SA, Flanagan KS, Bierman KL, Tu KM (2010) Friendships moderate psychosocial maladjustment in socially anxious early adolescents. J Appl Dev Psychol 31(1):15–26

Etkin A, Egner T, Kalisch R (2011) Emotional processing in anterior cingulate and medial prefrontal cortex. Trends Cogn Sci 15(2):85–93, http://dx.doi.org/10.1016/j.tics.2010.11.004

Faria, V., Åhs, F., Appel, L., Linnman, C., Banis, M., Betticas, P., et al. (2014). Amygdala-frontal couplings characterizing SSRI and placebo response in social anxiety disorder. *International Journal of Neuropsychopharmacology*, 17(08), 1149–1157. doi: http://dx.doi.org/10.1017/S1461145714000352

Fenigstein A, Scheier MF, Buss AH (1975) Public and private self-consciousness: assessment and theory. J Consult Clin Psychol 43(4):522–527, http://dx.doi.org/10.1037/h0076760

Flanagan KS, Erath SA, Bierman KL (2008) Unique associations between peer relations and social anxiety in early adolescence. J Clin Child Adolesc Psychol 37(4):759–769. doi:10.1080/15374410802359700

Fröjd S, Ranta K, Kaltiala-Heino R, Marttunen M (2011) Associations of social phobia and general anxiety with alcohol and drug use in a community sample of adolescents. Alcohol Alcohol 46(2):192–199. doi:10.1093/alcalc/agq096

Furmark T, Tillfors M, Marteinsdottir I, Fischer H, Pissiota A, Långström B et al (2002) Common changes in cerebral blood flow in patients with social phobia treated with citalopram or cognitive-behavioral therapy. Arch Gen Psychiatry 59(5):425–433, http://dx.doi.org/10.1001/archpsyc.59.5.425

Fyer AJ, Mannuzza S, Chapman TF, Martin LY, Klein DF (1995) Specificity in familial aggregation of phobic disorders. Arch Gen Psychiatry 52(7):564–573, http://dx.doi.org/10.1001/archpsyc.1995.03950190046007

Garcia-Lopez LJ (2013) Tratando…trastorno de ansiedad social [Treating…social anxiety disorder]. Piramide, Madrid in the References for that chapter

Garcia-Lopez LJ, Irurtia MJ, Caballo VE, Díaz-Castela MM (2011) Ansiedad social y abuso psicológico [Social anxiety and psychological abuse]. Behav Psycholy 19:223–236

Gorman JM, Kent JM, Sullivan GM, Coplan JD (2000) Neuroanatomical hypothesis of panic disorder, revised. Am J Psychiatr 157(4):493–505, http://dx.doi.org/10.1176/appi.ajp.157.4.493

Gross JJ (1998) The emerging field of emotion regulation: an integrative review. Rev Gen Psychol 2(3):271–299, http://dx.doi.org/10.1037//1089-2680.2.3.271

Harvey AG (2002) A cognitive model of insomnia. Behav Res Ther 40(8):869–893, http://dx.doi.org/10.1016/S0005-7967(01)00061-4

Harvey A, Watkins E, Mansell W, Shafran R (2004) Cognitive behavioral processes across psychological disorders: a transdiagnostic approach to research and treatment. Oxford University Press Inc., New York

Heatherton TF, Wagner DD (2011) Cognitive neuroscience of self-regulation failure. Trends Cogn Sci 15(3):132–139, http://dx.doi.org/10.1016/j.tics.2010.12.005

Hebert KR, Fales J, Nangle DW, Papadakis AA, Grover RL (2013) Linking social anxiety and adolescent romantic relationship functioning: indirect effects and the importance of peers. J Youth Adolesc 42(11):1708–1720. doi:10.1007/s10964-012-9878-0

Heiser NA, Turner SM, Beidel DC, Roberson-Nay R (2009) Differentiating social phobia from shyness. J Anxiety Disord 23(4):469–476. doi:10.1016/j.janxdis.2008.10.002

Herbert JD, Cardaciotto L (2005) An acceptance and mindfulness-based perspective on social anxiety disorder. In: Orsillo ISM, Roemer L (eds) Acceptance and mindfulness-based approaches to anxiety: conceptualization and treatment. Springer, New York, pp 189–212

Hettema JM, Prescott CA, Myers JM, Neale MC, Kendler KS (2005) The structure of genetic and environmental risk factors for anxiety disorders in men and women. Arch Gen Psychiatry 62(2):182–189, http://dx.doi.org/10.1001/archpsyc.62.2.182

Hudson JL, Rapee RM (2000) The origins of social phobia. Behav Modif 24(1):102–129, http://dx.doi.org/10.1177/0145445500241006

Jose PE, Brown E (2008) When does the gender difference in rumination begin? Gender and age differences in the use of rumination by adolescents. J Youth Adolesc 37(2):180–192, http://dx.doi.org/10.1007/s10964-006-9166-y

Kagan J (1999) The concept of behavioral inhibition. In: Schmidt LA, Schulkin J (eds) Extreme fear, shyness, and social phobia: origins, biological mechanisms, and clinical outcomes. Oxford University Press, Inc., New York, pp 3–13

Kagan J, Reznick SJ, Snidman N (1988) Biological bases of childhood shyness. Science 240:117–256

Kagan J, Snidman N, Arcus D (1993) On the temperamental categories of inhibited and uninhibited children. In: Rubin KH, Asendorpf JB (eds) Social withdrawal, inhibition, and shyness in childhood. Lawrence Erlbaum Associates, Inc., Hillsdale, pp 19–28

Kashdan TB (2007) Social anxiety spectrum and diminished positive experiences: theoretical synthesis and meta-analysis. Clin Psychol Rev 27(3):348–365

Kashdan TB, McKnight PE, Richey JA, Hofmann SG (2009) When social anxiety disorder co-exists with risk-prone, approach behavior: investigating a neglected, meaningful subset of people in the National Comorbidity Survey-Replication. Behav Res Ther 47(7):559–568

Kerr M, Tremblay RE, Pagani L, Vitaro F (1997) Boy's behavioral inhibition and the risk of later delinquency. Arch Gen Psychiatry 54:809–816

Kimbrel NA, Mitchell JT, Nelson-Gray RO (2010) An examination of the relationship between behavioral approach system (BAS) sensitivity and social interaction anxiety. J Anxiety Disord 24(3):372–378

La Greca AM, Harrison HM (2005) Adolescent peer relations, friendships, and romantic relationships: do they predict social anxiety and depression? J Clin Child Adolesc Psychol 34(1):49–61. doi:10.1207/s15374424jccp3401_5

La Greca A, Lopez N (1998) Social anxiety among adolescents: linkages with peer relations and friendships. J Abnorm Child Psychol 26(2):83–94. doi:10.1023/A:1022684520514

LeDoux JE (1996) The emotional brain: the mysterious underpinnings of emotional life. Simon & Schuster, New York

MacDonald G, Leary MR (2005) Why does social exclusion hurt? The relationship between social and physical pain. Psychol Bull 131(2):202–223, http://dx.doi.org/10.1037/0033-2909.131.2.202

Moffitt TE (1993) Adolescence-limited and life-course-persistent antisocial behavior: a developmental taxonomy. Psychol Rev 100(4):674–701

Moffitt TE, Caspi A (2001) Childhood predictors differentiate life-course persistent and adolescence-limited antisocial pathways among males and females. Dev Psychopathol 13:355–375

Ohayon MM, Roth T (2003) Place of chronic insomnia in the course of depressive and anxiety disorders. J Psychiatr Res 37(1):9–15, http://dx.doi.org/10.1016/S0022-3956(02)00052-3

Oschner KN, Gross JJ (2007) The neural architecture of emotion regulation. In: Gross JJ (ed) Handbook of emotion regulation. Guilford Press, New York, pp 87–109

Phan LK, Coccaro E-F, Angstadt M, Kreger KJ, Mayber HS, Liberzon I et al (2013) Cortico-limbic brain reactivity to social signals of threat before and after sertraline treatment in generalized social phobia. Biol Psychiatry 73(4):329–336. doi:10.1016/j.biopsych.2012.10.003
Ranta K, Kaltiala-Heino R, Pelkonen M, Marttunen M (2009) Associations between peer victimization, self-reported depression and social phobia among adolescents: the role of comorbidity. J Adolesc 32:77–93
Ranta K, Kaltiala-Heino R, Fröjd S, Marttunen M (2013) Peer victimization and social phobia: a follow-up study among adolescents. Soc Psychiatry Psychiatr Epidemiol 48:533–544
Rapee RM, Heimberg RG (1997) A cognitive behavioral model of anxiety in social phobia. Behav Res Ther 35(8):741–756, http://dx.doi.org/10.1016/S0005-7967(97)00022-3
Rapee RM, Spence SH (2004) The etiology of social phobia: empirical evidence and an initial model. Clin Psychol Rev 24(7):737–767. doi:10.1016/j.cpr.2004.06.004
Ray RD, Ochsner KN, Cooper JC, Robertson ER, Gabrieli JD, Gross JJ (2005) Individual differences in trait rumination and the neural systems supporting cognitive reappraisal. Cogn Affect Behav Neurosci 5(2):156–168, http://dx.doi.org/10.3758/CABN.5.2.156
Robinson JL, Kagan J, Reznick JS, Corley R (1992) The heritability of inhibited and uninhibited behavior: a twin study. Dev Psychol 28(6):1030–1037, http://dx.doi.org/10.1037//0012-1649.28.6.1030
Rose AJ (2002) Co-rumination in the friendships of girls and boys. Child Dev 73(6):1830–1843, http://dx.doi.org/10.1111/1467-8624.00509
Rose AJ, Carlson W, Waller EM (2007) Prospective associations of co-rumination with friendship and emotional adjustment: considering the socioemotional trade-offs of co-rumination. Dev Psychol 43(4):1019–1031, http://dx.doi.org/10.1037/0012-1649.43.4.1019
Rubin KH, Wojslawowicz JC, Rose-Krasnor L, Booth-LaForce C, Burgess KB (2006) The best friendships of shy/withdrawn children: prevalence, stability, and relationship quality. J Abnorm Child Psychol 34(2):143–157. doi:10.1007/s10802-005-9017-4
Rubin KH, Coplan RJ, Bowker JC (2009) Social withdrawal in childhood. Annu Rev Psychol 60(1):141–171. doi:10.1146/annurev.psych.60.110707.163642
Rubin KH, Root AK, Bowker J (2010) Parents, peers, and social withdrawal in childhood: a relationship perspective. New Dir Child Adolesc Dev 2010(127):79–94. doi:10.1002/cd.264
Sareen J, Stein MB, Cox BJ, Hassard ST (2004) Understanding comorbidity of anxiety disorders with antisocial behavior: findings from two large community surveys. J Nerv Ment Dis 192(3):178–186. doi:10.1097/01.nmd.0000116460.25110.9f
Sebastian C, Viding E, Kipling D, Blakemore S-J (2010) Social brain development and the affective consequences of ostracism in adolescence. Brain Cogn 72(1):134–145, http://dx.doi.org/10.1016/j.bandc.2009.06.008
Siegel RS, La Greca AM, Harrison HM (2009) Peer victimization and social anxiety in adolescents: prospective and reciprocal relationships. J Youth Adolesc 38(8):1096–1109
Sommerville LH, Jones RM, Casey BJ (2010) A time of change: behavioral and neural correlates of adolescent sensitivity to appetitive and aversive environmental cues. Brain Cogn 72(1): 124–133, http://dx.doi.org/10.1016/j.bandc.2009.07.003
Stein MB, Gorman JM (2001) Unmasking social anxiety disorder. J Psychiatry Neurosci 26(3):185–189
Steinberg L, Morris AS (2001) Adolescent development. Annu Rev Psychol 52:83–110. doi:10.1146/annurev.psych.52.1.83
Stöber J, Borkovec TD (2002) Reduced concreteness of worry in generalized anxiety disorder: findings from a therapy study. Cogn Ther Res 26(1):89–96. doi:10.1023/A:1013845821848
Stoeckli G (2010) The role of individual and social factors in classroom loneliness. J Educ Res 103(1):28–39. doi:10.1080/00220670903231169
Storch EA, Brassard MR, Masia-Warner CL (2003) The relationship of peer victimization to social anxiety and loneliness in adolescence. Child Study J 33(1):1–18
Thompson RA, Goodman M (2010) Development of emotion regulation. In: Kring AM, Sloan DM (eds) Emotion regulation and psychopathology: a transdiagnostic approach to etiology and treatment. The Guilford Press, New York, pp 38–58

Tillfors M (2004) Why do some individuals develop social phobia? A review with emphasis on the neurobiological influences. Nord J Psychiatry 58(4):267–276. doi:10.1080/08039480410005774

Tillfors M, Furmark T, Ekselius L, Fredrikson M (2001) Social phobia and avoidant personality disorder as related to parental history of social anxiety: a general population study. Behav Res Ther 39(3):289–298, http://dx.doi.org/10.1016/S0005-7967(00)00003-6

Tillfors M, El-Khouri B, Stein MB, Trost K (2009) Relationships between social anxiety, depressive symptoms, and antisocial behaviors: evidence from a prospective study of adolescent boys. J Anxiety Disord 23(5):718–724, http://dx.doi.org/10.1016/j.janxdis.2009.02.011

Tillfors M, Persson S, Willen M, Burk WJ (2012) Prospective links between social anxiety and adolescent peer relations. J Adolesc 35(5):1255–1263. doi:10.1016/j.adolescence.2012.04.008

Tillfors M, Mörtberg E, Van Zalk N, Kerr M (2013a) Inhibited and impulsive subgroups of socially anxious young adults: their depressive symptoms and life satisfaction. Open J Psychiatry 03(01):195–201. doi:10.4236/ojpsych.2013.31A016

Tillfors M, Van Zalk N, Kerr M (2013b) Investigating a socially anxious-impulsive subgroup of adolescents: a prospective community study. Scand J Psychol 54(3):267–273. doi:10.1111/sjop.12047

Van Ameringen M, Mancini C, Oakman JM, Farvolden P (1999) Selective serotonin reuptake inhibitors in the treatment of social phobia: the emerging gold standard. CNS Drugs 11(4): 307–315, http://dx.doi.org/10.2165/00023210-199911040-00006

Van der Helm E, Walker MP (2010) The role of sleep in emotional brain regulation. In: Kring AM, Sloan DM (eds) Emotion regulation and psychopathology: a transdiagnostic approach to etiology and treatment. The Guilford Press, New York, pp 38–58

Van Zalk N, Kerr M (2011) Shy adolescents' perceptions of parents' psychological control and emotional warmth: examining bidirectional links. Merrill-Palmer Q 57(4):375–401. doi:10.1353/mpq.2011.0021

Van Zalk, N., & Tillfors, M. (2014). Co-rumination moderates the link between social anxiety and depressive symptoms in early adolescence. *Manuscript Submitted For Publication*

Van Zalk, N., & Van Zalk, M. H. W. (in press). The importance of perceived support by fiends and parents for adolescent social anxiety. Journal of Personality. doi:10.1111/jopy.12108

Van Zalk N, Kerr M, Tilton-Weaver LC (2011a) Shyness as a moderator of the link between advanced maturity and early adolescent risk behavior. Scand J Psychol 52(4):341–353. doi:10.1111/j.1467-9450.2011.00877.x

Van Zalk N, Van Zalk M, Kerr M, Stattin H (2011b) Social anxiety as a basis for friendship selection and socialization in adolescents' social networks. J Pers 79(3):499–526. doi:10.1111/j.1467-6494.2011.00682.x

Van Zalk N, Van Zalk MHW, Kerr M (2011c) Socialization of social anxiety in adolescent crowds. J Abnorm Child Psychol 39(8):1239–1249. doi:10.1007/s10802-011-9533-3

Vermeiren R, Deboutte D, Ruchkin V, Schwab-Stone M (2002) Antisocial behaviour and mental health: findings from three communities. Eur Child Adolesc Psychiatry 11(4):168–175. doi:10.1007/s00787-002-0275-1

Wittchen H-U, Beesdo K, Bittner A, Goodwin RD (2003) Depressive episodes–evidence for a causal role of primary anxiety disorders? Eur Psychiatry 18(8):384–393

Wolfson AR, Carskadon MA (1998) Sleep schedules and daytime functioning in adolescents. Child Dev 69(4):875–887, http://dx.doi.org/10.1111/j.1467-8624.1998.tb06149.x

Zalta AK, Dowd S, Rosenfield D, Smits JA, Otto MW, Simon NM et al (2013) Sleep quality predicts treatment outcome in CBT for social anxiety disorder. Depress Anxiety 30(11): 1114–1120. doi:10.1002/da.22170

Zimmerman P, Wittchen HU, Hofler M, Pfister H, Kessler RC, Lieb R (2003) Primary anxiety disorders and the development of subsequent alcohol use disorders: a 4-year community study of adolescents and young adults. Psychol Med 33(7):1211–1222

Developmental Transitions in Adolescence and Their Implications for Social Anxiety

5

Annette M. La Greca and Klaus Ranta

Introduction

During adolescence, developmental changes and transitions occur across multiple areas and are most striking in the biological and social realms. Key biological changes involve the onset of puberty, with associated growth spurts and sexual development (Cole and Cole 2001). In the interpersonal realm, adolescents' lives undergo considerable reorganization that includes negotiating school transitions, establishing new relationships with peers, engaging in romantic relationships and in sexual activity, and negotiating greater autonomy and independence from the family (Cole and Cole 2001; Goodwin et al. 2012).

Adolescence is also a critical period for the emergence of social anxiety disorder (SAD). Studies reveal that the onset of SAD generally occurs in late childhood or mid-adolescence (Rosellini et al. 2013; Stein et al. 2001) and that the vast majority of individuals with SAD report its onset before age 18 years (Otto et al. 2001). The emergence of new cases of SAD in adulthood is rare unless they are secondary to another disorder such as major depression (Neufeld et al. 1999).

So, a key question emerges: Do the challenging developmental transitions that adolescents encounter contribute to the development of social anxiety symptoms or disorder? The purpose of the current chapter is to review what is currently known about the associations between the key biological and social transitions of adolescence and the development of SAD and/or elevated symptoms of social

A.M. La Greca, PhD, ABPP (✉)
Department of Psychology, University of Miami, Coral Gables, FL, USA
e-mail: alagreca@miami.edu

K. Ranta, MD, PhD
Department of Adolescent Psychiatry, Helsinki University Central Hospital, Helsinki, Finland

Department of Psychology, University of Turku, Turku, Finland
e-mail: klaus.ranta@hus.fi

K. Ranta et al. (eds.), *Social Anxiety and Phobia in Adolescents: Development, Manifestation and Intervention Strategies*, DOI 10.1007/978-3-319-16703-9_5

anxiety. Surprisingly, this is a neglected and understudied area of research, but one that has the potential to contribute to a better understanding of the etiology of SAD.

Developmental transitions are important because they may be viewed as stressors and, as such, can have an important impact on youths' psychological functioning (Grant et al. 2003, 2004). Developmental transitions often involve novel situations that adolescents must negotiate to develop more mature levels of social and emotional functioning; however, the novelty can bring uncertainty, opportunities for failure, and discomfort or distress. In fact, there is a substantial literature examining the impact of biological and social transitions on the emergence of adolescent depressive symptoms (e.g., Ge et al. 2001a, b; Mendle et al. 2007). Extending the study of developmental transitions to the emergence of significant symptoms of SAD in youth would appear to be an important and useful avenue for inquiry.

In the chapter sections below, we discuss pathways by which transitions might contribute to social anxiety and, in turn, why socially anxious youth might have trouble negotiating common developmental transitions. The specific adolescent transitions we discuss include the following: school transitions and their associated impact on peer relations; biological transitions such as the timing and onset of puberty and associated physical changes; the emergence of dating, romantic relationships, and sexual activity; and negotiating autonomy within the family. We end the chapter with a brief summary and recommendations for further research and clinical practice.

Developmental Transitions and Adolescent Social Anxiety

School Transitions and Peer Relations

During adolescence, most youth experience major school transitions, although the exact timing of the transitions may vary across countries. For example, in the United States, early adolescents typically transition from elementary to middle school (6th or 7th grade) around 12–13 years of age and enter high school (9th or 10th grade) around 14–15 years of age. After high school, older adolescents (18-year-olds) make another transition to college, vocational school, and/or work settings. A similar sequence of school transitions occurs in Japan (Center on International Education Benchmarking 2014a). In contrast, in Finland, youth remain in school through the 9th grade (about age 15 years), after which most (95 %) transition voluntarily to either academic or vocational upper secondary schools, with a small percentage of adolescents (5 %) leaving school to begin work (Center on International Education Benchmarking 2014b). School transitions typically involve a move to a different and often larger school, which can disrupt established peer groups but also provide opportunities for developing new friendships (Goodwin et al. 2012).

School or work transitions can have a substantial impact on adolescents' social lives, as they learn to interact with new peers and with adult authority figures (e.g., teachers, bosses). Adolescents who relocate to a new community are also faced with the prospect of making new friends and dealing with new teachers and other adults;

such adolescents may experience even greater challenges in making a successful school and social transition than those who are residentially stable (Vernberg 1990a, b; Vernberg et al. 2006).

It is not difficult to see why school transitions might contribute to social anxiety in youth, given the significant shifts that occur in adolescents' social lives and the myriad social challenges that adolescents must negotiate during school transitions. Adolescents typically experience uncertainty about their personal identity and how they "fit in" with others and place considerable importance on acceptance from peers and on companionship, intimacy, and emotional support from close friends (Furman et al. 2009; La Greca and Prinstein 1999). Peers, and especially close friends, become a key focus of adolescents' lives and represent a primary source of social support for adolescents (Furman et al. 2009; La Greca and Prinstein 1999). Across the adolescent years, the size of adolescents' peer groups increases, their close friendships become more intimate and intense, and adolescents spend more time with friends and peers than they do with parents or other adults (Brown 1990; Cole and Cole 2001; La Greca and Prinstein 1999). These significant friendships are disrupted during school transitions, leaving adolescents with the challenges of initiating and developing new friendships and of establishing close, intimate, supportive ties. In fact, adolescents facing community relocation often report concerns about making new friends and leaving close friendships behind (Vernberg and Randall 1997). The challenging social tasks that accompany school transitions can contribute to adolescents' feelings of social anxiety (La Greca and Lopez 1998). Moreover, adolescents who are already socially anxious may find relocation and school transitions especially challenging to negotiate (Vernberg et al. 2006).

The sparse literature on school transitions and social anxiety is consistent with the above perspective. Vernberg and colleagues (Vernberg 1990a, b; Vernberg et al. 1992) studied early adolescents (ages 12–14 years) who relocated to a new community within 3 months of the start of the school year and followed these youth at three time points (September, November, and May) over the course of their first year in a new school. In particular, Vernberg et al. (1992) examined bidirectional and prospective associations between adolescents' close friendship qualities and peer rejection experiences and their levels of social anxiety over the school year. In terms of the impact of peer experiences on social anxiety, Vernberg et al. (1992) found that adolescents with lower levels of companionship and intimacy in their close friendships at the start of the school year reported increased levels of social anxiety (i.e., fear of negative evaluations) over the fall; over the latter part of the school year, less intimacy in close friendships also predicted increased levels of social anxiety (i.e., social avoidance and distress). In addition, adolescents reporting higher levels of exclusion by peers (aka relational victimization; De Los Reyes and Prinstein 2004) over the fall reported increased social anxiety (i.e., fear of negative evaluation; social avoidance and distress, especially for girls); higher levels of social exclusion over the latter part of the school year also predicted increases in adolescents' social anxiety (i.e., generalized social avoidance and distress). These findings highlight the impact of close friendships and peer experiences on social anxiety during a school transition. Further, the findings also were consistent with the notion that social anxiety influences adolescents' friendship development, as adolescents with higher levels of social anxiety in September reported less companionship in their close friendships over the course of the fall.

In a larger follow-up to the above study, Vernberg et al. (2006) compared the peer experiences of 207 early adolescents who relocated and began their 7th or 8th grade in a new school with the experiences of 68 residentially stable adolescents. Most adolescents who relocated reported diminished levels of companionship and intimacy in their close friendships during the fall of the school year, but this effect was relatively short-lived, as the friendship qualities of relocated and stable adolescents were similar by the end of the school year. However, the degree of friendship disruption over the school year was significantly greater for socially anxious adolescents compared with less anxious peers.

It is unclear whether these findings for early adolescents also apply to older adolescents who undergo important school or work transitions. Studies of older adolescents' school transitions, such as from middle school to high school (typically around age 15 years in the United States) or from high school to college (typically around 18 years of age), have been lacking, at least with respect to the linkages between these transitions and adolescents' social anxiety. However, some information may be gleaned from several studies that examined related constructs, such as the impact of school transitions on social support or depressive symptoms. For example, Newman and colleagues (2007) followed adolescents over the transition from middle school to high school (8th to 9th grade), finding that parent and peer support declined over the transition period and that these declining support levels were associated with increasing symptoms of depression among adolescents. Further, a recent study by Goodwin et al. (2012) focused on adolescents' friendships over two school transitions (elementary to middle school and middle school to high school), finding that after each transition, adolescents selected friends with similar levels of depressive symptoms. These studies highlight the importance of school transitions for understanding adolescents' well-being and psychological adjustment.

Although not directly focused on school transitions, studies of older adolescents (e.g., 14–18 years of age) demonstrate that peer victimization experiences, especially those involving social exclusion or rejection by friends, are strongly associated with adolescent social anxiety, both concurrently and prospectively (e.g., Garcia-Lopez et al. 2011; La Greca and Harrison 2005; Siegel et al. 2009; Ranta et al. 2009, 2013; Storch and Masia-Warner 2004), and also that socially anxious adolescents are vulnerable to being social excluded by peers (Siegel et al. 2009) and report less social acceptance and support from classmates (La Greca and Lopez 1998). One implication of these findings is that school transitions are likely to be socially challenging for socially anxious youth and may exacerbate symptoms of social anxiety, especially if the transition does not go well or problems arise in establishing supportive friendships.

In summary, school transitions affect adolescents' social lives and increase their feelings of social anxiety, particularly because they value acceptance from peers and support from close friends, yet may be uncertain about how they "fit in" with others. Studies suggest that, for most adolescents, social transitions (e.g., moving and changing schools) have a short-term impact on adolescents' social lives and social anxiety; however, socially anxious youth may experience greater difficulty with social transitions than their peers. Further research examining the impact of social transitions, especially with older adolescents, will be important and desirable.

Biological Transitions

As youth transition from childhood to adulthood, roughly between the ages of 10–20 years, multiple and major changes occur across diverse biological system levels (e.g., endocrinological, neurological, reproductive). Many changes occur during puberty, although neurological changes extend to the later phases of the adolescent period (Blakemore and Choudhury 2006; Patton and Viner 2007). In this section, we review research on the associations between adolescents' heightened social anxiety or SAD and pubertal status and timing as well as body morphological and physiological transitions. The reader is referred to Chaps. 2 and 4 for further details on neurological development and social anxiety.

Pubertal Status and Pubertal Timing

The pubertal period refers collectively to biological changes induced by changes in the secretion of hypothalamic-pituitary-gonadal axis hormones, leading to marked acceleration in growth rate, sex-specific alterations in body muscle/fat proportions, and the development of secondary sex characteristics (Bordini and Rosenfield 2011). Two dimensions of puberty occur: pubertal status (i.e., the level of physical maturation reached by the individual) and pubertal timing (i.e., the individual's level of maturation relative to the majority of same-sex same-aged peers, which is considered to be early maturing, on time, or late maturing).

In longitudinal studies, both pubertal status and timing have been rather extensively investigated as factors contributing to concurrent or subsequent mental health outcomes (Ge et al. 2001b; Graber et al. 2004). In general, girls and boys who are "on time" experience the development of secondary sexual characteristics around ages 12 and 13 years, respectively (Tanner 1962). However, recent data also suggest that the average age of puberty onset is declining in the United States and other countries (e.g., Addo et al. 2014; Aksglaede et al. 2008; Jaruratanasirikul and Sriplung 2014), so pubertal changes may occur even earlier.

Although closely related to pubertal maturation per se, and likely interacting with maturation and other biological transition factors, girls' early pubertal timing has been associated with both depression and anxiety, including somatic anxiety symptoms, general anxiety, and panic attack symptoms (Aro and Taipale 1987; Ge et al. 2001a; Graber 2013; Hayward et al. 1997; Kaltiala-Heino et al. 2003; for a review see Reardon et al. 2009). Although less well researched, boys' early pubertal timing has likewise been associated with depression and generalized anxiety (Ge et al. 2001a; Natsuaki et al. 2009).

The role of pubertal maturation and/or timing in social anxiety and SAD has been examined in a number of studies (Blumenthal et al. 2009, 2011; Deardorff et al. 2007; Ge et al. 2006; Jones and Bayley 1971; Mathyssek 2014; Weingarden and Renshaw 2012), which are reviewed below. Overall, studies focused on the impact of early pubertal timing (rather than late timing) and examined pubertal effects separately for boys and girls.

A few studies observed significant effects for early-maturing girls, but not for early-maturing boys. For example, Deardorff et al. (2007) studied a sample of 9- to 11-year-old children and early adolescents with respect to either attaining puberty (i.e., Tanner stage II) or not (i.e., Tanner stage I) and self-reported social anxiety at age 11 years. They found an interaction between gender and pubertal status as predictors of social anxiety. Pubertal advancement was correlated with elevated symptoms of social anxiety in girls, but not in boys. However, no other psychopathology variables were controlled in this study. With regard to pubertal timing among 12- to 17-year-old adolescents, Blumenthal and colleagues (2011) found that early-maturing girls were at a higher risk of suffering from symptoms of social anxiety compared to on-time girls and early-maturing boys.

In contrast to the above studies, others have found effects for early-maturing boys but not for early-maturing girls. Specifically, in a sample of African-American early adolescents (10–12 years of age), Ge et al. (2006) observed that early-maturing boys showed higher social anxiety levels than boys whose puberty was not advanced; in girls, early pubertal timing (which largely coincided with pubertal advancement in this age range) did not have an effect on symptoms of social anxiety, but did on symptoms of general anxiety and depression. Furthermore, in a longitudinal study of 10- to 17-year-old Dutch youth, Mathyssek (2014) found no main effect for pubertal timing predicting symptoms of generalized anxiety, panic disorder, or social anxiety; however, an interaction between gender, age, and anxiety was observed. For boys aged 10–11 years, being ahead of other boys in pubertal development was associated with elevated anxiety symptom levels for each of the three anxiety domains, and the association was strongest for social anxiety. In contrast, for boys aged 14 years or older, pubertal development ahead of peers was associated with fewer anxiety symptoms in all three domains. Moreover, the researchers found no associations between pubertal timing and anxiety symptoms for girls.

Some of the equivocal findings across studies may be due to variables, such as peer relationship problems, that moderate associations between pubertal timing and social anxiety. For example, in a sample of 10- to 17-year-olds, Blumenthal et al. (2009) examined the interaction between peer relationship problems and pubertal timing in predicting social anxiety. They found no main effect for pubertal timing; however, early-maturing youth with problematic peer relationships were at heightened risk for social anxiety.

Only a few studies report findings pertinent to the impact of late pubertal timing and social anxiety. An early longitudinal study (Jones and Bayley 1971) observed higher social anxiety among late-maturing boys relative to early-maturing boys. The differences were evident across a 5-year period, but were most pronounced in mid-adolescence at age 16 years. In addition, in a retrospective population study using data (all female sample) from the National Comorbidity Survey Replication

(NCS-R; Kessler et al. 2004), Weingarden and Renshaw (2012) observed that both early and late perceived pubertal timing predicted increased risk of lifetime social anxiety disorder in adulthood. However, when the investigators controlled for comorbidity with other anxiety disorders, the association between early puberty and SAD disappeared, although late perceived puberty remained associated to SAD (the only anxiety disorder where an association was observed).

Thus, evaluating all the evidence, the findings appear equivocal, both for and against the notion that pubertal status and pubertal timing are associated with adolescent social anxiety. Some studies suggest a risk for early-maturing girls (Blumenthal et al. 2011; Deardorff et al. 2007), whereas others suggest a risk for early-maturing boys only (Ge et al. 2006; Mathyssek 2014); some studies even suggest that late maturation might be a risk factor for social anxiety (Jones and Bayley 1971; Weingarden and Renshaw 2012). The contradictory findings might reflect the presence of confounding factors (e.g., comorbid anxiety or depression) or important moderating variables (e.g., age, peer relationship quality) that could affect the associations between pubertal timing and social anxiety. Clearly, more controlled research is needed.

Body Morphological and Physiological Transitions

Related to the onset of puberty, and precipitated by underlying hormonal changes (e.g., Cameron 2004), marked changes occur in the shape, proportions, and functioning of the maturing adolescent body. In particular, changes occur in visible physical characteristics, such as height, subcutaneous fat, skin quality, and secondary sex characteristics; these changes may affect adolescents' feelings of comfort around others and have the potential to heighten social anxiety. Furthermore, although less well studied, it is likely that youth who are already socially anxious may be especially uncomfortable as visible bodily changes occur.

For example, during puberty, the increase in height during girls' growth spurt may arouse concerns about being stared at, heighten self-consciousness, and increase feelings of social anxiety (Booth 1988). On the other hand, boys' delayed growth may heighten their social anxiety (Huddleston and Ge 2003), as they may appear smaller or less muscular than their peers. Also, a radical increase in girls' subcutaneous fat (i.e., the fat spurt) may lead to significant fears of becoming fat and fears of negative evaluation (an aspect of social anxiety) and consequently raise the risk for maladaptive weight control behaviors and onset of an eating disorder (Attie and Brooks-Gunn 1989; Levinson and Rodebaugh 2011). Hormonally induced skin conditions, like acne, also raise appearance concerns and are associated with elevated levels of social anxiety in adolescents (Krowchuk et al. 1991). Similarly, the timing of the morphological changes in secondary sex characteristics (e.g., delayed breast development in girls; Carter et al. 2009), as well as changes in perspiration and body odor (Veale 2003; Eklund and Bianco 2000), are associated with adolescent social anxiety.

There are multiple reasons why bodily changes occurring during adolescence might contribute to social anxiety. In particular, bodily changes can affect adolescents' self-confidence as well as their peer relationships. For example, the significant variability in the timing of pubertal onset across adolescents of the same age as well as intraindividual asynchrony in the sequencing of pubertal changes (Hayward 2003) are likely to raise adolescents' doubts and anxiety over the normality of their own physical changes (Coleman 2001). Furthermore, physical appearance is related to adolescents' peer acceptance (Lerner et al. 1991), with considerable ecological evidence for adolescents' concerns of being excluded by peers if something is not right with their appearance. Teasing about physical appearance may occur (Kowalski 2000; Magin et al. 2008; Shapiro et al. 1991), which can have long-term consequences; in fact, appearance-related teasing in adolescence predicts subsequent social anxiety in adulthood (McCabe et al. 2003, 2010; Strawser et al. 2005). In addition, outright bullying directed at adolescents' general physical appearance (e.g., related to wearing unfashionable clothing) may intensify during adolescence (Keltner et al. 2001; Yoo and Johnson 2008), and such appearance-based victimization has been linked to social anxiety (e.g., Lavell et al. 2014).

For many adolescents, deviations from physical norms, as noted above, may interact with social pressures to be accepted and "fit in" (Cole and Cole 2001), potentially leading to fears of negative evaluation from peers and even feelings of humiliation. Indeed, by considering the social environment in which adolescents' physical changes occur, and by acknowledging the affective and cognitive transitions of adolescence, integrative developmental models of the onset and maintenance of SAD in adolescents can be constructed (Detweiler et al. 2010).

Several models of social anxiety may be pertinent to understanding the association between physical changes and adolescent social anxiety. In particular, the self-presentational theory of social anxiety (Leary 2010; Leary and Kowalski 1995) postulates that an individual experiences social anxiety when motivated to make a positive or desired impression on others, but is uncertain whether one is successful in this attempt. Other major models of SAD (e.g., Clark and Wells 1995; Heimberg et al. 2010; Rapee and Heimberg 1997) emphasize self-focused attention and/or hypothesized audience criticalness, and these conceptualizations also fit well with the adolescent experience (Detweiler et al. 2010).

The physical changes of adolescence also have substantial personal significance. For example, Harter (1999) found that adolescents' global self-esteem correlated highest with their physical appearance, after which factors like scholastic competence, social competence, and athletic competence came into play. Other findings demonstrate that low levels of perceived physical and global self-esteem raise the risk for social anxiety, trait anxiety, and eating disorder symptoms among adolescents (Obeid et al. 2013; Ohannessian et al. 1999).

In summary, adolescents experience dramatic bodily changes, many of which are precipitated by puberty onset and underlying hormonal changes. Such changes contribute to adolescents' feelings of social anxiety and to other related problems, such as eating disorders. Although less well studied, it is likely that bodily changes further heighten or exacerbate social anxiety in adolescents who are already prone to be socially anxious. Further research of a prospective nature would help to more clearly elucidate the potential pathways between the physical transitions of adolescence and adolescent social anxiety.

The Emergence of Romantic Relationships, Dating, and Sexual Activity

The emergence of romantic relationships is another important developmental transition that occurs during adolescence in Western cultures (Furman and Rose 2015). For example, in the United States, by age 16 years, most adolescents have had a romantic relationship (Carver et al. 2003), and the number continues to grow into early adulthood. Between ages 25 and 40 years, over 70 % of young men and women in the United States marry for the first time (Goodwin et al. 2009). A similar progression can be observed for involvement in sexual intercourse among US adolescents, although the prevalence rates are lower than for dating (Abma et al. 2004; see also Davila et al. in press).

For the most part, romantic relationships follow a typical developmental course (Furman and Rose 2015). During childhood, friendships predominantly occur between same-sex peers; however, puberty brings greater awareness of the other sex and of romantic attraction, which prompts interest and engagement in romantic activity (Bellis et al. 2006). During early adolescence, interest in members of the other sex and in "dating activities" often emerges within a group context (Shulman and Scharf 2000). As adolescence progresses, dyadic romantic relationships develop that involve increasing levels of support and intimacy (Davila et al. in press; La Greca et al. 2011; Shulman and Scharf 2000).

For most adolescents, dating and romantic relationships provide the context for engaging in sexual activities (Kuttler and La Greca 2004). Data from the 2013 survey of US adolescents (14–18 years) (Centers for Disease Control and Prevention 2014) reveal that 46.8 % of adolescents have had sexual intercourse (30 % for 9th graders, 64 % for 12th graders), 34 % had sexual intercourse within the previous 3 months (20 % for 9th graders, 49 % for 12th graders), and 5.6 % report having intercourse before age 13 years. Thus, engaging in romantic and sexual activity is a common and even normative activity among adolescents in the United States as well as in many other Western cultures (e.g., Skinner et al. 2008).

Romantic relationships may be beneficial to adolescents' emotional functioning, as such relationships provide social support, enhance self-esteem, and prepare adolescents for adult relationships (Collins 2003; Collins et al. 2009; Connolly and Goldberg 1999). Romantic experiences and relationships also help young people develop adaptive interpersonal skills (Seiffge-Krenke and Lang 2002), reduce anxiety (Glickman and La Greca 2004; La Greca and Harrison 2005), and contribute to healthy sexual development (Welsh et al. 2005).

Nevertheless, adolescent romantic relationships represent a significant interpersonal stressor that may cause distress, especially among adolescents who are just learning to navigate such relationships (Downey et al. 1999). Interactions with a romantic partner may involve criticism, conflict, and pressure, and negative interactions may be greater in adolescents' romantic relationships than in their close friendships, especially for girls (Kuttler and La Greca 2004; La Greca and Harrison 2005). Engaging in romantic relationships in early adolescence and romantic breakups are both associated with reports of depressive symptoms (Collins et al. 2009;

Davila 2008; Monroe et al. 1999). Involvement in dating and romantic relationships during adolescence, particularly if the involvement is frequent and includes sexual activity, is associated with negative affect and depressive symptoms among girls (see Davila et al. in press; La Greca et al. 2008).

The adolescent transition to dating and romantic relationships can be a challenging one for socially anxious adolescents, who show delays in romantic involvement. Specifically, adolescents with high levels of social anxiety (and/or dating anxiety, a related construct) are less likely than their peers to be romantically involved and more likely to report that they have never dated (La Greca and Harrison 2005; La Greca and Mackey 2007). This may be because such adolescents avoid or are uncomfortable in hetero-social situations that lead to opportunities for dating (Glickman and La Greca 2004). By avoiding romantic relationships, however, socially anxious youth miss out on the psychological benefits that romantic relationships can convey (e.g., social support, esteem enhancement).

Interpersonal impairments among socially anxious youth also may interfere with the development of romantic relationships. For example, Hebert and colleagues (2013) found that the interpersonal impairments of socially anxious youth limit their engagement in other-sex friendships that are precursors to romantic relationships and thus lead to interpersonal deficits in romantic relationships. Other data suggest that, once established, the qualities of romantic relationships are less skillful among socially anxious youth. Specifically, among adolescents who are romantically involved (and who are thus less likely to be socially anxious to begin with), higher levels of dating-related social anxiety are associated with fewer positive and more negative qualities in romantic relationships (La Greca and Mackey 2007). Similarly, young adults who are socially anxious display less emotional expression, fewer positive behaviors, less self-disclosure, and decreased intimacy in their romantic relationships (Sparrevohn and Rapee 2009; Wenzel et al. 2005). Such findings suggest that inhibition in close relationships might limit positive interactions within the romantic relationships of socially anxious adolescents and young adults.

Socially anxious youths' delays in developing romantic relationships and potential impairments in romantic functioning can extend into adulthood. Longitudinal studies find that shy and socially inhibited boys marry later in life than comparison youth (Caspi et al. 1988). Large-scale epidemiological studies also reveal that socially anxious adults are more likely to have been never married, separated, or divorced than their non-anxious counterparts (Lampe et al. 2003; Wittchen et al. 2000).

Because sexual activity often occurs within the context of dating or romantic relationships, one would expect socially anxious adolescents to be delayed in their sexual involvement. Consistent with this perspective, Thompson (1999) found that socially anxious adolescents were less likely to date or have friends who were sexually involved; in turn, less dating and having fewer sexually active friends predicted lower rates of adolescent sexual intercourse. However, once adolescents are romantically involved, evidence indicates that casual sexual activity (i.e., outside of a committed relationship) is linked with depression (e.g., Grello et al. 2003; see Davila et al. in press), although it is not clear whether such sexual activity is also linked with social anxiety.

The adolescent transition to the development of romantic relationships may lead to or exacerbate symptoms of social anxiety in youth. In general, the direction of causal pathways between adolescent social anxiety and romantic-relationship onset and qualities is not clear. One possibility is that adolescent social anxiety leads to social impairments and inhibited social behaviors that delay the onset of romantic (and sexual) relationships and reduce the intimacy and positive qualities of those relationships, once they are established (La Greca et al. 2011). Another possibility is that negative interactions in adolescents' romantic relationships contribute to or exacerbate feelings of distress and specifically social evaluative fears that are a key aspect of social anxiety (e.g., La Greca and Mackey 2007). This latter perspective is consistent with findings that adolescents demonstrate increased sensitivity to rejection from romantic partners (Downey et al. 1999). Also, the presence of frequent negative interactions with a romantic partner (e.g., criticism, pressure, conflict) and experiencing a break-up, both of which are fairly common among adolescents (Collins et al. 2009; Davila et al. in press), might directly contribute to adolescents' feelings of social anxiety.

Although research on adolescent romantic relationships is relatively new and gradually developing, most studies focus on adolescents with heterosexual romantic interests. Scant research has examined the developmental course of romantic relationships among sexual minority (i.e., gay, lesbian, or bisexual) youth, but this literature suggests that the initiation of romantic relationships for these youth does not follow the same progression as that for heterosexual adolescents (Davila et al. in press; Koch 1993; Savin-Williams 1994). Sexual minority youth may not feel comfortable initiating, or be able to safely initiate, romantic involvements (Davila et al. in press), especially in communities where few adolescents openly identify as sexual minorities (Collins et al. 2009). Sexual minority youth face challenges that may impact their psychological functioning and contribute to feeling of social anxiety; however, this area is not well studied at present and merits much closer attention.

Family Transitions and Increasing Adolescent Autonomy

The developmental transition of increasing adolescent autonomy and emotionally moving away from parents is an important aspect of adolescent development (Steinberg and Morris 2001). During childhood, parents represent the most important source of social support for youth; however, during adolescence, close friends take on increasing importance and in many cases exceed parents as a primary source of emotional support (Furman et al. 2009; Puklek Levpušček 2006). In general, the family environment, through antecedent socialization/child-rearing practices or concurrent family interactions, may facilitate or complicate this developmental shift.

As a whole, research on family factors in the development of anxiety disorders is quite extensive (see Bögels and Brechman-Toussaint 2006; Gar et al. 2005; Ginsburg et al. 2004; McLeod et al. 2007; Rapee 2012; van der Bruggen et al. 2008; Wood et al. 2003). Similarly, there is a relatively large body of research on early environmental and familial factors in SAD (Alden and Taylor 2004; Brook and Schmidt 2008; Garcia-Lopez et al. 2009, 2014; Knappe et al. 2009, 2012; Masia and Morris 1998; Rapee and Spence 2004; also see Chaps. 2 and 3, this volume).

Most studies on family contributions to adolescents' social anxiety have examined the roles of *earlier* child-rearing and family factors in the development of youths' symptoms of social anxiety. In the following section, we briefly review this research, concentrating on studies in which social anxiety or SAD has been assessed among adolescents. Then we review studies on the associations between social anxiety and SAD and concurrent family interactions (i.e., during the adolescent period).

Childhood Family Interpersonal Factors and Social Anxiety in Adolescence

Evidence suggests that parental overcontrol and rejection play a role in the development of adolescent social anxiety. Starting with an unselected, representative, epidemiological study, initial reports from the well-known prospective German Early Developmental Stages of Psychopathology (EDSP) study indicated that perceived parental overcontrol and rejection were associated with SAD in adolescents, even when parental psychopathology was controlled (Lieb et al. 2000). Following the adolescent sample 10 years later, and extending the time span of the study to cover the highest risk period for SAD, Knappe et al. (2009) again observed that perceived parental overcontrol and rejection, in addition to low emotional warmth, were associated with SAD in their offspring. However, there was an interaction with parental psychopathology, which revealed that their combined effect was significantly greater than the risk associated with child-rearing factors alone. In the third analysis from the EDSP sample, Knappe and colleagues (2012) distinguished between the contributions of maternal and paternal child rearing. They found that compared to other anxiety disorders, adolescents with SAD reported a pattern of maternal overprotection and paternal rejection and low emotional warmth. (Note that the measure of perceived parenting covered *past* parenting style.)

Other population-based studies also have addressed parenting issues using adolescents as informants. In a prospective study, Lewis-Morrarty et al. (2012) observed that maternal overcontrolling style of child rearing at age seven was associated with high rates of social anxiety symptoms and lifetime rates of SAD in adolescence. In this study, the temperamental characteristic of infant behavioral inhibition was associated with adolescent social anxiety only in interaction with age seven maternal overcontrol. Combining results from the adolescent studies with results from studies with follow-ups periods into adulthood (Knappe et al. 2010), it seems reasonable to conclude that overcontrol, rejection, and low warmth are associated with adolescent SAD; however, the interaction between these parenting factors and other offspring or parental factors has been insufficiently studied and warrants further examination.

Concurrent Parent-Adolescent Interactions

Associations between adolescents' social anxiety and familial interactions during the adolescent period have gained less attention than early familial factors, and there is a question of how distinguishable they are from earlier or even subsequent familial interactions. Recently, Yap et al. (2014) performed a meta-analysis of studies focusing on parenting during the adolescent period (between 12 and 18 years of age), with outcomes covering both anxiety disorders and depression. Using this meta-analysis and additional literature review, we identified seven studies relevant to the discussion of transitions during the adolescent period. Six studies (Bögels et al. 2001; Caster et al. 1999; Fisak and Mann 2010; Johnson et al. 2005; Rork and Morris 2009; Starr and Davila 2008) specifically focused on concurrent family interactions and adolescents' social anxiety/SAD and are reviewed below.

In a mixed group of clinically referred children and controls, with a mean age of 13 years, Bögels et al. (2001) found little support for the association of concurrent child-rearing practices and high social anxiety, aside from that attributable to family sociability (as measured by both offspring and maternal reports) and to offspring's perception of maternal overprotection. However, a comparison of clinically referred high socially anxious (SA), clinically referred low SA, and non-referred controls revealed that the clinical high SA group reported greater parental rejection, less emotional warmth, and less family sociability than did the controls; but the two clinical groups (high and low SA) did not differ, suggesting that those parenting factors were not specific to social anxiety.

In a slightly younger sample of early adolescents (age 10–13 years), Rork and Morris (2009) found both maternal and paternal overprotection and parental negative commanding style (i.e., telling their child what not to do) were associated with offspring's social anxiety; however low parental sociability and low warmth were not related to youths' social anxiety. These results partly confirmed (i.e., with regard to overprotection), but partly differed from (i.e., with regard to parental warmth and sociability), the findings of Bögels et al.

Caster et al. (1999) examined adolescents' and parents' perceptions of family interactions and their concurrent association with adolescent social anxiety in a large sample of youth (grades 7 to 11th). Adolescents who reported high social anxiety perceived their parents as being more socially isolating, excessively concerned about other people's opinions, ashamed of their shyness and poor performance, and less socially active than did youth reporting lower levels of social anxiety. The parents, however, did not differ in their perceptions of child-rearing styles and family environment for the socially anxious and non-anxious youth.

Johnson et al. (2005) also observed concurrent associations between social anxiety and adolescents' perceptions of parental sociability, shame, and dependency on others opinions, among youth in a large child-adolescent sample (mean age of 13.0 years). However, these perceived parental qualities were even higher for adolescents with depression or comorbid social anxiety and depression.

A further study by Fisak and Mann (2010) examined parental child-rearing practices relative to adolescent-reported social anxiety in a sample of 15- to 18-year-old adolescents. Adolescents with higher levels of social anxiety reported parental modeling of social fears and parental communication of shame to a greater degree than did adolescents with lower levels of social anxiety. The researchers did not, however, find differences between the high and low socially anxious adolescents in their levels of perceived parent sociability, as was found in the three abovementioned studies (Bögels et al. 2001; Caster et al. 1999; Johnson et al. 2005).

Finally, the study by Starr and Davila (2008) differs from the abovementioned studies in that the researchers measured parent-adolescent conflict as an indicator of familial interpersonal dysfunction rather than assessing parental child rearing, modeling, or parental communications; furthermore, they tried to disentangle the effects of depression from that of social anxiety and also assessed peer relationship competence and qualities. Using a sample of adolescent girls with a mean age of 13.5 years, they found that both social anxiety and depression were associated with parent-adolescent conflict and peer relationship competence in bivariate analyses. However, social anxiety was more strongly related to competence, trust, and communication in peer relationships (when controlling for depressive symptoms), whereas depressive symptoms were more strongly related to family variables such as low trust, alienation, and conflict in relationship with parents (when controlling for social anxiety). Comorbidity of social anxiety and depression was associated with both high levels of family conflict and low competence in peer relationships.

In summary, research mostly indicates that prior and concurrent parental overprotection, concurrent low parental sociability, and parental modeling of shame and dependency on others' opinions are associated with heightened social anxiety in adolescents. We found no studies that directly examined whether adolescents whose parents discourage their offspring's autonomous social behavior outside of family, especially in peer relationships, show a heightened risk for social anxiety. However, adolescents' social anxiety is associated with conceptually related parental behaviors (i.e., overprotection, low sociability, and modeling of shame). Thus, socially anxious adolescents' normative developmental transition to wider social contexts may be compromised by familial factors.

The contribution of adolescent-parent conflict or rejection to adolescents' concurrent social anxiety is less supported by research, but such family conflict may be more strongly associated with depression. However, despite the scarce evidence on the direct associations between concurrent family conflict and social anxiety in adolescents, there are two treatment studies which provide some indirect, tentative support that family conflict as assessed by parental expressed emotion (EE) (i.e., criticism, hostility, and emotional overinvolvement) may operate as maintaining factor in adolescent social anxiety. Socially anxious adolescents whose parents show high EE seem to benefit poorly from CBT, but treatment gains are reached when therapy is enhanced by adding parent training targeted at reducing the high EE (Garcia-Lopez et al. 2009, 2014).

In contrast, social anxiety seems to be more effected by the quality of adolescents' peer relationships. More research is needed to specify mechanisms behind observed associations between parental behavior and youths' social anxiety: for example, is overprotection primarily a parental factor that affects offspring, or does social anxiety in the offspring elicit parental overprotection?

Summary and Conclusions

As the literature reviewed in this chapter illustrates, developmental transitions occurring during adolescence have implications for the development or maintenance of social anxiety in youth. Although less often studied, evidence also suggests that socially anxious youth may encounter more difficulties than their less anxious peers during key developmental transitions, especially those involving changes in peer and romantic relationships.

In general, little research has examined the impact of significant school and peer transitions on adolescent social anxiety or how socially anxious adolescents handle social and school transitions. At this point, research has focused mainly on adolescent depression (rather than social anxiety) or on school transitions in the context of community relocation (Goodwin et al. 2012; Vernberg et al. 1992, 2006). Thus, there is a need for future studies to evaluate the interplay between school transitions and adolescent social anxiety. Adolescents who do not negotiate school transitions well, and who are socially anxious, may be at risk for absenteeism and poor academic achievement (e.g., Chalita et al. 2012; Ingul and Nordahl 2013). Future studies that examine the impact of such transitions on socially anxious youth and that evaluate youths' social and emotional functioning before and after significant school transitions would be useful and informative.

With respect to biological transitions, evidence is mixed regarding the associations between pubertal status, pubertal timing, and adolescent social anxiety. However, visible bodily changes (e.g., in height, subcutaneous fat, secondary sex characteristics), which are precipitated by puberty onset and underlying hormonal changes, do appear to contribute to adolescent social anxiety and other related problems, such as eating disorders. At this point, however, we know little about how these biological and physical changes heighten anxiety among adolescents who are already socially anxious. Prospective studies that examine bidirectional pathways between adolescent social anxiety and physical/biological transitions are needed.

Research is also sparse with respect to the interplay between adolescent social anxiety and the onset and course of romantic relationships. Socially anxious adolescents appear to begin dating and to have romantic relationship activities later than nonsocially anxious youth and to have poorer quality relationships. Problems within romantic relationships may also heighten adolescents' feelings of social anxiety, although this hasn't been examined directly.

Finally, in the family realm, little research has directly addressed the impact of increasing adolescent autonomy and decreasing family involvement on adolescent social anxiety. Although it is likely that family factors, such as parental overcontrol and low parental sociability, prepare the adolescent poorly to functioning in wider social contexts, there is a gap in the research addressing the possible impact of family factors and parenting style on adolescents' increasing autonomy and orientation toward social functioning in peer contexts. Most of the research linking family functioning (e.g., child-rearing practices, levels of support or rejection, family conflict, etc.) with anxiety has been conducted with preadolescent youth. To better understand the process of how family transitions affect adolescents' social anxiety over time or how socially anxious youth negotiate family transitions (especially with respect to gaining increased autonomy), multi-wave prospective studies are needed.

Across all the above transitions, it will be important to examine the key moderating variables that influence the associations between the developmental transition and social anxiety. In particular, gender appears to be an important variable to consider. For example, adolescent boys and girls display marked differences in (a) social functioning with peers (e.g., girls have more friends and more positive friendship qualities than boys; La Greca and Harrison 2005); (b) biological transitions (e.g., girls mature earlier than boys and early-maturing girls may experience more emotional difficulties than boys; Blumenthal et al. 2011; Deardorff et al. 2007; Huddleston and Ge 2003); and (c) romantic relationships (e.g., adolescent girls are more likely to date and have more positive qualities in their romantic relationships than boys; Kuttler and La Greca 2004; La Greca and Harrison 2005). Adolescent girls also may report more social anxiety than adolescent boys (La Greca and Lopez 1998; Ingles et al. 2010; Ranta et al. 2012), so the processes linking developmental transitions to social anxiety could potentially differ by gender.

Age is another important moderating variable to examine. The impact of school/peer, biological, romantic, and family transitions may differ depending on adolescent age or developmental status. For example, it would be valuable to evaluate the impact of school and peer transitions in late adolescence (e.g., during the transition to college or work settings) as available studies on school and peer transitions have focused predominantly on early adolescents. Moreover, the emotional impact of initiating or maintaining romantic (and sexual) relationships may be very different during early versus late adolescence (see Davila et al. in press).

Moderating variables that are specific to the area of developmental transition may also be important to evaluate. For example, school and social transitions may be the most anxiety provoking for adolescents who are already experiencing peer difficulties; similarly, family transitions and increasing adolescent autonomy may be most difficult for teens when high levels of parental overprotection or family conflict are present.

Finally, future research would benefit from using multi-wave, prospective research designs. Such methodologies would enable investigators to better evaluate the bidirectional interplay between key developmental transitions and adolescent social anxiety. Efforts of this kind are needed to better inform clinical prevention and intervention efforts to reduce social anxiety in youth.

References

Abma JC, Martinez GM, Mosher WD, Dawson BS (2004) Teenagers in the United States: sexual activity, contraceptive use, and childbearing, 2002. Vital and Health Statistics 23(24). National Center for Health Statistics, Hyattsville

Addo OY, Miller BS, Lee PA, Hediger ML, Himes JH (2014) Age at hormonal onset of puberty based on luteinizing hormone, inhibin B, and body composition in preadolescent US girls. Pediatr Res 76(6):564–570. doi:10.1038/pr.2014.131

Aksglaede L, Olsen LW, Sorensen TI, Juul A (2008) Forty years trends in timing of pubertal growth spurt in 157,000 Danish school children. PLoS One 3:e2728. Published online Jul 16, 2008. doi:10.1371/journal.pone.0002728
Alden LE, Taylor CT (2004) Interpersonal processes in social phobia. Clin Psychol Rev 24:857–882
Aro H, Taipale V (1987) The impact of timing of puberty on psychosomatic symptoms among fourteen- to sixteen-year-old Finnish girls. Child Dev 58:261–268
Attie I, Brooks-Gunn J (1989) Development of eating problems in adolescent girls: a longitudinal study. Dev Psychol 25:70–79
Bellis MA, Downing J, Ashton JR (2006) Adults at 12? Trends in puberty and their public health consequences. J Epidemiol Community Health 60:910–911
Blakemore SJ, Choudhury S (2006) Development of the adolescent brain: implications for executive function and social cognition. J Child Psychol Psychiatry 47:296–312
Blumenthal H, Leen-Feldner EW, Trainor CD, Babson KA, Bunaciu L (2009) Interactive roles of pubertal timing and peer relations in predicting social anxiety symptoms among youth. J Adolesc Health 44:401–403
Blumenthal H, Leen-Feldner EW, Babson KA, Gahr JL, Trainor CD, Frala JL (2011) Elevated social anxiety among early maturing girls. Dev Psychol 47:1133–1140
Bögels SM, Brechman-Toussaint ML (2006) Family issues in child anxiety: attachment, family functioning, parental rearing and beliefs. Clin Psychol Rev 26:834–856
Bögels SM, van Oosten A, Muris P, Smulders D (2001) Familial correlates of social anxiety in children and adolescents. Behav Res Ther 39:273–287
Booth ND (1988) The relationship between height and self-esteem, and the mediating effects of self-consciousness. The University of Arizona, Ann Arbor
Bordini B, Rosenfield RL (2011) Normal pubertal development: Part I: The endocrine basis of puberty. Pediatr Rev 32:223–229
Brook CA, Schmidt LA (2008) Social anxiety disorder: a review of environmental risk factors. Neuropsychiatr Dis Treat 4:123–143
Brown BB (1990) Peer groups and peer cultures. In: Feldman SS, Elliot GR (eds) At the threshold: the developing adolescent. Harvard University Press, Cambridge, MA, pp 171–196
Caglar E, Bilgili N, Karaca A, Ayaz S, Asci FH (2010) The psychological characteristics and health related behavior of adolescents: the possible roles of social physique anxiety and gender. Span J Psychol 13:741–750
Cameron JL (2004) Interrelationships between hormones, behavior, and affect during adolescence: understanding hormonal, physical, and brain changes occurring in association with pubertal activation of the reproductive axis. Introduction to part III. Ann N Y Acad Sci 1021:110–123
Carter R, Jaccard J, Silverman WK, Pina AA (2009) Pubertal timing and its link to behavioral and emotional problems among 'at-risk' African American adolescent girls. J Adolesc 32:467–481
Carver K, Joyner K, Udry JR (2003) National estimates of adolescent romantic relationships. In: Florsheim P (ed) Adolescent romantic relationships and sexual behavior: theory, research, and practical implications. Cambridge University, New York, pp 291–329
Caspi A, Elder GH, Bem DJ (1988) Moving away from the world: life-course patterns of shy children. Dev Psychol 24:824–831
Caster JB, Inderbitzen HM, Hope D (1999) Relationship between youth and parent perceptions of family environment and social anxiety. J Anxiety Disord 13:237–251
Center on International Education Benchmarking (2014a) Japan: instructional systems. http://www.ncee.org/programs-affiliates/center-on-international-education-benchmarking/top-performing-countries/japan-overview/japan-instructional-systems/
Center on International Education Benchmarking (2014b) Finland: instructional systems. Available from: http://www.ncee.org/programs-affiliates/center-on-international-education-benchmarking/top-performing-countries/finland-overview/finland-instructional-systems/
Centers for Disease Control and Prevention (2014) Youth risk behavior surveillance – United States, 2013. MMWR Morb Mortal Wkly Rep 57:SS-4

Chalita PJ, Palacios L, Cortes JF, Landeros-Weisenberger A, Panza KE, Bloch MH (2012) Relationship of Dropout and Psychopathology in a High School Sample in Mexico. Frontiers in Psychiatry 3:20. doi:10.3389/fpsyt.2012.00020
Clark DM, Wells A (1995) A cognitive model of social phobia. In: Heimberg R, Liebowitz M, Hope DA, Schneier FR (eds) Social phobia: diagnosis, assessment and treatment. Guilford Press, New York, pp 69–93
Cole M, Cole SR (2001) The development of children, 4th edn. Worth Publishers, New York
Coleman J (2001) Meeting the health needs of young people. J Epidemiol Community Health 55:532–533
Collins WA (2003) More than myth: the developmental significance of romantic relationships during adolescence. J Res Adolesc 13:1–24
Collins WA, Welsh DP, Furman W (2009) Adolescent romantic relationships. Annu Rev Psychol 60:631–652
Connolly JA, Goldberg A (1999) Romantic relationships in adolescence: the role of friends and peers in their emergence and development. In: Furman W, Brown BB, Feiring C (eds) The development of romantic relationships in adolescence. Cambridge University Press, New York, pp 266–290
Davila J (2008) Depressive symptoms and adolescent romance: theory, research, and implications. Child Dev Perspect 2:26–31
Davila J, Capaldi DM, La Greca AM (in press) Adolescent/young adult romantic relationships and psychopathology. In: Cicchetti D (ed) Developmental psychopathology. Wiley, New York
Deardorff J, Hayward C, Wilson KA, Bryson S, Hammer LD, Agras S (2007) Puberty and gender interact to predict social anxiety symptoms in early adolescence. J Adolesc Health 41:102–104
Detweiler MF, Comer JS, Albano AM (2010) Social anxiety in children and adolescents: biological, developmental, and social considerations. In: Hofmann SG, DiBartolo PM (eds) Social anxiety. Clinical, developmental, and social perspectives, 2nd edn. Elsevier, Burlington, pp 223–270
De Los Reyes A, Prinstein MJ (2004) Applying depression-distortion hypotheses to the assessment of peer victimization in adolescents. J Clin Child Adolesc Psychol 33(2):325–335
Downey G, Bonica C, Rincon C (1999) Rejection sensitivity and adolescent romantic relationships. In: Furman W, Brown BB, Feiring C (eds) The development of romantic relationships in adolescence. Cambridge University Press, New York, pp 148–174
Eklund RC, Bianco T (2000) Social physique anxiety and physical activity among adolescents. Recl Child Youth 9:139–142
Fisak B, Mann A (2010) The relation between parent rearing practices and adolescent social anxiety: a factor analytic approach. Int J Adolesc Youth 15:303–317
Furman W, Rose AJ (2015) Friendships, romantic relationships, and other dyadic peer relationships in childhood and adolescence: a unified relational perspective. In: Lerner R (series ed), Lamb ME, Coll CG (volume eds) The handbook of child psychology and developmental science, 7th edn, vol 3, Social and emotional development. Wiley, Hoboken
Furman W, McDunn C, Young B (2009) The role of peer and romantic relationships in adolescent affective development. In: Allen N, Sheeber L (eds) Adolescent emotional development and the emergence of depressive disorders. Cambridge University Press, New York, pp 299–317
Gar NS, Hudson JL, Rapee RM (2005) Family factors and the development of anxiety disorders. In: Hudson JL, Rapee RM (eds) Psychopathology and the family. Elsevier, Amsterdam, pp 125–145
Garcia-Lopez L-J, Muela JM, Espinosa-Fernandez L, Diaz-Castela M (2009) Exploring the relevance of expressed emotion to the treatment of social anxiety disorder in adolescence. J Adolesc 32:1371–1376
Garcia-Lopez LJ, Irurtia MJ, Caballo VE, Díaz-Castela MM (2011) Ansiedad social y abuso psicológico [Social anxiety and psychological abuse]. Behav Psycholy 19:223–236
Garcia-Lopez L-J, Diaz-Castela M, Muela-Martinez JA, Espinosa-Fernandez L (2014) Can parent training for parents with high levels of expressed emotion have a positive effect on their child's social anxiety improvement? J Anxiety Disord 28:812–822

Ge X, Conger RD, Elder GH Jr (2001a) Pubertal transition, stressful life events, and emergence of gender differences in adolescent depressive symptoms. Dev Psychol 37:404–417

Ge X, Conger RD, Elder GH Jr (2001b) The relation between puberty and psychological distress in adolescent boys. J Res Adolesc 11:49–70

Ge X, Brody GH, Conger RD, Simons RL (2006) Pubertal maturation and African American children's internalizing and externalizing symptoms. J Youth Adolesc 35:531–540

Ginsburg GS, Siqueland L, Masia-Warner C, Hedtke KA (2004) Anxiety disorders in childhood: family matters. Cogn Behav Pract 11:28–43

Glickman AR, La Greca AM (2004) The dating anxiety scale for adolescents: scale development and associations with adolescent functioning. J Clin Child Adolesc Psychol 33:566–578

Goodwin P, McGill B, Chandra A (2009) Who marries and when? Age at first marriage in the United States, 2002, vol 19, NCHS data brief. National Center for Health Statistics, Hyattsville

Goodwin NP, Mrug S, Borch C, Cillessen AH (2012) Peer selection and socialization in adolescent depression: the role of school transitions. J Youth Adolesc 41:320–332

Graber JA (2013) Pubertal timing and the development of psychopathology in adolescence and beyond. Horm Behav 64:262–269

Graber JA, Seeley JR, Brooks-Gunn J, Lewinsohn PM (2004) Is pubertal timing associated with psychopathology in young adulthood. J Am Acad Child Adolesc Psychiatry 43:718–726

Grant KE, Compas BE, Stuhlmacher A, Thurm AE, McMahon S, Halpert J (2003) Stressors and child/adolescent psychopathology: moving from markers to mechanisms of risk. Psychol Bull 129:447–466

Grant K, Compas B, Thurm A, McMahon S, Gipson P (2004) Stressors and child and adolescent psychopathology: measurement issues and prospective effects. J Clin Child Adolesc Psychol 33:412–425

Grello CM, Welsh DP, Harper MS, Dickson JW (2003) Dating and sexual relationship trajectories and adolescent functioning. Adolesc Fam Health 3:103–112

Harter S (1999) The construction of the self: a developmental perspective. Guilford, New York

Hayward C (2003) Methodological concerns in puberty-related research. In: Hayward C (ed) Gender differences at puberty. Cambridge University Press, Cambridge, pp 1–14

Hayward C, Killen JD, Wilson D, Hammer LD, Litt I, Kraemer HC et al (1997) Psychiatric risk associated with early puberty in adolescent girls. J Am Acad Child Adolesc Psychiatry 36:255–262

Hebert KR, Fales J, Nangle DW, Papadakis AA, Grover RL (2013) Linking social anxiety and adolescent romantic relationship functioning: indirect effects and the importance of peers. J Youth Adolesc 42:1708–1720

Heimberg RG, Brozovich FA, Rapee RM (2010) A cognitive behavioral model of social anxiety disorder: update and extension. In: Hofmann SG, DiBartolo PM (eds) Social anxiety. Clinical, developmental, and social perspectives, 2nd edn. Elsevier, Burlington, pp 395–422

Huddleston J, Ge X (2003) Boys at puberty: psychosocial implications. In: Hayward C (ed) Gender differences at puberty. Cambridge University Press, Cambridge, pp 113–134

Ingles CJ, La Greca AM, Marzo JC, Garcia-Lopez LJ, Garcia-Fernandez JM (2010) Social anxiety scale for adolescents: factorial invariance and latent mean differences across gender and age in spanish adolescents. J Anxiety Disord 24:847–855

Ingul JM, Aune T, Nordahl HM (2013) A randomized controlled trial of individual cognitive therapy, group cognitive behaviour therapy and attentional placebo for adolescent social phobia. Psychother Psychosom 83(1):54–61. doi: 10.1159/000354672. Epub 2013 Nov 19

Jaruratanasirikul S, Sriplung H (2014) Secular trends of growth and pubertal maturation of school children in Southern Thailand. Ann Hum Biol 18:1–8

Johnson HS, Inderbitzen-Nolan HM, Schapman AM (2005) A comparison between socially anxious and depressive symptomatology in youth: a focus on perceived family environment. J Anxiety Disord 19:423–442

Jones MC, Bayley N (1971) Physical maturing among boys as related to behavior. In: Jones MC, Bayley N, MacFarlane JW, Honzik MP (eds) The course of human development. Xerox College Publishing, Waltham, pp 252–257

Kaltiala-Heino R, Marttunen M, Rantanen P, Rimpelä M (2003) Early puberty is associated with mental health problems in middle adolescence. Soc Sci Med 57:1055–1064

Keltner D, Capps L, Kring AM, Young RC, Heerey EA (2001) Just teasing: a conceptual analysis and empirical review. Psychol Bull 127:229–248. doi:10.1037//0033-2909.127.2.229

Kessler RC, Berglund P, Chiu WT, Demler O, Heeringa S, Hiripi E, Zheng H (2004) The US national comorbidity survey replication (NCS-R): design and field procedures. Int J Methods Psychiatr Res 13:69–92

Knappe S, Lieb R, Beesdo K, Fehm L, Low NCP, Gloster AT (2009) The role of parental psychopathology and family environment for social phobia in the first three decades of life. Depress Anxiety 26:363–370

Knappe S, Beesdo-Baum K, Wittchen H-U (2010) Familial risk factors in social anxiety disorder: calling for a family-oriented approach for targeted prevention and early intervention. Eur Child Adolesc Psychiatry 19:857–871

Knappe S, Beesdo-Baum K, Fehm L, Lieb R, Wittchen H-U (2012) Characterizing the association between parenting and adolescent social phobia. J Anxiety Disord 26:608–616

Koch PB (1993) Promoting healthy sexual development during early adolescence. In: Lerner R (ed) Early adolescence: perspectives on research, policy, and intervention. Lawrence Erlbaum, Hillsdale, pp 293–307

Kowalski RM (2000) "I was only kidding!": victims' and perpetrators' perceptions of teasing. Pers Soc Psychol Bull 26:231–241

Krowchuk DP, Stancin T, Keskinen R, Walker R, Bass J, Anglin TM (1991) The psychosocial effects of acne on adolescents. Pediatr Dermatol 8:332–338

Kuttler AF, La Greca AM (2004) Adolescents' romantic relationships: do they help or hinder close friendships? J Adolesc 27:395–414

La Greca AM, Harrison HW (2005) Adolescent peer relations, friendships and romantic relationships: do they predict social anxiety and depression? J Clin Child Adolesc Psychol 34: 49–61

La Greca AM, Lopez N (1998) Social anxiety among adolescents: linkages with peer relations and friendships. J Abnorm Child Psychol 26:83–94

La Greca AM, Mackey ER (2007) Adolescents' anxiety in dating situations: do friends and romantic partners contribute? J Clin Child Adolesc Psychol 34:522–533

La Greca AM, Prinstein MJ (1999) Peer group. In: Silverman WK, Ollendick TH (eds) Developmental issues in the clinical treatment of children. Allyn & Bacon, Needham Heights, pp 171–198

La Greca AM, Davila J, Siegel R (2008) Peer relations, friendships, and romantic relationships: implications for the development and maintenance of depression in adolescents. In: Allen NB, Sheeber LB (eds) Adolescent emotional development and the emergence of depressive disorders. Cambridge University Press, New York, pp 318–336

La Greca AM, Davila J, Landoll RR, Siegel R (2011) Dating, romantic relationships and social anxiety in young people. In: Alfano CA, Beidel DC (eds) Social anxiety disorder in adolescents and young adults: translating developmental research into practice. American Psychological Association, Washington, DC

Lampe L, Slade T, Issakidis C, Andrews G (2003) Social phobia in the Australian National Survey of Mental Health and Well-Being (NSMHWB). Psychol Med 33:637–646

Lavell CH, Zimmer-Gembeck MJ, Farrell LJ, Webb H (2014) Victimization, social anxiety, and body dysmorphic concerns: appearance based rejection sensitivity as a mediator. Body Image 11:391–395

Leary MR (2010) Social anxiety as an early warning system: a refinement and extension of the self-presentation theory of social anxiety. In: Hofmann SG, DiBartolo PM (eds) Social anxiety. Clinical, developmental, and social perspectives, 2nd edn. Elsevier, Burlington, pp 471–486

Leary MR, Kowalski RM (1995) The self-presentational model of social phobia. In: Heimberg RG, Liebowitz MR, Hope DA, Schneier FR (eds) Social phobia: diagnosis, assessment, and treatment. Guilford, New York, pp 94–112

Lerner RM, Lerner JV, Hess LE, Schwab J, Jovanovic J, Talwar R et al (1991) Physical attractiveness and psychosocial functioning among early adolescents. J Early Adolesc 11:300–320
Levinson CA, Rodebaugh TL (2011) Validation of the social appearance anxiety scale: factor, convergent, and divergent validity. Assessment 18:350–356
Lewis-Morrarty E, Degnan KA, Chronis-Tuscano A, Rubin KH, Cheah CSL, Pine DS, Henderon HA, Fox NA (2012) Maternal over-control moderates the association between early childhood behavioral inhibition and adolescent social anxiety symptoms. J Abnorm Child Psychol 40:1363–1373
Lieb R, Wittchen H, Höfler M, Fuetsch M, Stein MB, Merikangas KR (2000) Parental psychopathology, parenting styles, and the risk of social phobia in offspring: a prospective-longitudinal community study. Arch Gen Psychiatry 57:859–866
Magin P, Adams J, Heading G, Pond D, Smith W (2008) Experiences of appearance-related teasing and bullying in skin diseases and their psychological sequelae: results of a qualitative study. Scand J Caring Sci 22:430–436. doi:10.1111/j.1471-6712.2007.00547.x
Masia CL, Morris TL (1998) Parental factors associated with social anxiety: methodological limitations and suggestions for integrated behavioral research. Clin Psychol Sci Pract 5:211–228
Mathyssek C (2014) The development of anxiety symptoms in adolescents. University of Rotterdam, Rotterdam
McCabe RE, Antony MM, Summerfeldt LJ, Liss A, Swinson RP (2003) Preliminary examination of the relationship between anxiety disorders in adults and self-reported history of teasing or bullying experiences. Cogn Behav Ther 32:187–193. doi:10.1080/16506070310005051
McCabe RE, Miller JL, Laugesen N, Antony MM, Young L (2010) The relationship between anxiety disorders in adults and recalled childhood teasing. J Anxiety Disord 24:238–243
McLeod BD, Wood JJ, Weisz JR (2007) Examining the association between parenting and childhood anxiety: a meta-analysis. Clin Psychol Rev 27:155–172
Mendle J, Turkheimer E, Emery RE (2007) Detrimental psychological outcomes associated with early pubertal timing in adolescent girls. Dev Rev 27:151–171
Monroe SM, Rohde P, Seeley JR, Lewinsohn PM (1999) Life events and depression in adolescence: relationship loss as a prospective risk factor for first onset of major depressive disorder. J Abnorm Psychol 108:606–614
Natsuaki MN, Klimes-Dougan B, Ge X, Shirtcliff EA, Hastings PD, Zahn-Waxler C (2009) Early pubertal maturation and internalizing problems in adolescence: sex differences in the role of cortisol reactivity to interpersonal stress. J Clin Child Adolesc Psychol 38:513–524
Neufeld KJ, Swartz KL, Bienvenu OJ, Eaton WW, Cai G (1999) Incidence of DIS/DSM-IV social phobia in adults. Acta Psychiatr Scand 100:186–192
Newman BM, Newman PR, Griffen S, O'Connor K, Spas J (2007) The relationship of social support to depressive symptoms during the transition to high school. Adolescence. Fall 42(167):441–59.
Obeid N, Buchholz A, Boerner KE, Henderson KA, Norris M (2013) Self-esteem and social anxiety in an adolescent female eating disorder population: age and diagnostic effects. Eat Disord 21:140–153
Ohannessian CM, Lerner RM, Lerner JV, von Eye A (1999) Does self-competence predict gender differences in adolescent depression and anxiety? J Adolesc 22:397–411
Otto MW, Pollack MH, Maki KM, Gould RA, Worthington JL, Smoller JW, Rosenbaum JF (2001) Childhood history of anxiety disorders among adults with social phobia: rates, correlates, and comparisons with patients with panic disorder. Depress Anxiety 14(209–213):2001
Patton GC, Viner R (2007) Adolescent health: pubertal transitions in health. Lancet 369:1130–1139
Puklek Levpušček M (2006) Adolescent individuation in relation to parents and friends: age and gender differences. Eur J Dev Psychol 3:238–264
Ranta K, Kaltiala-Heino R, Pelkonen M, Marttunen M (2009) Associations between peer victimization, self-reported depression and social phobia among adolescents: the role of comorbidity. J Adolesc 32:77–93

Ranta K, Junttila N, Laakkonen E, Uhmavaara A, La Greca AM, Niemi PM (2012) Social anxiety scale for adolescents (SAS-A): measuring social anxiety among Finnish adolescents. Child Psychiatry Hum Dev 43:574–591

Ranta K, Kaltiala-Heino R, Fröjd S, Marttunen M (2013) Peer victimization and social phobia: a follow-up study among adolescents. Soc Psychiatry Psychiatr Epidemiol 48:533–544

Rapee RM (2012) Family factors in the development and management of anxiety disorders. Clin Child Fam Psychol Rev 15:69–80

Rapee RM, Heimberg RG (1997) A cognitive-behavioral model of anxiety in social phobia. Behav Res Ther 35:741–756

Rapee RM, Spence SH (2004) The etiology of social phobia: empirical evidence and an initial model. Clin Psychol Rev 24:737–767

Reardon LE, Leen-Feldner EW, Hayward C (2009) A critical review of the empirical literature on the relation between anxiety and puberty. Clin Psychol Rev 29:1–23

Rork KE, Morris TL (2009) Influence of parenting factors on childhood social anxiety: direct observation of parental warmth and control. Child Fam Behav Ther 31:220–235. doi:10.1080/07317100903099274

Rosellini AJ, Rutter LA, Bourgeois ML, Emmert-Aronson BO, Brown TA (2013) The relevance of age of onset to the psychopathology of social phobia. J Psychopathol Behav Assess 35:356–365

Savin-Williams RC (1994) Dating those you can't love and loving those you can't date. In: Montemayor R, Adams GR, Gullatta TP (eds) Advances in adolescent development personal relationships during adolescence, vol 6. Sage, Thousand Oaks, pp 168–195

Seiffge-Krenke I, Lang J (2002) Forming and maintaining romantic relations from early adolescence to young adulthood: evidence of a developmental sequence. In: Shulman S, Seiffge-Krenke I (co-chairs) Antecedents of the quality and stability of adolescent romantic relationships. Symposium at the conference of the Society for Research on adolescence, New Orleans

Shapiro JP, Baumeister RF, Kessler JW (1991) A three-component model of children's teasing: aggression, humor, and ambiguity. J Soc Clin Psychol 10:459–472. doi:10.1521/jscp.1991.10.4.459

Shulman S, Scharf M (2000) Adolescent romantic behaviors and perceptions: age- and gender-related differences, and links with family and peer relationships. J Res Adolesc 10:99–118

Siegel R, La Greca AM, Harrison HM (2009) Peer victimization and social anxiety in adolescents: prospective and reciprocal relationships. J Youth Adolesc 38:1096–1109

Skinner SR, Smith J, Fenwick J, Fyfe S, Hendriks J (2008) Perceptions and experiences of first sexual intercourse in Australian adolescent females. J Adolesc Health 43:593–599

Sparrevohn RM, Rapee RM (2009) Self-disclosure, emotional expression and intimacy within romantic relationships of people with social phobia. Behav Res Ther 47:1074–1078

Starr LR, Davila J (2008) Differentiating interpersonal correlates of depressive symptoms and social anxiety in adolescence: implications for models of comorbidity. J Clin Child Adolesc Psychol 37:337–349

Stein MB, Chavira DA, Jang KL (2001) Bringing up bashful baby: developmental pathways to social phobia. Psychiatr Clin North Am 24:661–675

Steinberg L, Morris AS (2001) Adolescent development. Annu Rev Psychol 52:83–110

Storch EA, Masia-Warner C (2004) The relationship of peer victimization to social anxiety and loneliness in adolescent females. J Adolesc 27:351–362

Strawser MA, Storch EA, Roberti JW (2005) The teasing questionnaire–revised: measurement of childhood teasing in adults. J Anxiety Disord 19:780–792

Tanner JM (1962) Growth at adolescence: with a general consideration of the effects of hereditary and environmental factors upon growth and maturation from birth to maturity. Blackwell Scientific Publications, Oxford

Thompson KM (1999) The role of social anxiety in the sexual involvement of ethnically diverse adolescents with chronic medical conditions. Dissertations from ProQuest. Paper 3740. http://scholarlyrepository.miami.edu/dissertations/3740

van der Bruggen CO, Stams GJ, Bögels SM (2008) Research review: the relation between child and parent anxiety and parental control: a meta-analytic review. J Child Psychol Psychiatry 49:1257–1269. doi:10.1111/j.1469-7610.2008.01898.x
Veale D (2003) Treatment of social phobia. Adv Psychiatr Treat 9:258–264
Vernberg EM (1990a) Psychological adjustment and experiences with peers during early adolescence: reciprocal, incidental, or unidirectional relationships? J Abnorm Child Psychol 18:187–198
Vernberg EM (1990b) Experiences with peers following relocation during early adolescence. Am J Orthopsychiatry 60:466–472
Vernberg EM, Randall CJ (1997) Homesickness after relocation during early adolescence. In: Van Tilburg M, Vingerhoets A (eds) Home is where the heart is: the psychological aspects of permanent and temporary geographical moves. Tilburg University Press, Tilburg, pp 165–180
Vernberg EM, Abwender DA, Ewell KK, Beery SH (1992) Social anxiety and peer relationships in early adolescence: a prospective analysis. J Clin Child Psychol 21:189–196
Vernberg EM, Greenhoot AF, Biggs BK (2006) Intercommunity relocation and adolescent friendships: who struggles and why? J Consult Clin Psychol 74:511–523
Weingarden H, Renshaw KD (2012) Early and late perceived pubertal timing as risk factors for anxiety disorders in adult women. J Psychiatr Res 46:1524–1529
Welsh DP, Haugen PT, Widman L, Darling N, Grello CM (2005) Kissing is good: a developmental investigation of sexuality in adolescent romantic couples. Sex Res Soc Policy 2(4):32–41
Wenzel A, Graff-Dolezal J, Macho M, Brendle JR (2005) Communication and social skills in socially anxious and nonanxious individuals in the contest of romantic relationships. Behav Res Ther 43:505–519
Wittchen HU, Fuetsch M, Sonntag H, Muller N, Liebowitz M (2000) Disability and quality of life in pure and comorbid social phobia: findings from a controlled study. Eur Psychiatry 15:46–58
Wood JJ, McLeod BD, Sigman M, Hwang W, Chu BC (2003) Parenting and childhood anxiety: theory, empirical findings, and future directions. J Child Psychol Psychiatry 44:134–151
Yap MB, Pilkington PD, Ryan SM, Jorm AF (2014) Parental factors associated with depression and anxiety in young people: a systematic review and meta-analysis. J Affect Disord 156:8–23
Yoo JJ, Johnson KK (2008) Self-objectification and appearance-based teasing during adolescence. J Fam Cons Sci Educ 26:14–28

Part II

Recognition and Manifestations of Adolescent Social Anxiety and Phobia in Diverse Settings

Assessment of Social Anxiety in Adolescents

6

Luis-Joaquin Garcia-Lopez, Maria do Ceu Salvador, and Andres De Los Reyes

Introduction

Effective treatment of social anxiety disorder (SAD) and clinical research in this area require a thorough assessment, using reliable and valid assessment instruments (Tulbure et al. 2012). The appropriate and effective assessment of SAD in adolescence involves a multilevel, multi-procedure, and multi-informant process, which captures the essence of the disorder as well as other personal and family characteristics and functioning (Silverman and Ollendick 2005). In addition, the need for shortened versions of self-report measures has increased in recent years as a result of the increased importance of mental health screening by primary health-care providers, school counselors, and psychologists (Garcia-Lopez et al. 2008c). Having a screening protocol would help the scientific community to increase the awareness and detection of SAD in adolescents, particularly if the protocol was brief, valid, and reliable and demonstrated appropriate sensitivity and specificity.

In this chapter, we review clinical assessment procedures for SAD in adolescents and provide suggestions to conduct a thorough and psychometrically sensitive assessment. The chapter begins with a review of clinician assessment methods, followed by self-report measures. Next, we discuss multi-informant and

L.-J. Garcia-Lopez, PhD (✉)
Department of Psychology, University of Jaen, Jaen, Spain (Europe)
e-mail: ljgarlo@cop.es; ljgarcia@ujaen.es

M. do Ceu Salvador, PhD
Department of Psychology, University of Coimbra, Coimbra, Portugal (Europe)

A. De Los Reyes, PhD
Department of Psychology, University of Maryland at College Park, College Park, MD, USA

K. Ranta et al. (eds.), *Social Anxiety and Phobia in Adolescents: Development, Manifestation and Intervention Strategies*, DOI 10.1007/978-3-319-16703-9_6

context-sensitive clinical assessment, physiological assessment methods, and observational and role-play procedures. Finally, we present some issues regarding the future of assessment of social anxiety in adolescents.

Clinician Assessment

Clinician assessment consists of clinical interviews, ratings of adolescent social anxiety, and general ratings of overall functioning. We briefly present each type of measure in the following sections.

Clinician-Administered Interviews

General Clinical Interviews

Clinical interviews, either structured or more general in nature, are one of the most important sources of information gathering. Although a structured interview may be preferred to establish a reliable diagnosis, general interviews will cover other topics pertinent to adolescent SAD. Important topics include: physiological, cognitive, and behavioral symptoms of SAD; impact of the symptomatology on everyday life; information to rule out other diagnoses or to establish comorbid disorders; life stressors; coping skills; level of functioning in important areas (school, family, hobbies, etc.); etiological factors; maintenance factors; developmental history; the adolescent's and family's health status; and the family and cultural context (Kearney 2005).

Despite the fact that developing good rapport is an important requisite in assessment, this is particularly true with adolescents with SAD (Garcia-Lopez 2013). On one hand, adolescents may not be aware of social distress and difficulties that are associated with the disorder. They may view the condition as part of who they are, adapt their lifestyle to accommodate avoidance of social and/or performance situations in a way that camouflages their distress, and rationalize this avoidance. For all these reasons, adolescents with SAD tend to report fewer social anxiety symptoms relative to other informants (e.g., parents; see De Los Reyes et al. 2012). Furthermore, identification of social anxiety by parents and teachers is often difficult (see section "Multi-informant and context-sensitive clinical assessment" of this chapter), at least until underachievement or school refusal is identified. Lack of identification of SAD by parents is critical as especially younger adolescents depend on their parents to be taken to therapy. Finally, the very nature of SAD may interfere with the therapeutic relationship (and therefore with the assessment process). For example, adolescents may be afraid of being negatively evaluated by the therapist or interviewer (i.e., they may think that their problems are unique and that they must be weird to have them) and are vigilant for signs of disapproval. The attitude of the clinician, particularly in the first meeting, is therefore critical. The clinician's task will be to create a warm, uncritical, and understanding atmosphere, where the adolescent feels comfortable discussing his/her fears and worries.

Several strategies may be used to establish a good rapport in an initial session with an adolescent with SAD (Herbert et al. 2010). One consists of the clinician talking first about some general topic and asking the adolescent some general questions (e.g., age, school, friends, hobbies). This will break the ice and give the adolescent time to feel more at ease and comfortable in the therapy room. Also extremely important is that the clinician avoids any signs of disapproval throughout the interview. Finally, the interviewer should provide normalizing psychoeducation, emphasizing how common the adolescent's social or performance problems are, acknowledging that they must be difficult to handle sometimes, and clearly stating that there are effective treatments for such a condition. Usually, the pace of the interview will be slower, and the interview may take longer than with adolescents exhibiting other primary concerns (e.g., depression, generalized anxiety disorder).

Structured and Semistructured Interviews

Structured and semistructured interviews are important tools that guide the clinician through the diagnostic decision-making process, leading to more reliable diagnoses. Additionally, they not only allow the categorical assessment of disorders but also the evaluation of the severity, impairment, and course of disorders. Diagnostic interviews also have the advantage of being open to evaluation of their psychometric properties and decreasing the variability inherent in clinical judgment. However, they are not without limitations. Three of the most important limitations of diagnostic interviews are that almost all require significant training to administer reliably, may be time consuming due to their length, and may be difficult to score (e.g., Beidel and Turner 2007).

There are several well-established structured and semistructured interview schedules based on DSM criteria that include an assessment of adolescents' social fears and that are used to collect information about symptomatology and additional diagnoses. Before describing the most common interviews, we would like to emphasize that the adolescent may view the interview situation as artificial and uncomfortable. For example, adolescents may answer "no" to the interview questions, particularly if they realize that this will lead to the interviewer skipping several pages (i.e., due to "skip out" rules linked to diagnostic criteria). To counteract this tendency, the clinician should ensure that a good rapport is established prior to the interview, the interview is not approached as an interrogation, and the interview begins with an informal conversation about school, friends, and hobbies. Furthermore, suggesting a break during the interview can also improve the adolescent's cooperation (Beidel and Turner 2007).

The *Anxiety Disorders Interview Schedule for DSM-5: Child and Parent Versions* (ADIS-5-C/P; Albano and Silverman 2014) is the most widely used interview to assess anxiety disorders in youth 6–17 years, is derived from the adult ADIS (Brown and Barlow 2013), and is organized according to anxiety disorders in the Diagnostic and Statistical Manual of Mental Disorders (5th ed. [DSM-5]; American Psychiatric Association, 2013). The ADIS-5-C/P consists of comparable but separate parent and child interviews and offers a comprehensive assessment for an adolescent with SAD. Although designed specifically to diagnose anxiety disorders, the ADIS-5-C also assesses affective disorders and attention-deficit/hyperactivity disorder (ADHD). Additionally, it includes screening questions for a range of other disorders (substance abuse, schizophrenia, eating disorders, somatoform disorders). It also includes questions about school and the ways that youth connect with others (including texting and social media) that are relevant for an adolescent with SAD. The parent version (ADIS-5-P) includes the additional diagnostic categories of conduct disorder and oppositional defiant disorder, as well as screening questions for several other disorders, including enuresis, pervasive developmental disorders, and learning disorders. For each diagnosis, there are several questions to assess specific symptoms (on a 3-point scale, "yes," "no," and "other," or in a 9-point scale, "not at all" to "very, very much"). There are also questions to assess the disorder's duration and interference in everyday life, using a 9-point Likert-type scale; in order to be coded as a final diagnosis, a rating of at least 4 (moderate impairment) must be given by the adolescent or the parent.

All these criteria combined allow confirming or excluding a diagnosis. To derive a combined diagnosis from child and parent reports, a diagnosis is assigned if either one or the other indicates the presence of the disorder. At the end of the interview, a composite profile of diagnoses resulting from the information of the interviews is obtained, and each diagnosis is associated with a clinician severity rating (CSR) (from 0 to 8). These ratings are used to classify the diagnoses as principal (the most impairing one), coprincipal (other diagnoses that may share the same highest clinician severity rating), or additional (any other diagnosis with a lower severity rating). This classification is used to prioritize the disorder that causes greatest distress and impairment and that may be addressed first in treatment. The SAD section includes a list of situations that have to be rated according to the degree of anxiety and avoidance it provokes.

Administration of the whole interview, either the child or parent version, usually takes longer (about 60–120 min in total) than a typical clinical session (March and Albano 2002). However, if time is limited and a particular case involves assessing the presence of SAD (or performance anxiety), the clinician may decide to administer only the SAD section (or other relevant sections) to obtain important information about the problem and its interference (Kearney 2005).

The ADIS-IV-C/P (Silverman and Albano 1996) has demonstrated excellent test–retest reliability, excellent reliability for deriving combined diagnosis of separation anxiety disorder, SAD, specific phobia, and generalized anxiety disorder, and is highly reliable for deriving the same diagnoses with either child or parent information (Silverman et al. 2001). Its concurrent validity has also been established, particularly for the SAD, separation anxiety disorder, and panic disorder (Wood et al. 2002). Another study (Lyneham et al. 2007) explored interrater agreement, indicating that the ADIS-IV-C/P provided consistent diagnostic results across different clinicians.

Another commonly used interview is the *Schedule for Affective Disorders and Schizophrenia for School Age Children-Present and Lifetime Version* (K-SADS-PL; Kaufman et al. 1997). The K-SADS was designed to assess present and past episodes of 33 mental disorders and their interference (either in a paper and pencil format or using a computerized version) according to the DSM-IV (APA 1994). Three DSM-IV compatible versions of the K-SADS are in general use, all providing a current diagnostic assessment: one present state (K-SADS-P IVR) and two epidemiological editions (the K-SADS-E (Epidemiological Version) and the K-SADS-PL (Present and Lifetime Version)). The K-SADS-P IVR also evaluates the worst past episode during the previous year, while the K-SADS-E and the K-SADS-PL provide a lifetime diagnosis. Furthermore, the K-SADS-E and the K-SADS PL are primarily categorical diagnostic interviews; however, the K-SADS-P IVR also measures symptom severity, thus allowing its use to monitor treatment response (for more details, see Ambrosini 2000). All versions of this interview are semistructured integrated parent–child interviews where the clinician records data from parents and youth on a common answer sheet. Diagnoses are assigned by synthesizing parent and child data (Kaufman 1997).

The K-SADS demonstrated good concurrent validity, good to excellent test–retest reliability for present and lifetime diagnoses, and high interrater agreement in a sample of children, adolescents, and their parents (Kaufman 1997). Reviewing the various past and current K-SADS editions and respective literature, Ambrosini (2000) concluded that all editions had good interrater reliability, noting, nevertheless, that the quality of the validating data was limited.

The *Structured Clinical Interview for DSM-IV Childhood Diagnoses* (KID-SCID; Hien et al. 1994) is a semistructured interview to assess childhood DSM-IV diagnoses, based on the Structured Clinical Interview for DSM-IV for adults (First et al. 1994). Its structure consists of questions for each DSM-IV criterion, and the interviewer rates the presence of each criterion using a three-point rating scale (absent, possibly present, or present). Both child and parent(s) provide answers that the interviewer combines to rate a "best" score. Next, the number of symptoms rated as "present" is counted, and if the required number of symptoms according DSM-IV symptom-criterion is met, the interviewer asks about other DSM criteria, such as age of onset and interference. Finally, a KID-SCID diagnosis is obtained if all DSM-IV criteria are met. Several studies support the validity of the KID-SCID (Matzner 1994; Matzner et al. 1997; Smith et al. 2005; Trimbremont et al. 2004). Additionally, two studies reported very good interrater reliability (Hien et al. 1994; Trimbremont et al. 2004) and another study (Matzner et al. 1997) showed fair to excellent test–retest reliability.

The *Diagnostic Interview for Children and Adolescents* (DICA; Reich 1998) is another widely used diagnostic interview for children and adolescents under 18 years. The DICA has a child version (DICA-C) for children aged 8–12 years, an adolescent version (DICA-A; 13–17 years), and a parent version that contains the same categories as the child and adolescent versions with the addition of two categories to solicit information on prenatal health (pregnancy/birth) and early child development. The DICA-IV offers a screening for a broad range of clinical symptoms and it also includes the Stein-Reich critical items listing. These items identify high-risk features that can alert the clinician for dangerous behavior (e.g., suicidal thoughts and behavior, drug abuse). The DICA has been computerized, allowing both an interviewer-administrated and a self-administrated version (Reich et al.

1997). Weldner et al. (1987) reported high reliability and high interrater agreement between DICA-C diagnoses and clinician's diagnoses and moderate to good parent–child agreement for most diagnoses. After reviewing administration procedures, psychometric properties, and comparisons with other measures, Reich (2000) concluded that this interview had good reliability and could serve as a valid tool for assessing psychiatric information in children and adolescents. Sala et al. (2005) have applied factor analysis to the DICA-IV responses provided by a sample of Spanish children/adolescents and parents and obtained a two-dimensional model (internalizing–externalizing) with good internal consistency and validity. These authors concluded that the DICA-IV could be used to obtain both categorical and dimensional indicators.

The *Diagnostic Interview Schedule for Children Version IV* (DISC-IV; Shaffer et al. 2000) is a highly structured diagnostic interview that consists of a series of close-ended questions to evaluate more than 30 psychiatric disorders in children and adolescents. The DISC-IV also collects information about several aspects of school functioning as well as information about the child/adolescent relationships with family, peers, and teachers. It has a version for children or adolescents (DISC-Y; from 9 to 17 years), a version for parents (DISC-P; from 6 to 17 years), and a version for teachers (DISC-T); the teacher version is limited to disorders whose symptoms might be expected to be observed in a school setting (e.g., disruptive disorders). The DISC-IV assesses the presence of diagnoses in three different moments in time: the previous 4 weeks, the previous year, and "whole life." Its format and structure (either in paper and pencil or computer format) allows the DISC-IV to be administered by lay interviewers after a minimal training period. Previous versions of the DISC have shown moderate to good criterion validity across a number of diagnoses (Schwab-Stone et al. 1996), moderate to substantial test–retest reliability (Jensen et al. 1995), and good reliability and acceptability (Shaffer et al. 1996). However, Lewczyk et al. (2003) reported that, compared to clinician diagnosis, the DISC-IV had a significantly higher prevalence of ADHD, disruptive behavior disorders, and anxiety disorders and a significantly lower prevalence of mood disorders.

The *Child and Adolescent Psychiatric Assessment* (CAPA; Angold and Costello 2000) is a structured interview for use with children/adolescents (ages 9–17) and their parents. The CAPA includes several sections: psychiatric symptoms, functional impairment, demographics, and family structure and dynamics. Included in this interview are three sections that specifically assess social fears: shyness with peers, social anxiety in interaction contexts, and fears of activities in public. The CAPA also has a glossary providing operationalized symptom definitions and application rules. The time frame is the three previous months, but duration of symptoms is in line with diagnostic frameworks. Results from the study of Angold and Costello (2000) confirmed the CAPA's test–retest reliability and validity.

The Mini International Neuropsychiatric Interview for Children and Adolescents (MINI-KID; Sheehan et al. 1998) is a short structured clinical diagnostic interview designed to assess the presence of psychiatric disorders according to DSM-IV and ICD-10 criteria. The MINI-KID was based on the adult version of the interview (MINI; Lecrubier et al. 1997; Sheehan et al. 1997, 1998) and is intended to be used with children and adolescents aged 6–17 years without mental retardation. It is organized in diagnostic modules with screening questions for each disorder that, if they are endorsed, will be followed by additional symptoms questions. Twenty-four disorders are screened, excluding organic mental disorders and specific learning disabilities. Current and lifetime suicide risk is additionally screened. Sheehan and collaborators (2010) found that the MINI-KID presented substantial to excellent agreement to the K-SADS-PL (Kaufman et al. 1997) on every disorder, except psychotic disorder, where results were more modest. The same authors reported substantial sensitivity, excellent specificity, and almost perfect interrater agreement and test–retest reliability. Also, the concordance of the parent version (MINI-KID-P) with the standard MINI-KID was good. Finally, the MINI-KID took a third of the time to be administered compared to the K-SADS.

Clinician-Administered Scales

In addition to clinical interviews, clinician-administered measures include scales for social anxiety assessment, scales that assess anxiety and include a section for social anxiety, and ratings of the overall level of adolescent functioning.

Clinician-Administered Social Anxiety Scales

There are two clinician-administered measures to specifically assess social anxiety in children and adolescents, which are described below.

The *Liebowitz Social Anxiety Scale for Children and Adolescents* (LSAS-CA; Masia-Warner et al. 2003), based on its adult version (Liebowitz 1987), is a 24-item clinician-administered rating scale that assesses youths' anxiety and avoidance for both social and performance situations. Twelve items describe interaction situations and the other 12 describe performance situations. For each item, the clinician asks for a separate rating for anxiety and avoidance, using a 0–3 Likert scale, but these ratings may also be adjusted based on clinical judgment, further inquiry, and behavioral observation of the youth. Items are then summed in two subscales assessing social interactions and performance situations. Six scores may be obtained: total anxiety, social anxiety, performance anxiety, total avoidance, social avoidance, and performance avoidance. Masia-Warner et al. (2003) reported high internal consistency (both for the full sample and for a SAD group), high test–retest reliability (for the total and subscales), stronger positive associations with measures of social anxiety and general impairment than with a measure of depression, and sensitivity to discriminate youth with SAD from youth with other anxiety disorder and from healthy controls. However, factor analysis of the LSAS-CA indicated that anxiety and avoidance ratings were better explained by a two-factor solution that measures social anxiety and avoidance in social or school performance situations (Storch et al. 2006). These two factors—social and school performance—obtained high internal consistency and acceptable validity (Storch et al. 2006). The LSAS-CA has been used in several treatment studies and has demonstrated sensitivity to treatment effects (Masia-Warner et al. 2005; Wagner et al. 2004). It has also been useful as a self-report measure (see "Social anxiety measures specifically designed for adolescents" section of this chapter).

The *Kutcher Generalized SAD Scale for Adolescents* (K-GSADS-A; Brooks and Kutcher 2004) is a clinician-rated scale designed to assess the severity of SAD and to measure treatment outcome in adolescents (i.e., monitoring the severity of symptoms over time). The K-GSADS-A is divided in three sections, each reflecting different aspects of SAD. Section A includes 18 items related to fear and avoidance of social situations, each rated on two 4-point scales (i.e., from "none" to "severe" on anxiety and from "none" to "total" on avoidance.) Section B asks the adolescent to choose the three most feared social situations and then rate them using the same 4-point system; these three items will be rerated on repeated administrations of the K-GSADS-A. Section C includes 11 items that describe affective distress and somatic distress symptoms, rated from 0 ("never") to 3 ("severe") according to how strongly each symptom occurs in most social situations. This section allows the evaluation of whether a particular treatment has differential effects on affective and somatic symptoms (Brooks and Kutcher 2004). Four subscales can then be calculated: fear and anxiety (the sum of section A's discomfort ratings), avoidance (the sum of section A's avoidance items), affective distress (the sum of section C's affective items), and somatic distress (the sum of Section C's somatic items). Finally, the sum of these four subscales comprises the K-GSADS-A Total Score. Brooks and Kutcher (2004) explored and supported the scale's internal consistency, test–retest reliability, and convergent and divergent validity. The K-GSADS-A's sensitivity to treatment outcomes has also been established (Brooks and Kutcher 2004; Wagner et al. 2004).

Ratings of Global Level of Functioning

Finally, global clinician ratings are useful measures of the youth's overall level of functioning or of his/her treatment progress. These instruments are applicable across all psychiatric disorders and treatments and were designed for easy use. If the clinician has enough information available, the measures only take a few minutes to complete. Two of these instruments are briefly reviewed.

The *Clinical Global Impression Scale* (CGI; Guy 1976) was developed to provide a brief, stand-alone assessment of the clinician's view of the individual's global functioning prior to and after treatment, taking into account all available information on the person's history, psychosocial circumstances, symptoms, behavior, and interference (Busner and Targum 2007). The CGI consists of two subscales, rated in a 7-point scale: Severity of Illness (CGI-S), which rates illness severity (ranging from 1 = "normal not at all ill" to 7 = "among the most extremely ill patients"), and Global Improvement (CGI-I), which assesses improvement relative to treatment baseline (ranging from 1 = "very much improved since the initiation of treatment" to 7 = "very much worse since the initiation of treatment"). The CGI has been shown to correlate with other well-known treatment efficacy scales across a wide range of psychiatric disorders in adults, including SAD (Bandelow et al. 2006; Zaider et al. 2003). The CGI has also demonstrated sensitivity to treatment effects in children and adolescents with SAD (Compton et al. 2001).

The *Children's Global Assessment Scale* (CGAS; Shaffer et al. 1983) is an adaptation from the Global Assessment Scale for Adults (GAS; Endicott et al. 1976). It contains numeric scale (from 1 = most impaired to 100 = least impaired) to assess overall functioning during the previous month for children under the age of 18 years. It is easy to use and it takes only a few minutes to complete. Shaffer et al. (1983) found the CGAS to be reliable between raters and across time and also reported concurrent and discriminant validity. The psychometric characteristics of the CGAS are well documented, its utility is well established in nationwide clinical settings, and it has been used in treatment outcome studies of childhood psychopathology (see Schorre and Vandvik 2004 for a review).

Self-Report Measures

Scales Designed or Adapted to Measure Social Anxiety in Adolescents

Social Anxiety Measures Specifically Designed for Adolescents

The *Social Anxiety Scale for Children-Revised* (SASC-R; La Greca and Stone 1993; La Greca 1999) was designed to assess levels of social anxiety in children aged 7–13 years (elementary school). The SASC-R contains 18 items (plus 4 filler items) and evaluates three aspects of social anxiety: Fear of Negative Evaluation from Peers (FNE = 8 items), Social Avoidance and Distress specific to new situations or unfamiliar peers (SAD-New = 6 items), and Generalized Social Avoidance and Distress (SAD-General = 4 items). Items are rated on a 5-point Likert scale and summed across relevant items to obtain total SASC-R scores and scores for each of the three subscales. The total score can range from 18 to 90. In addition to the findings of La Greca and colleagues, good psychometric properties have been found in Finnish, Dominican, Puerto Rican, Portuguese, Japanese, Spanish, US, and Norwegian children (e.g., Kristensen and Torgersen 2006; Kuusikko et al. 2009; Martins et al. 2014; Okajima et al. 2009; Reijntjes et al. 2007; Sandin et al. 1999; Storch et al. 2003).

The *Social Anxiety Scale for Adolescents* (SAS-A; La Greca and Lopez 1998) was adapted from the SASC-R to assess adolescents' levels of social anxiety. The SAS-A is suitable for adolescents ages 13–18 years (middle and high school). As with the SASC-R, the SAS-A contains 22 items (including 4 filler items) and evaluates FNE (range: 8–40), SAD-New (range: 6–30), and SAD-General (range: 4–20). A total score can also be computed (range: 18–90). The rating scale for each item ranges from 1 (never) to 5 (always). In line with the original study, research carried out by Inderbitzen-Nolan and Walters (2000) and Myers et al. (2002) confirmed the three-factor structure in US adolescents. Similarly, studies in countries such as Finland, Turkey, Spain, Portugal, China, Japan, and Latin America have reported excellent psychometric properties for this measure of social anxiety in adolescents (Aydin and Sütcü 2007; Cunha et al. 2004; Garcia-Lopez et al. 2005, 2009, 2014b; Jimenez-Lopez et al. 2013; La Greca et al. (in press); Okajima et al.

2009; Olivares et al. 2005; Ranta et al. 2012a). In addition, Olivares et al. (2002) suggested a cutoff score of 44, rather than the score of 50 proposed by the original authors. Furthermore, Ingles et al. (2010) and La Greca et al. (2014) have found factorial invariance for the scale.

Social Phobia and Anxiety Inventory for Children (SPAI-C; Beidel et al. 1995). The SPAI-C evaluates the somatic, cognitive, and behavioral aspects of social anxiety in children between the ages of 8 and 14. The SPAI-C consists of 26 items with a 3-point (0–2) Likert rating format. The scale has been used in Brazil, Norway, Finland, Spain, Italy, and the USA (Aune et al. 2008; Beidel et al. 2000a, b; Gauer et al. 2005; Inderbitzen-Nolan et al. 2004; Kuusikko et al. 2009; Ogliari et al. 2012; Olivares et al. 2010; Storch et al. 2004). Kuusikko et al. (2009) recommended a cutoff score of 18 for a Finnish adolescent population. A meta-analysis conducted by Scaini et al. (2012) found that SPAI-C presents with good cross-cultural validity.

The *Liebowitz Social Anxiety Scale for Children and Adolescents* (LSAS-CA; Masia et al. 1999) is based on the adult version (LSAS; Liebowitz 1987). The LSAS-CA is a 24-item scale with a 4-point (0–3) Likert rating format, designed for children over the age of 7 years. This measure rates the following: total fear, fear of social interaction, fear of performance, total avoidance, avoidance of social interaction, and avoidance of performance. Although it was originally conceptualized as a clinician-administered scale (see section "Clinician-administered social anxiety scales"), a self-report version (LSAS-CA_SR) has been developed, with appropriate psychometric properties for French- and Spanish-speaking adolescents (Olivares et al. 2009; Schmits et al. 2014).

Social Anxiety Questionnaire for Children (SAQ-C; Caballo et al. 2012) assesses social anxiety in children between the ages of 9 and 14 years. It consists of 24 items grouped into six factors or dimensions (4 items for factor): (1) speaking in public/interactions with teachers, (2) interactions with strangers, (3) interactions with the opposite sex, (4) criticism and embarrassment, (5) assertive expression of annoyance or disgust, and (6) performing in public. Each item is answered on a 4-point Likert scale to indicate how much the child feels afraid, embarrassed, or nervous in response to each social situation: 1 (none), 2 (a little), 3 (quite a lot), and 4 (a lot). Available psychometric properties are limited to the study published by authors.

Escala para la Detección de Ansiedad Social (EDAS; *Social Anxiety Screening Scale*, SASS; Olivares and Garcia Lopez 1998; Olivares & Piqueras, 2005). This measure consists of 10 items: 2 are dichotomous and the remaining 8 have three-independent-factor structure (avoidance, distress, and interference). Validation of the scale is limited to Hispanic populations (Olivares & Piqueras, 2005; Olivares et al. 2004b; Piqueras et al. 2011, 2012b, c; Vera-Villarroel et al. 2007).

Social Anxiety and Avoidance Scale for Adolescents (SAASA; Cunha et al. 2008; Salvador, 2009). The primary aims of this instrument are: (1) to identify possible dimensions of social fears in a specific developmental context; (2) to serve as an assessment measure for adolescents at risk for developing SAD; (3) to be a helpful tool in the clinical assessment of adolescents with SAD, identifying the intensity and frequency of anxiety and avoidance responses to feared situations; and (4) to be a useful instrument for tailoring an intervention and assessing its outcome. The scale consists of 34 items, with each item score ranging from 1 to 5. The total score for each of the SAASA subscales (the distress/anxiety subscale and the avoidance subscale) varies between 34 and 170. A total score may also be obtained by calculating the mean of the two subscales.

Social Anxiety Scale for Adolescents (SASA; Puklek 1997a, b). The SASA was developed in Slovenia to measure anxiety in social situations that typically evoke uneasiness, worry, and avoidant behavior in adolescents. The work conducted by Puklek and colleagues (Puklek Levpuscek 2004; Puklek and Vidmar 2000) revealed that Watson and Friend's (1969) two components of social anxiety were also evident in Slovene adolescents. Specifically, the SASA has 28 items (Likert range: 1–5) and a two-factor structure: (a) Apprehension and Fear of Negative Evaluation (AFNE), consisting of 15 items that assess the adolescent's fears, worries, and anticipations of possible negative evaluation by their peers and audience, and (b) Tension and Inhibition in Social Contact (TISC), consisting of 13 items that assess social tension/relaxation, speech or behavior inhibition, and readiness to exposure in social interactions. Further papers have confirmed the psychometric properties of the scale in Slovenia (Puklek Levpuščček and Videc 2008). This scale also has the same factor structure and test–retest reliability in Spanish adolescents (Garcia-Lopez et al. 2011b).

Social Anxiety Measures Adapted for Adolescents

Fear of Negative Evaluation (FNE) and Social Avoidance and Distress Scale (SAD). Watson and Friend (1969) developed these scales to measure social-evaluative anxiety and social anxiety/distress and avoidance of social situations among college students prior to the DSM-III recognition of social phobia or SAD as a diagnostic entity. The FNE is a 30-item scale and the SAD is a 28-item scale, both of which employ a true–false format. Studies have demonstrated the reliability and validity of the scales in a Spanish-speaking adolescent sample (Garcia-Lopez et al. 2001).

The *Social Phobia Inventory* (SoPhI; Moore and Gee 2003) is a 21-item scale that measures social anxiety according to DSM-IV-TR criteria (American Psychiatric Association 2000). Items are rated on a 5-point scale (1–5). This is the only scale that includes an item to tap DSM duration criteria for SAD, stating that social anxiety symptomatology must be present for at least 6 months. The SoPhI has been validated in Spain by Bermejo et al. (2011).

Social Phobia Inventory (SPIN; Connor et al. 2000). This 17-item questionnaire measures behavioral, physiological, and cognitive symptoms associated with social phobia. Six of its items assess fear in social situations, seven measure avoidance of performing in social situations, and four items assess physiological discomfort in social situations. Adolescents are asked to rate the frequency with which they experienced each symptom over the last week, using a five-point Likert-type scale (0–4). Thus, total scores can range from 0 to 68. Although initially developed for adults, research has also demonstrated its validity and reliability in adolescent populations in countries such as the USA, Finland, Canada, Germany, Spain, and Brazil (Antony et al. 2006; Garcia-Lopez et al. 2010; Johnson et al. 2006; Pereira et al. 2004; Ranta et al. 2007a, b; Sosic et al. 2008; Vilete et al. 2004).

Mini-Social Phobia Inventory (Mini-SPIN; Connor et al. 2001) is a 3-item scale derived from the SPIN. Recently, Ranta et al. (2012b) and Garcia-Lopez and Moore (2015) found it to be a valid and reliable measure for screening socially anxious adolescents in Spain and Finland.

Self-Statements During Public Speaking Scale (SSPS; Hofmann & DiBartolo, 2000) was designed to specifically assess typical negative and positive self-statements related to public speaking situations. This measure contains 10 items, and each self-statement is rated on a 0–5-point scale. Factor analytic studies have reliably identified a 5-item subscale assessing negative self-statements (SSPS-N) and a 5-item subscale measuring positive self-statements (SSPS-P). Rivero et al. (2010) found that this scale, and particularly the SPSS-N, is a valid and reliable self-statement measure of public speaking anxiety for adolescents.

Social Phobia and Anxiety Inventory (SPAI; Turner et al. 1989). In the late 1980s, these authors developed a self-report inventory that assesses behavioral, physiological, and cognitive symptoms associated with SAD. The SPAI is comprised of two scales: the 32-item Social Phobia subscale (Likert-type scale: 1–7) and the 13-item Agoraphobia subscale. The difference score is calculated by subtracting the Social Phobia subscale from the Agoraphobia subscale. Research has demonstrated that the SPAI is a valid and reliable measure for use with English and Spanish-speaking adolescent populations (Clark et al. 1994; Garcia-Lopez et al. 2001, 2005; Olivares et al. 1999). A cutoff score of 70 on the Social Phobia subscale has been shown to produce the highest agreement rate among Spanish adolescents (Olivares et al. 2002). Olivares et al. (2004a) found that FNE, SAD, SAS-A, and SPAI are invariant among samples, and all of them assess a single higher-order factor, labeled as "social anxiety," although each measure appears to tap different symptomatology. In this study, data revealed SPAI and SAS-A are better predictors of social phobia than FNE and SAD. As a result, these authors recommended the SPAI and the SAS-A as first-line assessment measures to assess adolescents' social anxiety.

The *Social Phobia and Anxiety Inventory-Brief* (SPAI-B; Garcia-Lopez et al. 2008a) stems from the SPAI and assesses both interactional and performance situations, and the three-response system approach (Lang 1968). It is a brief version of the SPAI, albeit different in terms of the Likert scale format used, the number of items, and avoidance of heterocentric language, as recently proposed by Weiss et al. (2013). Unlike SPAI, SPAI-B is a short self-report, particularly useful when screening for social anxiety. It consists of 16 items using a 5-point Likert scale (1–5). For example, "I feel nervous when I have to speak in public." Items 15 and 16 are comprised of sub-items related to cognitive and somatic symptoms; hence item 15 is scored as the average of 4 sub-items, and item 16 as the average of 5 sub-items. Therefore, decimals can be obtained. The SPAI-B score is the sum of item ratings minus 16. As a result, a total score can also be computed (range: 0–64). Although originally developed to screen for adolescents with social anxiety, Piqueras et al. (2012a) found it to be useful for young adults. Vieira et al. (2011; 2013) have confirmed its excellent psychometric properties in a Portuguese adolescent population. Finally, Piqueras et al. (2012a) have revealed that SPAI-B can be administered using online or paper and pencil formats and is a sensitive measure of treatment outcome (Garcia-Lopez et al. 2009; 2014; 2015).

Anxiety Scales Including Social Anxiety Measures

The *Multidimensional Anxiety Scale for Children* (MASC; March 1998; March et al. 1997) assesses the presence of symptoms related to anxiety disorders in youth aged 8–19 years. The MASC consists of 39 items (score range: 1–4) distributed across four major factors, three of which can be parsed into two subfactors. Main and subfactors include: (1) physical symptoms (tense/restless and somatic/autonomic), (2) social anxiety (humiliation/rejection and public performance fears), (3) harm avoidance (perfectionism and anxious coping), and (4) separation anxiety. Good psychometric properties in the social anxiety subscale have been found for adolescents (Anderson et al. 2009; Gastel and Ferdinand 2008; Grills-Taquechel et al. 2008; Wood et al. 2002).

The *Screen for Child Anxiety-Related Disorder* (SCARED; Birmaher et al. 1997) measures anxiety symptomatology in children and adolescents ranging from 8 to 18 years. It contains 41 items, using a 3-point Likert format (0–2). The SCARED is a screening instrument that purports to measure five child and adolescent anxiety disorder symptom dimensions. Four of the five factors (generalized anxiety disorder, panic disorder, separation anxiety disorder, and SAD) are clearly related to DSM-IV-TR anxiety disorders. The fifth anxiety symptom dimension of the SCARED is school anxiety (or school refusal). The SCARED has been validated for use among Cypriot, German, Italian, Spanish, Indian, Chinese, UK, South African, and Dutch adolescents (Crocetti et al. 2009; Essau et al. 2002, 2013; Hale et al. 2005, 2013; Linyan et al. 2008; Muris and Merkelbach 2000; Su et al. 2008; Vigil-Colet et al. 2009). A cutoff of 21 has been suggested as the optimal score to screen for adolescents with anxiety disorders (Swamidhas et al. 2013).

Spence Children's Anxiety Scale (SCAS; Spence 1998). The SCAS assesses six domains of anxiety covering generalized anxiety, panic/agoraphobia, social phobia, separation anxiety, obsessive–compulsive disorder, and physical injury fears. Each symptom is scored on a 4-point (0–3) frequency scale. This measure contains 44 items, 38 of which reflect specific anxiety symptoms and 6 are positive filler items to reduce negative response bias. In addition to the data provided by Spence and colleagues (Spence 1997, 1998; Spence et al. 2003) in an Australian population, the scale has proven to be valid and reliable measure in countries such as Japan, Germany, Cyprus, Spain, the Netherlands, and Mexico (Essau et al. 2004, 2011; Godoy et al. 2011; Hernandez-Guzman et al. 2010; Muris & Merckelbach, 2000; Orgiles et al. 2012). Parent versions have been developed with norms for 6–18-year-olds (Nauta et al. 2004.)

Multi-Informant and Context-Sensitive Clinical Assessment

Properly assessing social anxiety among adolescents involves structuring assessments with the idea that not all individuals express social anxiety in the same way. For example, some individuals may experience clinically significant social anxiety concerns but only within structured performance contexts such as public speaking, whereas others may experience concerns across these performance contexts and also in unstructured social contexts (e.g., asking a stranger for directions) (Bögels et al. 2010). This key component of adolescents' clinical presentations—the potential for significant variations in the contexts in which social concerns may occur—necessitates a comprehensive assessment approach. This approach involves obtaining self-reports from adolescents as well as reports from significant others in adolescents' lives, such as parents and teachers (Silverman and Ollendick 2005). These informants observe adolescents in different contexts (e.g., home vs. school vs. peer interactions); thus, not surprisingly, their reports often yield different conclusions as to adolescents' social anxiety concerns (i.e., *informant discrepancies*; De Los Reyes 2013; De Los Reyes & Kazdin, 2005; Hoffman & Chu, 2015).

One interesting observation involves comparing patterns of informant discrepancies across clinic and community samples. Specifically, in a recent large-scale study of cross-informant correspondence across community samples in 25 societies, adolescents tended to self-report greater anxiety concerns than parents reported about adolescents (Rescorla et al. 2013), whereas in previous work with clinic samples, adolescents have tended to self-report lower concerns relative to parent reports (e.g., De Los Reyes et al. 2012; De Los Reyes et al. 2010). These differences in patterns of informant discrepancies have led many mental health professionals to assume that, when adolescents self-report fewer concerns than adult informants (e.g., parents), in clinical settings, the adolescent is providing unreliable and invalid self-reports (for a review, see De Los Reyes et al. 2011).

However, two key pieces of evidence-based assessment research contradict this interpretation of patterns of informant discrepancies, particularly in terms of adolescent patients' self-reports. First, decades of research attest to the reliability and validity of adolescent self-reports of social anxiety concerns (Silverman and Ollendick 2005). Second, the strong psychometric support for adolescent self-reports extends to circumstances in which one observes large discrepancies between adolescents' self-reports and reports from other informants. For instance, on well-researched, established clinical instruments, even when adolescents' self-reported anxiety concerns evidence low correspondence with parents' reports about adolescents' concerns, both reports nonetheless exhibit the same factor structure (for a review, see De Los Reyes 2013). Further, De Los Reyes and colleagues (2012) recruited a group of adolescents referred for a clinical evaluation for social anxiety concerns, as well as an age- and gender-matched community control group. In this study, clinic-referred adolescents self-reported fewer social anxiety concerns than parents reported about the adolescents, and adolescents' self-reports exhibited very low correspondence with objective measures of their baseline physiological regulation. Yet, adolescents' self-reports nonetheless evidenced high internal consistency, convergent validity, and could significantly distinguish adolescents on referral status (i.e., clinic-referred vs. community control).

Observational and Role-Playing Assessment

Behavioral observation of anxious youth can occur in more or less structured contexts, involving only the adolescent or including the family. Since observation in the natural environment (especially with adolescents) is usually very difficult, structured or unstructured role-play procedures in various situations have become widely used.

The *Behavioral Assessment Tests* (BATs), sometimes also called behavioral avoidance tasks/tests or behavioral approach tasks/tests, are structured role-play procedures commonly used in the behavioral assessment of anxiety disorders. Despite a long history in the assessment of other anxiety disorders, BATs use in the assessment of SAD in children and adolescents were rare until recently. In BATs, the adolescent is exposed to anxiety-provoking situations (included in the adolescent's fear and avoidance list or hierarchy), while the approach or avoidance of the situation and related behaviors are rated, which can be very useful to assess the presence and nature of social fears.

BATs can consist of several types of tasks. Some BATs explore the presence of social skills, using role-plays and asking the adolescent to engage in a simulated social encounter, where a trained confederate plays the role of an interpersonal partner in different scenarios (e.g., having a conversation, giving or receiving a compliment) (e.g., Spence et al. 1999). In a recent study, Mesa et al. (2014) have used a novel social interaction task in which the adolescent played a video game with an unfamiliar confederate. The BAT tasks usually have a set time (e.g., 10 min), during which subjects are instructed to behave as they would if they were actually in that situation, and the confederate may have certain instructions regarding the interaction. Other BATs may be more focused on the ability to perform in front of an audience or in front of a camera, like giving an impromptu speech. In both types of situations, the adolescent may be audiotaped or videotaped, and his/her performance is scored by the confederate and/or by an independent observer for various indicators of social anxiety and social skills (e.g., eye contact, posture, appropriate verbal content). Additionally, before, during, or after the performance of the task, several measures can be employed. These measures include the adolescent's ratings of distress (e.g., 0–100 Subjective Units of Distress Scale), thought-listing procedures, or, if possible, measures of physiological reactions. Cartwright-Hatton et al. (2003) have developed an eight-item Performance Questionnaire to be used in behavioral assessment, which consists of a child version (PQ-C) and an observer version (PQ-O), and that has demonstrated acceptable inter-item and interrater reliability. Although the authors have used this scale with children, it can easily be used with adolescents.

One specific BAT is the *Revised Behavioral Assertiveness Test for Children* (BAT-CR; Ollendick 1981; Ollendick et al. 1985). The BAT-CR, derived from the

Behavioral Assertiveness Test-Revised (Eisler et al. 1975) and from the Behavioral Assertiveness Test for Children (Bornstein et al. 1977), is a measure of children's social skills and social competence that assesses responses to both positive and negative assertion situations with peers. The child/adolescent is required to participate in a series of 12 role-plays, of which 6 require positive assertion (e.g., giving a compliment) and the other 6 require negative assertion (e.g., refusing unreasonable requests). The role-plays are videotaped for later scoring of assertiveness by a trained independent observer (from −2 = very submissive to 2 = very aggressive). The total assertiveness score, obtained by adding the absolute value of the 12 role-play assertiveness ratings, reflects the deviation of the responses from assertion.

Coding categories include eye contact, response latency, response length, and verbal content (Ollendick et al. 1985). The BAT-CR has been found to demonstrate high interrater reliability (Ollendick et al. 1985, 1986; Spence et al. 1999, 2000) and validity (Ollendick 1981; Ollendick et al. 1986). Although this task was not originally developed to be used with children, several studies have used it both with children and with young adolescents (8–14 years; e.g., Spence et al. 1999, 2000).

Structured role-play procedures have been used with children and adolescents in treatment outcome research to assess social anxiety and social skills (e.g., Beidel et al. 2005; Compton et al. 2001; Herbert et al. 2009; Spence et al. 2000). Further research is needed to standardize these procedures and allow comparisons across studies and investigations on their validity and reliability.

Although BATs are useful assessment tools in research, they may not be easy to use in everyday clinical practice due to their time requirements and complexity: an analogue situation has to be created, an appropriate confederate has to be found (same age, same gender) and sometimes trained, and a coding system must be used. However, BATs adapted to clinical use can provide important information on the adolescent's behavior when in social situations. Asking the adolescent to engage in a brief role-play with the clinician (adapted for a relevant situation), or to engage in a performance situation (a reading aloud task, giving a brief speech, or an oral presentation), either in front of an audience or videotaped, can give the clinician important information on his/her baseline anxiety and behavior. This information will help the clinician to decide on the best treatment targets and treatment options and can also help the clinician to evaluate treatment outcome (Beidel and Turner 2007; Kearney 2005).

Naturalistic observations of behavior can also be used for the assessment of social anxiety. Situations to be observed may include ordering food at a restaurant or cafe, buying an article in a store, asking for information, and so on. Although a formal coding of behavioral categories in these observations may not be feasible, it is possible to obtain other types of ratings. For example, adolescents could rate their anxiety before, during, and after the observation; rate their desire to escape the situation; or use a think aloud or thought-listing procedure to express their fears. On the other hand, certain behaviors can be observed in session or in the waiting room. General appearance, fidgeting or other signs of nervousness, lack of eye contact, facial expressions, body posture, or level of other social skills may be identified and can be highly informative (Kearney 2005). Also, parent–child interactions can also be observed. Clinicians should pay attention to instances of conflict, overprotectiveness, or parent reinforcement of anxious/fearful and avoidance behavior.

Physiological Assessment

An interesting area for future research involves developing paradigms for integrating physiological measures into clinical assessments of adolescent social anxiety (for a review, see De Los Reyes and Aldao 2015). That is, can we integrate physiological measures with our traditional clinical tools (e.g., clinical interviews, multi-informant assessments, and/or behavioral observations) in a way that improves clinical decision-making? Some recent work indicates potential for advancements on these issues. For example, using functional magnetic resonance imaging (fMRI), researchers have identified neural circuits that relate to how adolescents process fearful and rewarding stimuli (e.g., social rejection vs. social approval), and this work may inform us of the biological factors that predispose some adolescents to develop social anxiety, particularly within the context of exposure to aversive social experiences (e.g., humiliating peer interactions; Caouette and Guyer 2014). Recently, Myllyneva, Ranta, Hietanen (in press) have found psychophysiological responses (i.e., enhanced autonomic and self-evaluated arousal, attenuated relative left-sided frontal cortical activity) to eye contact in adolescents with social anxiety disorder. Further, with relatively inexpensive and noninvasive modalities for assessing physiology (e.g., heart rate monitors), one can reliably elicit biological markers of stress reactivity (e.g., low heart rate variability) within widely used clinical tasks (e.g., public speaking tasks) (Thomas et al. 2012). Yet, although researchers have fruitfully leveraged fMRI to begin investigating possible neurobiological mechanisms underlying adolescent social anxiety (Caouette and Guyer 2014), as a whole fMRI research is relatively underdeveloped in terms of demonstrating the ability of these assessments for incrementally predicting "real-world" clinical outcomes (e.g., diagnostic status and treatment response) above and beyond our traditional clinical tools (Berkman and Falk 2013). For that matter, the same can be said for relatively less expensive physiological measures (e.g., electroencephalography, heart rate monitors, and salivary assays; see Youngstrom and De Los Reyes 2015).

Using heart rate monitors and indicators of adolescent arousal and/or physiological regulation (e.g., heart rate and heart rate variability), researchers have sought to provide "proof-of-concept" support for the ability of physiological measures to inform clinical decision-making in assessments of adolescent social anxiety. For instance, in two recent studies, researchers integrated physiological measures with informants' reports of adolescents' social anxiety to understand whether physiological measures provide incremental information regarding adolescents' diagnostic status (Anderson and Hope 2009) and clinical referral status (De Los Reyes et al. 2012). In another recent study, researchers demonstrated that personnel without a background in physiology (i.e., undergraduate research assistants) could reliably and accurately interpret graphical representations of adolescents' physiological arousal during a social stressor task (i.e., whether adolescents' heart rates rose above clinical norms of resting heart rate) (De Los Reyes et al. 2015). Collectively, this recent work indicates the potential for physiological measures to yield fruitful information within clinical assessments of adolescent social anxiety, and paradigms exist that might allow assessors without a background in physiology to interpret these data. In line with this recent work, future research might involve examining whether paradigms can be developed for leveraging physiological data to understand the specific contexts in which adolescents experience biological responses linked to social anxiety (e.g., cardiovascular and brain responses to aversive social experiences; see also De Los Reyes and Aldao 2015). Such paradigms might have important clinical implications, as they might allow mental health professionals to identify whether treatment changes an important component of clinical models of social anxiety (i.e., physiological arousal; for a review, see Thomas et al. 2012).

The Future of Assessment of Social Anxiety in Adolescents

Significant progress in the assessment of adolescents with SAD has been made over the last decades. More adolescents with SAD are being identified and accurately diagnosed. A number of psychometrically sound assessment measures are available for adolescents, parents, teachers, and clinicians to report on socially anxious adolescents (Garcia-Lopez and Storch 2008). However, many questions remain to be answered about how to efficiently detect adolescent population who is suffering or at risk of suffer SAD. Screening adolescents for SAD in schools has its own characteristics. Masia-Warner and Garcia-Lopez's teams have implemented two-step screening approaches, consisting of administering self-report measures or nominations by school personnel, followed by phone or personal interviews. Evidence supports using self-report measures (but not school staff nominations) in the first step to screen for socially anxious adolescents and interviews as second step for the identification of adolescents with SAD (Garcia-Lopez et al. 2001, 2006, 2009; 2014; Masia-Warner et al. 2005, 2007; Olivares & Garcia-Lopez, 2001; Sweeney et al. 2015). Using this two-step screening approach developed in mid-1990s, Garcia-Lopez and Moore (2015) have examined the performance of a number of brief social anxiety measures validated for Spanish adolescents, namely, the SPIN, SAS-A, SASA, LSAS-CA, SPAI-B, Mini-SPIN, SoPhI, and EDAS. Findings reveal all scales were accurate in detecting socially anxious adolescents, but the SPAI-B cut-off score yielded the best balance between sensitivity and specificity and the highest Youden Index. Depending on the purpose of the study, SAS-A may be especially useful for reducing false negatives and SPAI-B for false positives. Given that effective treatments are available, useful screening can contribute to no longer say SAD is an under-detected condition. Finally, it is crucial to develop a screening protocol in the school system, including strategies for obtaining data from underrepresented populations such as immigrant and minority groups.

Despite the need for multimethod assessment, agreement on symptoms of social anxiety is rare. In light of recent work in evidence-based assessment (see section "Multi-informant and context-sensitive clinical assessment" of this chapter), the key question for future research is not: *Which informants provide psychometrically sound reports about adolescent social anxiety*? Rather, the key question is: *How can assessors maximize the value of multi-informant assessments*? That is, discrepancies among informants' reports may meaningfully reflect differences in the contexts in which adolescents express social anxiety (De Los Reyes et al. 2013b). To this end, future work might involve using independent behavioral assessments to corroborate the discrepancies observed within multi-informant assessments. This approach may allow mental health professionals to use informant discrepancies as tools for understanding the specific contexts in which adolescents evidence social anxiety. As an example of this approach, consider that in recent work with adult social anxiety patients, convergence between patients' self-reports and clinician reports about patients' internalizing symptoms tended to occur when patients expressed social skills deficits across multiple standardized social interactions (e.g., one-on-one social interactions and public speaking in front of strangers; De Los Reyes et al. 2013a). If these effects generalize to assessments with adolescent patients, contextually sensitive clinical assessments may inform treatment planning and plans for monitoring treatment response (see also De Los Reyes 2013).

In addition, Garcia-Lopez et al. (2011a) revealed that socially anxious adolescents' language can be used as a complementary treatment outcome measure, using a Corpus Linguistic methodology. These authors found that the linguistic analysis of adolescents' discourse is useful when evaluating the efficacy of treatment, as a close relationship between the sensitivity of treatment outcome and adolescents' use of language was revealed. Further, Garcia-Lopez and Diez-Bedmar (2008) found there is different linguistic pattern to discriminate between adolescents with social anxiety disorder in comparison with a control group. These authors suggested an additional linguistic measure could be used when some discrepancy between self-report and clinician is observed. This is particularly important as adolescents are likely to minimize their social anxiety symptomatology during assessment in an attempt to make a good impression on the diagnostician.

Finally, to target the size and burden of SAD, it seems crucial not only to obtain data from different sources other than the youth themselves, such as teachers and parents, but also to analyze and evaluate data from a multidisciplinary approach. Further, safety behaviors or avoidance on a covert level in adolescents with SAD (eg, "shadow friend"; Garcia-Lopez, 2013) should be assessed. Until now, screening protocols to detect SAD have been designed from traditional approaches and considered only a single perspective, which clearly limits the impact of findings. Further, screening protocols rarely cover the full spectrum of emotional problems and rarely include risk factors. Given the fast expansion of new technologies across world, Information and Communication Technologies and Computerized-Adaptive Testing-based (ICT- and CAT-based) methods of surveying may offer flexibility in the collection of information from different sources and contexts and cost-effectiveness in both implementation and maintenance. This may be especially true in populations such as children and adolescents, who are familiar with the use of electronic devices such as computers, laptops, smartphones, or tablets. Future work could examine potential role of these methodologies in the assessment process. ICT- and CAT-based screening protocols may serve as a feasible, acceptable, and multifaceted delivery method because they can provide assessment at a relatively low cost in large groups of youths. Identification of variables affecting early detection of adolescents at risk for SAD from a comprehensive, multidisciplinary perspective may be the next step in assessment of SAD in adolescents.

References

Albano AM, Silverman WK (2015) The anxiety disorders interview schedule for children for DSM-5, child and parent versions. Oxford University Press, New York

Ambrosini E (2000) Historical development and present status of the Schedule for Affective Disorders and Schizophrenia for School-Age Children (K-SADS). J Am Acad Child Adolesc Psychiatry 39:49–58

American Psychiatric Association (1994) *Diagnostic and statistical manual of mental disorders (4th ed.)*. American Psychiatric Association, Washington, DC

American Psychiatric Association (2013) *Diagnostic and statistical manual of mental disorders* (5th ed.). American Psychiatric Association, Washington, DC

Anderson ER, Hope DA (2009) The relationship among social phobia, objective and perceived physiological reactivity, and anxiety sensitivity in an adolescent population. J Anxiety Disord 23:18–26. doi:10.1016/j.janxdis.2008.03.011

Anderson ER, Jordan JA, Smith AJ, Inderbitzen-Nolan HM (2009) An examination of the MASC social anxiety scale in a non-referred sample of adolescents. J Anxiety Disord 23:1098–1105

Angold A, Costello EJ (2000) The Child and Adolescent Psychiatric Assessment (CAPA). J Am Acad Child Adolesc Psychiatry 39:39–48

Antony MM, Coons MJ, McCabe RE, Ashbaugh A, Swinson RP (2006) Psychometric properties of the social phobia inventory: further evaluation. Behav Res Ther 44:1177–1185

Aune T, Stiles TC, Svarva K (2008) Psychometric properties of the Social Phobia and Anxiety Inventory for Children using a non-American population-based sample. J Anxiety Disord 22:1075–1086

Aydin A, Sütcü ST (2007) Validity and reliability of Social Anxiety Scale for Adolescents (SAS-A). Turk J Child Adolesc Ment Health 14:79–89

Bandelow B, Baldwin DS, Dolberg OT, Andersen HF, Stein DJ (2006) What is the threshold for symptomatic response and remission for major depressive disorder, panic disorder, social anxiety disorder, and generalized anxiety disorder? J Clin Psychiatry 67:1428–1434

Beidel DC, Turner SM (2007) Shy children, phobic adults: nature and treatment of social anxiety disorder, 2nd edn. American Psychological Association, Washington, DC

Beidel DC, Turner SM, Hamlin K, Morris TL (2000a) The Social Phobia and Anxiety Inventory for Children (SPAI-C): external and discriminative validity. Behav Ther 31:75–87

Beidel DC, Turner SM, Morris TL (2000b) The Social Phobia and Anxiety Inventory for Children. Psychol Assess 7:73–79

Beidel, D.C., Turner, S.M., & Morris, T.L. (1995). A new inventory to assess child social phobia: The Social Phobia and Anxiety Inventory for Children. Psychological Assessment, 7:73–79

Beidel DC, Turner SM, Young B, Paulson A (2005) Social effectiveness therapy for children: three-year follow-up. J Consult Clin Psychol 73:721–725

Berkman ET, Falk EB (2013) Beyond brain mapping: using neural measures to predict real-world outcomes. Curr Dir Psychol Sci 22:45–50. doi:10.1177/0963721412469394

Bermejo RM, Garcia-Lopez LJ, Hidalgo MD, Moore KA (2011) The Social Phobia Inventory (SoPhI): validity and reliability in an adolescent population. Ana Psicol 27:342–349

Birmaher B, Khetarpal S, Brent D, Cully M, Balach L, Kaufman J, & cols (1997) The Screen for Child Anxiety Related Emotional Disorders (SCARED): scale construction and psychometric characteristics. J Am Acad Child Adolesc Psychiatry 36:545–553

Bögels SM, Alden L, Beidel DC, Clark LA, Pine DS, Stein MB, Voncken M (2010) Social anxiety disorder: questions and answers for the DSM-V. Depress Anxiety 27:168–189. doi:10.1002/da.20670

Bornstein MR, Bellack AS, Hersen M (1977) Social-skills training for unassertive children: a multiple baseline analysis. J Appl Behav Anal 10:183–195

Brooks SJ, Kutcher S (2004) The Kutcher Generalized Social Anxiety Disorder Scale for Adolescents: assessment of its evaluative properties over the course of a 16-week pediatric psychopharmacotherapy trial. J Child Adolesc Psychopharmacol 14:273–286

Brown T, Barlow DH (2013) Anxiety disorders interview schedule for DSM-5. Oxford University Press, New York

Busner J, Targum SD (2007) The clinical global impression scale: applying a research tool in clinical practice. Psychiatry 4:28–37

Caballo VE, Arias B, Salazar IC, Calderero M, Irurtia MJ, Ollendick TH (2012) A new self-report assessment measure of social phobia/anxiety in children: the Social Anxiety Questionnaire for Children (SAQ-C24). Behav Psychol 20:485–503

Caouette JD, Guyer AE (2014) Gaining insight into adolescent vulnerability for social anxiety from developmental cognitive neuroscience. Dev Cogn Neurosci 8:65–76. doi:10.1016/j.dcn.2013.10.003

Cartwright-Hatton S, Hodges L, Porter J (2003) Social anxiety in childhood: the relationship with self and observer rated social skills. J Child Psychol Psychiatry 44:737–742

Clark DB, Turner SM, Beidel DC, Donovan JE, Kirisci L, Jacob RG (1994) Reliability and validity of the social phobia and anxiety inventory for adolescents. Psychol Assess 6:135–140

Compton SN, Grant PJ, Chrisman AK, Gammon PJ, Brown VL, March JS (2001) Sertraline in children and adolescents with social anxiety disorder: an open trial. J Am Acad Child Adolesc Psychiatry 40:564–571

Connor KM, Davidson JRT, Churchill LE, Sherwood A, Foa E, Weisler RH (2000) Psychometric properties of the Social Phobia Inventory (SPIN). Br J Psychiatry 176:379–386

Connor KM, Kobak KA, Churchill LE, Katzelnick D, Davidson JR (2001) Mini-SPIN: a brief screening assessment for generalized social anxiety disorder. Depress Anxiety 14:137–140

Crocetti E, Hale WW III, Fermani A, Raaijmakers Q, Meeus W (2009) Psychometric properties of the Screen for Child Anxiety Related Emotional Disorders (SCARED) in the general Italian adolescent population: a validation and a comparison between Italy and The Netherlands. J Anxiety Disord 23:824–829

Cunha M, Pinto-Gouveia J, Alegre S, Salvador MC (2004) Avaliação da Ansiedade Social na Adolescência. A versão portuguesa da SAS-A [Assessment od social anxiety in adolescence. The Portuguese version of the SAS-A]. Psychologica 35:249–263

Cunha M, Pinto-Gouvieia JP, Salvador MC (2008) Social fears in adolescence: The Social Anxiety and Avoidance Scale for Adolescents. Eur Psychol 13:197–213

De Los Reyes A (2013) Strategic objectives for improving understanding of informant discrepancies in developmental psychopathology research. Dev Psychopathol 25:669–682. doi:10.1017/S0954579413000096

De Los Reyes A, Aldao A (2015) Introduction to the special issue: Toward implementing physiological measures in clinical child and adolescent assessments. J Clin Child Adolesc Psychol 44: 221–237. doi:10.1080/15374416.2014.891227

De Los Reyes A, Kazdin AE (2005) Informant discrepancies in the assessment of childhood psychopathology: a critical review, theoretical framework, and recommendations for further study. Psychol Bull 131:483–509. doi:10.1037/0033-2909.131.4.483

De Los Reyes A, Alfano CA, Beidel DC (2010) The relations among measurements of informant discrepancies within a multisite trial of treatments for childhood social phobia. J Abnorm Child Psychol 38:395–404. doi:10.1007/s10802-009-9373-6

De Los Reyes A, Youngstrom EA, Swan AJ, Youngstrom JK, Feeny NC, Findling RL (2011) Informant discrepancies in clinical reports of youths and interviewers' impressions of the reliability of informants. J Child Adolesc Psychopharmacol 21:417–424. doi:10.1089/cap.2011.0011

De Los Reyes A, Aldao A, Thomas SA, Daruwala SE, Swan AJ, Van Wie M, Lechner WV (2012) Adolescent self-reports of social anxiety: can they disagree with objective psychophysiological measures and still be valid? J Psychopathol Behav Assess 34:308–322. doi:10.1007/s10862-012-9289-2

De Los Reyes A, Bunnell BE, Beidel DC (2013a) Informant discrepancies in adult social anxiety disorder assessments: links with contextual variations in observed behavior. J Abnorm Psychol 122:376–386. doi:10.1037/a0031150

De Los Reyes A, Thomas SA, Goodman KL, Kundey SMA (2013b) Principles underlying the use of multiple informants' reports. Annu Rev Clin Psychol 9:123–149. doi:10.1146/annurev-clinpsy-050212-185617
De Los Reyes A, Augenstein TM, Aldao A, Thomas SA, Daruwala SE, Kline K, Regan T (2015) Implementing psychophysiology in clinical assessments of adolescent social anxiety: use of rater judgments based on graphical representations of psychophysiology. J Clin Child Adolesc Psychol 44. Advance online publication. doi:10.1080/15374416.2013.859080
Eisler RM, Hersen M, Miller PM, Blanchard EB (1975) Situational determinants of assertive behaviors. J Consult Clin Psychol 43:330–340
Endicott J, Spitzer RL, Fleiss JL, Cohen J (1976) The global assessment scale. A procedure for measuring overall severity of psychiatric disturbance. Arch Gen Psychiatry 33:766–771
Essau CA, Muris P, Ederer EM (2002) Reliability and validity of the Spence Children's Anxiety Scale and the Screen for Child Anxiety Related Emotional Disorders in German children. J Behav Ther Exp Psychiatry 33:1–18
Essau CA, Sakano Y, Ishikawa S, Sasagawa S (2004) Anxiety symptoms in Japanese and in German children. Behav Res Ther 42:601–612
Essau CA, Anastassiou-Hadjicharalambous X, Muñoz LC (2011) Psychometric properties of the Spence Children's Anxiety Scale (SCAS) in Cypriot children and adolescents. Child Psychiatry Hum Dev 42:557–568
Essau CA, Anastassiou-Hadjicharalambous X, Muñoz LC (2013) Psychometric properties of the Screen for Child Anxiety Related Emotional Disorders (SCARED) in Cypriot Children and Adolescents. Eur J Psychol Assess 29:19–27
First MB, Spitzer RL, Gibbon M, Williams JBW (1994) Structured clinical interview for DSM-IV Axis I disorders. Biometric Research Department, New York State Psychiatric Institute, New York
Garcia-Lopez LJ (2013) Tratando…trastorno de ansiedad social [Treating…social anxiety disorder]. Piramide, Madrid
Garcia-Lopez LJ, Diez-Bedmar MB (2008). Can Corpus Linguistics add some input to clinical psychology by distinguishing adolescents with and without social anxiety disorder? Oral paper presented at the XIth EARA conference, Turin
Garcia-Lopez LJ, Moore H (2015) The Mini-Social Phobia Inventory: psychometric properties in an adolescent general and clinical population. PLOS One (in press)
Garcia-Lopez LJ, Olivares J, Beidel D, Albano AM, Turner S, Rosa AI. (2006). Efficacy of three treatment protocols for adolescents with social anxiety disorder: a 5-year follow-up assessment. J Anxiety Disord. 20:175–191
Garcia-Lopez LJ, Storch EA (2008) Recent advances in anxiety disorders in childhood. Foreword. Behav Psychol 16:361–363
Garcia-Lopez LJ, Olivares J, Hidalgo MD, Beidel DC, Turner SM (2001) Psychometric Properties of the Social Phobia and Anxiety Inventory, the Social Anxiety Scale for Adolescents, the Fear of Negative Evaluation Scale, and the Social Avoidance and Distress Scale in an Adolescent Spanish-Speaking Sample. J Psychopathol Behav Assess 23:51–59
Garcia-Lopez LJ, Beidel DC, Hidalgo MD, Olivares J, Turner S (2008a) Brief form of the Social Phobia and Anxiety Inventory (SPAI-B) for adolescents. Eur J Psychol Assess 24:150–156
Garcia-Lopez LJ, Ingles CJ, Garcia-Fernandez JM (2008b) Exploring the relevance of gender and age differences in the assessment of social fears in adolescence. Soc Behav Pers 36:385–390
Garcia-Lopez LJ, Piqueras JA, Diaz-Castela MM, Ingles CJ (2008c) Social anxiety disorder in childhood and adolescents: current trends, advances, and future directions. Behav Psychol 16:501–533
Garcia-Lopez LJ, Muela JA, Espinosa-Fernández L, Diaz-Castela MM (2009) Exploring the relevance of expressed emotion to the treatment of social anxiety disorder in adolescence. J Adolesc 32:1371–1376. doi:10.1016/j.adolescence.2009.08.001
Garcia-Lopez LJ, Bermejo RM, Hidalgo MD (2010) The Social Phobia Inventory: screening and cross-cultural validation in Spanish adolescents. Span J Psychol 13:970–980
Garcia-Lopez LJ, Diez-Bedmar MB, Perez-Paredes P, Tornero E (2011a) Treatment change in adolescents with social anxiety disorder: Insights from corpus linguistics. Ansiedad Estres Anxiety Stress 17:149–155

Garcia-Lopez LJ, Ingles CJ, Garcia-Fernandez JM, Hidalgo MD, Bermejo R, Puklek Levpušček M (2011b) Psychometric properties and clinical cut-off scores of the Spanish version of the Social Anxiety Scale for Adolescents. J Pers Assess 93:474–482

Garcia-Lopez LJ, Beidel DC, Muela-Martinez JM (2015) Optimal cut-off score for detecting social anxiety disorder and DSM-5 specifier with the Social Phobia and Anxiety Inventory-Brief form. Eur J Psychol Assess (in press)

Garcia-Lopez LJ, Diaz-Castela MM, Muela-Martinez JA, Espinosa-Fernandez L (2014) Can parent training for parents with high levels of expressed emotion have a positive effect on their child's social anxiety improvement? J Anxiety Disord 28:812–822. doi:10.1016/j.janxdis.2014.09.001

Garcia-Lopez LJ, Saez-Castillo A, Beidel DC, La Greca AM (in press). Brief measures to screen for social anxiety in Spanish adolescents. J Dev Behav Pediatr

Garcia-Lopez LJ, Moore H 2015. The Mini-Social Phobia Inventory: psychometric properties in an adolescent general and clinical population. PLOS ONE (in press)

Gastel W, Ferdinand RF (2008) Screening capacity of the Multidimensional Anxiety Scale for Children (MASC) for DSM-IV anxiety disorders. Depress Anxiety 25:1046–1052

Gauer GJC, Picon P, Vasconcellos SJL, Turner SM, Beidel DC (2005) Validation of the Social Phobia and Anxiety Inventory for Children (SPAI-C) in a sample of Brazilian children. Braz J Med Biol Res 38:795–800

Godoy A, Gavino A, Carrillo F, Cobos MP, Quintero C (2011) Composición factorial de la versión española de la Spence Children Anxiety Scale (SCAS). [Factor structure of the Spanish version of the Spence Children Anxiety Scale (SCAS)]. Psicothema 23:289–294

Grills-Taquechel G, Ollendick TH, Fisak B (2008) Reexamination of the MASC factor structure and discriminant ability in a mixed clinical outpatient sample. Depress Anxiety 25:942–950

Guy W (ed) (1976) ECDEU assessment manual for psychopharmacology. US Department of Health, Education, and Welfare Public Health Service Alcohol, Drug Abuse, and Mental Health Administration, Rockville

Hale WW III, Raaijmakers QAW, Muris P, Meeus W (2005) Psychometric properties of the Screen for Child Anxiety Related Emotional Disorders (SCARED) in the general adolescent population. Am Acad Child Adolesc Psychiatry 44:283–290

Hale WW III, Raaijmakers QAW, Garcia-Lopez LJ, Espinosa-Fernandez L, Muela JA, Diaz-Castela MM (2013) Psychometric properties of the SCARED for socially anxious and non-anxious Spanish adolescents. Span J Psychol 16:1–7

Herbert JD, Gaudiano BA, Rheingold AA, Moitra E, Myers VH, Dalrymple KL, Brandsma LL (2009) Cognitive behavior therapy for generalized social anxiety disorder: a randomized controlled trial. J Anxiety Disord 23:167–177

Herbert JD, Rheingold AA, Brandsma LL (2010) Assessment of social anxiety and social phobia. In: Hofmann SG, DiBartolo PM (eds) Social anxiety: clinical developmental and social perspectives. Elsevier, London, pp 23–64

Hernandez-Guzman L, Bermudez-Ornelas G, Spence SH, Gonzalez MJ, Martínez-Guerrero JI, Aguilar J, Gallegos J (2010) Versión en español de la Escala de Ansiedad para Niños de Spence (SCAS) [Spanish versión of the Spence Children's Anxiety Scale]. Rev Latinoam Psicol 42:13–24

Hien D, Matzner FJ, First MB, Spitzer RL, Gibbon M, Williams JBW (1994) Structured clinical interview for DSM–IV –Child edition (Version 1.0). Columbia University, New York

Hofmann, S. G. & DiBartolo, P. M. (2000). An instrument to assess self-statements during public speaking: Scale development and preliminary psychometric properties. Behavior Therapy, 31:499–515

Hoffman LJ and Chu BC (2015). Target problem (mis) matching: Predictors and consequences ofparent–youth agreement in a sample of anxious youth. J Anxiety Disord 31: 11-19

Inderbitzen-Nolan HM, Walters KS (2000) Social Anxiety Scale for Adolescents: normative data and further evidence of construct validity. J Clin Child Psychol 29:360–371

Inderbitzen-Nolan HM, Davies CA, McKean NE (2004) Investigating the construct validity of the SPAI-C. Comparing the sensitivity and specifity of the SPAI-C and SAS-A. J Anxiety Disord 18:547–560

Ingles CJ, La Greca AM, Marzo JC, Garcia-Lopez LJ, García-Fernández JM (2010) Social Anxiety Scale for Adolescents: factorial invariance and latent mean differences across gender and age in Spanish adolescents. J Anxiety Disord 24:847–855
Jensen ES, Roper M, Fisher P, Piacentini J, Canino G, Richters J, Davies M (1995) Test-retest reliability of the Diagnostic Interview for Children (DISC 2.1): parent, child, and combined algorithms. Arch Gen Psychiatry 52:61–71
Jimenez-Lopez LM, Sanchez Aragon R, Valencia-Cruz A (2013) Escala de Ansiedad Social para Adolescentes: confiabilidad y validez en una muestra mexicana [Scale of Social Anxiety for Adolescents: Reliability and validity in a Mexican sample]. Psicol Iberoam 21:72–84
Johnson HS, Inderbitzen-Nolan HM, Anderson ER (2006) The Social Phobia Inventory: validity and reliability in an adolescent community sample. Psychol Assess 18:269–277
Kaufman J, Birmaher B, Brent D, Rao U, Flynn C, Moreci P, Ryan N (1997) Schedule for Affective Disorders and Schizophrenia for School-Age Children-Present and Lifetime Version (K-SADS-PL): initial reliability and validity data. J Am Acad Child Adolesc Psychiatry 39:980–988
Kearney CA (2005) Social anxiety and social phobia in youth: characteristics, assessment, and psychological treatment. Springer, New York
Kristensen H, Torgersen S (2006) Social anxiety disorder in 11-12-years-old children: the efficacy of screening and issues in parent–child agreement. Eur Child Adolesc Psychiatry 15:163–171
Kuusikko S, Pollock-Wurman R, Ebeling H, Hurtig T, Joskitt L, Mattila ML, Jussila K, Moilanen I (2009) Psychometric evaluation of social phobia and anxiety inventory for children (SPAI-C) and social anxiety scale for children-revised (SASC-R). Eur Child Adolesc Psychiatry 18:116–124
La Greca AM (1999) Manual for the social anxiety scales for children and adolescents. Author, Miami
La Greca AM, Lopez N (1998) Social anxiety among adolescents: linkages with peer relations and friendship. J Abnorm Child Psychol 26:83–94
La Greca AM, Stone WL (1993) Social Anxiety Scale for Children-Revised: factor structure and concurrent validity. J Clin Child Psychol 22:17–27
La Greca AM, Ingles CJ, Lai BS, Marzo JC (2014, 2015) Social Anxiety Scale for Adolescents: factorial invariance across gender and age in Hispanic-American adolescents. Assessment, 22:224–232
Lang PJ (1968) Fear reduction and fear behavior: problems in treating a construct. In: Shlien JM (ed) Research in psychotherapy, vol 3. American Psychological Association, Washington, DC, pp 90–102
Lecrubier Y, Sheehan DV, Weiller E, Amorim P, Bonora I, Sheehan KH, Dunbar GC (1997) The Mini International Neuropsychiatric Interview (MINI). A short diagnostic structured interview: reliability and validity according to the CIDI. Eur Psychiatry 12:224–231
Lewczyk CM, Garland AF, Hurlburt MS, Gearity J, Hough RL (2003) Comparing DISC-IV and clinician diagnoses among youths receiving public mental health services. J Am Acad Child Adolesc Psychiatry 42:349–356
Liebowitz MR (1987) Social Phobia. Mod Probl Pharmacopsychiatry 22:141–173
Linyan S, Kai W, Fang F, Yi S, Xueping G (2008) Reliability and validity of the screen for child anxiety related emotional disorders (SCARED) in Chinese children. J Anxiety Disord 22:612–621
Lyneham HJ, Abbott MJ, Rapee RM (2007) Interrater reliability of the Anxiety Disorders Interview Schedule for DSM-IV: child and parent version. J Am Acad Child Adolesc Psychiatry 46:731–736
March JS (1998) Manual for the Multidimensional Anxiety Scale for Children (MASC). Multi-Health Systems, Toronto
March JS, Albano AM (2002) Anxiety disorders in children and adolescents. In: Stein DJ, Hollander E (eds) Textbook of anxiety disorders. American Psychiatric Publishing, Washington, DC, pp 415–427
March JS, Parker JDA, Sullivan K, Stallings P, Conners K (1997) The Multidimensional Anxiety Scale for Children (MASC): factor structure, reliability and validity. J Am Acad Child Adolesc Psychiatry 36:554–565

Martins AC, Almeida JP, Viana V (2014) Social Anxiety Disorder in Childhood and Pre-Adolescence: adaptation of the SASC-R for European Portuguese. Psicol Reflex Crit 27:300–307. doi:10.1590/1678-7153.201427210
Masia CL, Hofmann SG, Klein RG, Liebowitz MR (1999) The Liebowitz Social Anxiety Scale for Children and Adolescents (LSAS-CA). Available from Carrie Masia-Warner, NYU Child Study Center, 215 Lexington Avenue, 13th floor, New York, NY 10016
Masia-Warner C, Storch EA, Pincus DB, Klein RG, Heimberg RG, Liebowitz MR (2003) The Liebowitz social anxiety scale for children and adolescents: an initial psychometric investigation. J Am Acad Child Adolesc Psychiatry 42:1076–1084
Masia-Warner C, Klein RG, Dent H, Fisher PH, Alvir J, Albano AM, Guardino M (2005) School-based intervention for adolescents with social anxiety disorder: results of a controlled study. J Abnorm Child Psychol 33:707–722
Masia-Warner, C., Fisher, P. H., Shrout, P. E., Rathor, S., & Klein, R. G. (2007). Treating Adolescents with Social Anxiety Disorder in school: an attention control trial. Journal of Child Psychology and Psychiatry, 48:676–686
Matzner F (1994) Videotapes as training tools for the development of the KID-SCID. Paper presented at the scientific proceedings of the American Academy of Child and Adolescent Psychiatric Association, 42nd annual meeting. Washington, DC
Matzner F, Silva R, Silvan M, Chowdhury M, Nastasi L (1997) Preliminary test-retest reliability of the KID-SCID. Paper presented at the scientific proceedings of the American Academy of Child and Adolescent Psychiatric Association, 150th annual meeting. Washington, DC
Mesa F, Beidel DC, Bunnell BE (2014) An examination of psychopathology and daily impairment in adolescents with social anxiety disorder. PLoS One 9:e93668. doi:10.1371/journal.pone.0093668
Moore KA, Gee DL (2003) The reliability, validity, discriminant and predictive properties of the Social Phobia Inventory (SoPhI). Anxiety Stress Coping 16:109–117
Muris P, Mayer B, Bartelds E, Tierney S, Bogie N (2001). The revised version of the Screen for Child Anxiety Related Emotional Disorders (SCARED-R): Treatment sensitivity in an early intervention trial for childhood anxiety disorders. British Journal of Clinical Psychology, 40:323–336
Muris P, Merckelbach H (2000) Correlations among two self-report questionnaires for measuring DSM-defined anxiety disorder symptoms in children: the Screen for Child Anxiety Related Emotional Disorders and the Spence Children's Anxiety Scale. Pers Individ Differ 28:333–346
Muris P, Schmidt H, Engelbrecht P, Perold M (2002) DSM-IV-defined anxiety disorder symptoms in South African children. J Am Acad Child Adolesc Psychiatry 41:1360–1368
Myers MG, Stein MB, Aarons G (2002) Cross validation of the Social Anxiety Scale for Adolescents in a high school sample. J Anxiety Disord 16:221–232
Myllyneva A, Ranta K, Hietanen JK (in press). Psychophysiological responses to eye contact in adolescents with social anxiety disorder. Biol Psychol. doi:10.1016/j.biopsycho.2015.05.005
Nauta MH, Scholing A, Rapee RM, Abbott M, Spence SH, Waters A (2004) A parent report measure of children's anxiety. Behav Res Ther 42:813–839
Ogliari A, Scaini S, Kofler MJ, Lampis V, Zanoni A, Pesenti-Gritti P, Spatola CAM, Battaglia M, Beidel DC (2012) Psychometric properties of the Social Phobia and Anxiety Inventory for Children (SPAI-C). A sample of Italian School-Aged Children from the general population. Eur J Psychol Assess 28:51–59
Okajima I, Fukuhara S, Yamada S, Sakano Y, La Greca AM (2009) Development and validation of a Japanese version of the social anxiety scale for children-revised (SASC-R) and the social anxiety scale for adolescents (SAS-A). Jpn J Child Adolesc Psychiatry 50:457–468
Olivares J, Garcia Lopez LJ (1998) Escala para la Detección de la Ansiedad Social [Social Anxiety Screening Scale, SASS]. Universidad de Murcia, Murcia
Olivares J, Piqueras JA (2005) Escala para la Detección de la Ansiedad Social (EDAS) [Social Anxiety Screening Scale, SASS]. En Vera-Villaroel P, Oblitas L (Coords.). Manual de Escalas, & Cuestionarios Iberoamericanos en Psicología Clínica, & de la Salud [Handbook

of Iberoamerican scales and tests in Health and Clinical Psychology]. Psicom Editores, Colombia. p 350

Olivares J, Garcia-Lopez LJ, Hidalgo MD, Turner SM, Beidel DC (1999) The Social Phobia and Anxiety Inventory: reliability and validity in an adolescent Spanish population. J Psychopathol Behav Assess 21:67–78

Olivares, J. & Garcia-Lopez, L. J. (2001). Un nuevo tratamiento multicomponente para adolescentes con fobia social generalizada: Resultados de un estudio piloto. (A new multicomponent treatment for adolescents with generalized social phobia: Results of a pilot study). Psicologia Conductual, 9:247–254

Olivares J, Garcia-Lopez LJ, Hidalgo MD, La Greca AM, Turner SM, Beidel DC (2002) A pilot study on normative data for two social anxiety measures: The Social Phobia and Anxiety Inventory and the Social Anxiety Scale for Adolescents. Int J Clin Health Psychol 2:467–476

Olivares J, Garcia-Lopez LJ, Hidalgo MD, Caballo VE (2004a) Relationships among social anxiety measures and its invariance: a confirmatory factor analysis. Eur J Psychol Assess 20:172–179

Olivares J, Piqueras JA, Sánchez-García R (2004b) Escala para la Detección de la Ansiedad Social (EDAS): estructura factorial, & fiabilidad en una muestra de adolescentes entre 14 y18 años [Social Anxiety Screening Scale: factorial structure and reliability in Adolescents]. Psicol Conductual 12:251–268

Olivares J, Ruiz J, Hidalgo MD, Garcia-Lopez LJ, Rosa AI, Piqueras JA (2005) Social Anxiety Scale for Adolescents (SAS-A): psychometric properties in a Spanish-speaking population. Int J Clin Health Psychol 5:85–97

Olivares J, Sanchez-Garcia R, Lopez-Pina JA (2009) The Liebowitz social anxiety scale for children and adolescents. Psicothema 21:486–491

Olivares J, Sanchez-Garcia R, Lopez-Pina JA, Rosa-Alcazar AI (2010) Psychometric properties of the Social Phobia and Anxiety Inventory for Children in a Spanish Sample. Span J Psychol 13:961–969

Ollendick TH (1981) Assessment of social interaction skills in school children. Behav Couns Q 1:227–243

Ollendick TH, Hart KJ, Francis G (1985) Social validation of the revised behavioral assertiveness test for children (BAT-CR). Child Fam Behav Ther 7:17–33

Ollendick TH, Meador AE, Villanis C (1986) Relationship between the Children's Assertiveness Inventory (CAI) and the Revised Behavioral Assertiveness Test for Children (BAT-CR). Child Fam Behav Ther 8:27–36

Orgiles M, Méndez X, Spence SH, Ruedo-Medina TB, Espada JP (2012) Spanish validation of the Spence Children's Anxiety Scale. Child Psychiatry Hum Dev 43:271–281

Pereira LM, Freire EDS, De Vasconcellos IL (2004) Confiabilidade da versão em Português do Inventário de Fobia Social (SPIN) entre adolescentes estudantes do Município do Rio de Janeiro. Cad Saúde Pública (Rio de Janeiro) 20:89–99

Piqueras JA, Olivares J, Hidalgo MD, Vera-Villarroel P, Marzo JC (2011) Psychometric update of the Social Anxiety Screening Scale (SASS/EDAS) in a Spanish adolescent population. Span J Psychol 14:977–989

Piqueras JA, Espinosa-Fernández L, Garcia-Lopez LJ, Beidel DC (2012a) Validación del Inventario de Ansiedad, & Fobia Social-Forma Breve en jóvenes adultos españoles [Validation of the SPAI-B in young adults]. Behav Psychol 20:505–528

Piqueras JA, Olivares J, Hidalgo MD (2012b) Screening utility of the Social Anxiety Screening Scale in Spanish speaking adolescents. Span J Psychol 15:710–723

Piqueras JA, Olivares J, Vera-Villarroel P, Marzo JC, Kuhne W (2012c) Invarianza factorial de la Escala para la Detección de Ansiedad Social (EDAS) en adolescentes españoles, & chilenos [Factorial invariance of Social Anxiety Screening Scale in Chilean and Spanish adolescents]. Ana psicol 28:203–214

Puklek M (1997a) Sociocognitive aspects of social anxiety and its developmental trend in adolescence. Universidad de Ljubljana, Eslovenia

Puklek M (1997b) Sociocognitive aspects of social anxiety in adolescence. Horiz Psychol 13:27–40

Puklek Levpušček, M. (2004). Development of the two forms of social anxiety in adolescence. Horizons of Psychology, 13:27–40

Puklek Levpušček M, Videc M (2008) Psychometric properties of the Social Anxiety Scale for Adolescents (SASA) and its relation to positive imaginary audience and academic performance in Slovene adolescents. Stud Psychol 50:49–65

Puklek M, Vidmar G (2000) Social Anxiety in Slovene Adolescents: Psychometric properties of a new measure, age differences and relations with self-consciousness and perceived incompetence. Eur Rev Appl Psychol 50:249–258

Ranta K, Kaltiala-Heino R, Koivisto AM, Tuomisto MT, Pelkonen M, Marttunen M (2007a) Age and gender differences in social anxiety symptoms during adolescence: The Social Phobia Inventory (SPIN) as a measure. Psychiatry Res 153:261–270

Ranta K, Katiala-Heino R, Rantanen P, Tuomisto MT, Marttunen M (2007b) Screening social phobia in adolescents from general population: the validity of the Social Phobia Inventory (SPIN) against a clinical interview. Eur Psychiatry 22:244–251

Ranta K, Junttila N, Laakkonen E, Uhmavaara A, La Greca AM, Niemi PM (2012a) Social Anxiety Scale for Adolescents (SAS-A): measuring social anxiety among Finnish adolescents. Child Psychiatry Hum Dev 43:574–591

Ranta K, Kaltiala-Heino R, Rantanen P, Marttunen M (2012b) The Mini-Social Phobia Inventory: psychometric properties in an adolescent general population sample. Compr Psychiatry 53:630–637

Reich W (1998) The Diagnostic Interview for Children and Adolescents (DICA): DSM.IV version. Washington University School of Medicine, St. Louis

Reich W (2000) Diagnostic Interview for Children and Adolescents (DICA). J Am Acad Child Adolesc Psychiatry 39:59–66

Reich W, Leacock N, Shanfeld K (1997) DICA-IV Diagnostic Interview for children and Adolescents-IV [Computer software]. Multi-Health Systems, Inc., Toronto

Reijntjes A, Dekovic M, Telch MJ (2007) Support for the predictive validity of the SASC-R. Linkages with reactions to an in vivo peer evaluation manipulation. J Anxiety Disord 21:903–917

Rescorla LA, Ginzburg S, Achenbach TM, Ivanova MY, Almqvist F, Begovac I, Verhulst FC (2013) Cross-informant agreement between parent-reported and adolescent self-reported problems in 25 societies. J Clin Child Adolesc Psychol 42:262–273. doi:10.1080/15374416.2012.717870

Rivero R, Garcia-Lopez LJ, Hofmann SG (2010) The Spanish version of the Self-Statements during Public Speaking Scale. Validation in adolescents. Eur J Psychol Assess 26:129–135

Sala R, Granero R, Ezpeleta L (2005) Dimensional analysis of a categorical diagnostic interview: the DICA-IV. Psicothema 18:123–129

Salvador MC (2009) Ser eu próprio entre os outros: um novo protocolo de intervenção para adolescentes com fobia social generalizada [To be myself among the others: a new intervention protocol for adolescentes with generalized social phobia]. Unpublished doctoral dissertation. Faculty of Psychology and Education Sciences, Coimbra University

Sandin B, Chorot P, Valiente RM, Sanchez MA, Sanchez-Arribas C (1999) Estructura factorial de la escala de ansiedad social para niños-revisada (SASC-R) [Factor structure of the SASC-R]. Rev Psicopatol Psicol Clin 4:105–113

Scaini S, Battaglia M, Beidel DC, Ogliari A (2012) A meta-analysis of the cross-cultural psychometric properties of the Social Phobia and Anxiety Inventory for Children (SPAI-C). J Anxiety Disord 26:182–188

Schmits E, Heeren A, Quertemont E (2014) The self-report version of the LSAS-CA: Psychometric properties of the French version in a non-clinical adolescent sample. Psychol Belg 54:181–198

Schorre BEH, Vandvik IH (2004) Global assessment of psychosocial functioning in child and adolescent psychiatry: a review of three unidimensional scales (CGAS, GAF, GAPD). Eur Child Adolesc Psychiatry 13:273–286

Schwab-Stone ME, Shaffer D, Dulcan MK, Jensen PS, Fisher P, Bird HR, Rae DS (1996) Criterion validity of the NIMH Diagnostic Interview Schedule for Children version 2.3 (DISC 2.3). J Am Acad Child Adolesc Psychiatry 35:878–888

Shaffer D, Gould MS, Brasic J, Ambrosini P, Fisher P, Bird H, Aluwahlia S (1983) A children's global assessment scale (CGAS). Arch Gen Psychiatry 40:1228–1231

Shaffer D, Fisher E, Dulcan MK, Davies M, Piacentini J, Schwab-Stone M, Lahey B, Bourdon K, Jensen E, Bird H, Canino G, Regier D (1996) The NIMH Diagnostic Interview Schedule for Children Version 2.3 (DISC-2.3): Description, acceptability, prevalence rates, and performance in the MECA study. J Am Acad Child Adolesc Psychiatry 35:865–877

Shaffer D, Fisher P, Lucas CP, Dulcan MK, Schwab-Stone ME (2000) NIMH Diagnostic Interview Schedule for Children Version IV (NIMH DISC-IV): Description, differences from previous versions, and reliability of some common diagnosis. J Am Acad Child Adolesc Psychiatry 39:8–39

Sheehan DV, Lecrubier Y, Sheehan KH, Janavs JY, Weiller E, Keskiner A, Dunbar GC (1997) The validity of the Mini International Neuropsychiatric Interview (MINI). According to the SCID-P and its reliability. Eur Psychiatry 12:232–241

Sheehan DV, Lecrubier Y, Sheehan KH, Amorim P, Janavs J, Weiller E, Dunbar GC (1998) The Mini International Neuropsychiatric Interview (M.I.N.I.): the development and validation of a structured diagnostic psychiatric interview for DSM-IV and ICD-10. J Clin Psychiatry 59:22–33

Sheehan DV, Sheehan KH, Shytle RD, Janavs J, Bannon Y, Rogers JE, Wilkinson B (2010) Reliability and validity of the Mini International Neuropsychiatric Interview for Children and Adolescents (MINI-KID). J Clin Psychiatry 71:313–326

Silverman WK, Albano AM (1996) Anxiety Disorders Interview Schedule for Children for DSM-IV, child and parent version. Oxford University Press, London

Silverman WK, Ollendick TH (2005) Evidence-based assessment of anxiety and its disorders in children and adolescents. J Clin Child Adolesc Psychol 34:380–411. doi:10.1207/s15374424jccp3403_2

Silverman WK, Saavedra LM, Pina AA (2001) Test-retest reliability of anxiety symptoms and diagnoses with the Anxiety Disorders Interview Schedule for DSM-IV: Child and Parent Versions. J Am Acad Child Adolesc Psychiatry 40:937–944

Smith DC, Huber DL, Hall JA (2005) Psychometric evaluation of the structured clinical interview for DSM-IV childhood diagnoses (KID-SCID). J Hum Behav Soc Environ 11:1–21

Sosic Z, Gieler U, Stangier U (2008) Screening for social phobia in medical in-and outpatients with the German version of the Social Phobia Inventory (SPIN). J Anxiety Disord 22:849–859

Spence SH (1997) Structure of anxiety symptoms among children: a confirmatory factor-analytic study. J Abnorm Psychol 106:280–297

Spence SH (1998) A measure of anxiety symptoms among children. Behav Res Ther 35: 545–566

Spence SH, Donovan C, Brechman-Toussaint M (1999) Social skills, social outcomes, and cognitive features of childhood social phobia. J Abnorm Psychol 108:211–221

Spence SH, Donovan C, Brechman-Toussaint M (2000) The treatment of childhood social phobia: the effectiveness of a social skills training-based, cognitive-behavioural intervention, with and without parental involvement. J Child Psychol Psychiatry 41:713–726

Spence SH, Barrett PM, Turner CM (2003) Psychometric properties of the Spence Children's Anxiety Scale with young adolescents. J Anxiety Disord 17:605–625

Storch EA, Eisenberg PS, Roberti JW, Barlas ME (2003) Reliability and Validity of the Social Anxiety Scale for Children-Revised for Hispanic children. Hisp J Behav Sci 25:410–422

Storch EA, Masia-Warner C, Dent HC, Roberti JW, Fisher PH (2004) Psychometric evaluation of the Social Anxiety Scale for Adolescents and the Social Phobia and Anxiety Inventory for Children: construct validity and normative data. J Anxiety Disord 18:665–679

Storch EA, Masia-Warner C, Heidgerken AD, Fisher PH, Pincus DB, Liebowitz MR (2006) Factor structure of the Liebowitz Social Anxiety Scale for Children and Adolescents. Child Psychiatry Hum Dev 37:25–37

Su L, Wang K, Fan F, Su Y, Gao X (2008) Reliability and validity of the Screen for Child Anxiety Related Emotional Disorders (SCARED) in Chinese children. J Anxiety Disord 22: 612–621

Swamidhas P, Nair MKC, Russell S, Shanmukham V, Zeena A, Nazeema S, George B (2013) ADad 2: the validation of the Screen for Child Anxiety Related Emotional Disorders for Anxiety Disorders among adolescents in a rural community population in India. Indian J Pediatry 1–5

Sweency, C., Masia-Warner C, Brice C, Stewart C, Ryan J, Loeb KL, & McGrathare RE (2015). Identification of social anxiety in schools: The utility of a two-step screening process. Manuscript submitted for publication.

Thomas SA, Aldao A, De Los Reyes A (2012) Implementing clinically feasible psychophysiological measures in evidence-based assessments of adolescent social anxiety. Prof Psychol Res Pract 43:510–519. doi:10.1037/a0029183

Trimbremont B, Braet C, Dreessen L (2004) Assessing depression in youth: relation between the children's depression inventory and a structured interview. J Clin Child Adolesc Psychol 33:149–157

Tulbure B, Szentagotai A, Dobrean A, David D (2012) Evidence based clinical assessment of child and adolescent social phobia: a critical review of rating scales. Child Psychiatry Hum Dev 43:795–820

Turner SM, Beidel DC, Costello A (1987) Psychopathology in the offspring of anxiety disorders patients. J Consult Clin Psychol 55:229–235

Turner SM, Beidel DC, Dancu CV, Stanley MA (1989) An empirically derived inventory to measure social fears and anxiety: the Social Phobia and Anxiety Inventory. Psychol Assess 1:35–40

Vera-Villarroel PE, Olivares J, Kuhne W, Rosa AI, Santibáñez C, López-Pina JA (2007) Propiedades psicométricas de la Escala para la Detección de la Ansiedad Social (EDAS) en una muestra de adolescentes chilenos. Int J Clin Health Psychol 7:795–806

Vieira S, Salvador MC, Matos AP, Garcia-Lopez LJ, Beidel D (2011) Validación de la versión breve del Inventario de ansiedad, & fobia social (SPAI-B) para adolescentes en población portuguesa [Validação da Versão Breve do Inventário de Ansiedade e Fobia Social (SPAI-B) para Adolescentes na população Portuguesa]. Psiquiatr Clin 32:139–147

Vieira S, Salvador MC, Matos AP, Garcia-Lopez LJ, Beidel D (2013) Inventario de Fobia, & Ansiedad Social- Versión Breve: Propiedades psicométricas en una muestra de adolescentes portugueses [SPAI-B: Psychometric properties in a sample of Portuguese adolescents]. Behav Psychol 21:25–38

Vigil-Colet A, Canals J, Cosí S, Lorenzo-Seva U, Ferrando PJ, Hernández-Martínez C, Jané C, Viñas F, Doménech E (2009) The factorial structure of the 41-item versión of the Screen for Child Anxiety Related Emotional Disorders (SCARED) in a Spanish population of 8 to 12 years-old. Int J Clin Health Psychol 9:313–327

Vilete LMP, Coutinho EAF, Figueira ILV (2004) Reliability of the Portuguese-language version of the Social Phobia Inventory (SPIN) among adolescent students in the city of Rio de Janeiro. Cad Saúde Pública 20:89–99

Wagner KD, Berard R, Stein MD, Wetherhold E, Carpenter DJ, Perera P, Machin A (2004) A multicenter, randomized, double-blind, placebo-controlled trial of paroxetine in children and adolescents with social anxiety disorder. Arch Gen Psychiatry 61:1153–1162

Watson D, Friend R (1969) Measurement of social-evaluative anxiety. J Consult Clin Psychol 33:448–457

Weiss BJ, Hope DA, Capozzoli MC (2013) Heterocentric language in commonly used measures of social anxiety: recommended alternate wording. Behav Ther 44:1–11

Weldner Z, Reich W, Herjanic B, Jung KG, Amado H (1987) Reliability, validity and parent–child agreement studies of the Diagnostic Interview for Children and Adolescents (DICA). J Am Acad Child Adolesc Psychiatry 26:649–653

Wood JJ, Piacentini JC, Bergman RL, McCracken J, Barrios V (2002) Concurrent validity of the anxiety disorders section of the Anxiety Disorders Interview Schedule for DSM-IV: child and parent Versions. J Clin Child Adolesc Psychol 31:335–342

Yen JY, Ko C-H, Yen C-F, Wu HY, Yang M-J (2007) The comorbid psychiatric symptoms of internet addiction: Attention Deficit and Hyperactivity Disorder (ADHD), depression, social phobia, and hostility. J Adolesc Health 41:93–98

Youngstrom EA, De Los Reyes A (2015) Commentary: Moving towards cost-effectiveness in using psychophysiological measures in clinical assessment: validity, decision-making, and adding value. J Clin Child Adolesc Psychol 44:352–361. doi: 10.1080/15374416.2014.913252

Zaider TI, Heimberg RG, Fresco DM, Schneier FR, Liebowitz MR (2003) Evaluation of the Clinical Global Impression Scale among individuals with social anxiety disorder. Psychol Med 33:11–22

Social Anxiety and the School Environment of Adolescents

7

Anke W. Blöte, Anne C. Miers, David A. Heyne, and P. Michiel Westenberg

During the school week, adolescents ordinarily spend somewhere between one-third and one-half of their waking time at school, necessitating a considerable degree of social interaction. As noted by McShane et al. (2004), the climate at secondary school is one of "forced and broad social interaction" (p. 54). In adolescence, peers also become a major influence in the life of the young person. As Eckert (1989) put it: "In secondary school, where the social structure of the student cohort dominates virtually all aspects of life in the institution, choices in all domains are restricted, not so clearly by adult judgment as by peer social boundaries" (p. 12). On the one hand, social interactions within school settings can be very stimulating for the developing adolescent and promote efficient and successful learning of the educational curriculum and life skills. On the other hand, these social interactions bring with them a less positive aspect, namely, the possibility that one will be negatively judged and evaluated.

Empirical findings show a normative increase in subjective and physiological sensitivity to negative evaluation from age peers during adolescence (Van den Bos et al. 2014; Westenberg et al. 2004). The inherently social nature of school combined with a developmental increase in sensitivity to negative evaluation highlights the potential influence of this setting on the adolescent. Being placed under the scrutiny of others in social situations can cause concern and worry and may increase or at least maintain social anxiety in some students.

Social anxiety occurs in degrees. Concern or apprehension about a social situation is described as being at the lower end of a continuum of social anxiety, with intense social anxiety at the upper end (Rapee and Spence 2004). A sizeable

A.W. Blöte, PhD (✉) • A.C. Miers, PhD •
D.A. Heyne, BA, Dip Ed Psych, M Psych, PhD • P.M. Westenberg, PhD
Developmental & Educational Psychology Unit,
Institute of Psychology, Faculty of Social and Behavioural Sciences,
Leiden University, Leiden, The Netherlands
e-mail: bloete@fsw.leidenuniv.nl

K. Ranta et al. (eds.), *Social Anxiety and Phobia in Adolescents: Development, Manifestation and Intervention Strategies*, DOI 10.1007/978-3-319-16703-9_7

group of adolescents are very anxious about social situations and potential negative evaluation from others (Gren-Landell et al. 2009). In these cases, a high level of anxiety for social situations may interfere with their daily functioning. Giving an oral presentation, answering questions in class, making friends, and participating in cliques or gangs are all potentially stressful for them. In these situations, they may be ridiculed, excluded, or even victimized. The socially anxious student may stop socializing with classmates and friends, stop attending certain classes, or even refuse to attend school altogether. This can have severe and detrimental consequences for their cognitive and social development as well as their academic achievements (Van Ameringen et al. 2003).

This chapter begins with a description of the way social anxiety manifests itself in the school setting. More specifically, we review situations which are distressful for and even avoided by socially anxious students. An extreme consequence of this distress and avoidance, school refusal, is also discussed. In the second part of the chapter, we describe the way in which socially anxious students' behavior, and the behavior of their peers or classmates, may contribute to the difficulty that socially anxious youth experience during social interactions at school. In addition to these behavioral and interpersonal factors, we pay attention to the negative social cognitions of socially anxious students. We discuss whether, and to what extent, these negative cognitions are biased or contain a kernel of truth (Norton and Hope 2001). Finally, we present some considerations for intervention and future research.

The Manifestation of Social Anxiety in the School Setting

Distress and Avoidance in Specific School Situations

What do we know about how adolescents with high levels of social anxiety experience social situations in school settings? Two studies focused on how socially anxious and non-anxious adolescents differed in their fear and avoidance of school-related social situations (Gren-Landell et al. 2009; Ranta et al. 2012). Two other studies investigated fear and avoidance of social situations in adolescents with clinical social anxiety levels only (Beidel et al. 2007; Rao et al. 2007), and three investigated adolescents from the general population (Essau et al. 1999; Ranta et al. 2007; Wittchen et al. 1999). The following overview begins with the two studies conducted with clinical samples.

In a sample of 150 children and adolescents with clinical social anxiety levels, Rao et al. (2007) used the Anxiety Disorders Interview Schedule for Children (ADIS-C; Silverman and Albano 1996) to investigate distress and avoidance related to 20 different social situations. More than 80 % of adolescents (13–17 years) diagnosed with Social Anxiety Disorder (SAD) reported moderate-to-severe distress in the school situations focused on "giving oral reports/presentations" and "asking teacher a question." These two situations were also frequently avoided. Respectively, 71.1 and 73.7 % of adolescents reported at least moderate avoidance. Fewer adolescents reported at least moderate distress or avoidance in other school situations focused on "taking tests" and "participating in gym class." Across all situations adolescents reported significantly greater fear and more avoidance than did children. Specifically, a significantly higher percentage of adolescents than children reported moderate-to-severe distress and at least moderate avoidance in the school situations "asking teacher a question" and "writing on chalkboard." Children and adolescents did not differ in distress or avoidance for the situations "giving oral reports/presentations" or "taking tests" (Rao et al. 2007). In the Beidel et al. (2007) study, which also used the ADIS-C in a study of 63 adolescents (aged 13–16 years) with social anxiety disorder, very similar results were reported. The school situations "oral reports or reading aloud" and "asking the teacher a question or asking for help" were again two of the most distressing social situations reported by adolescents. The percentages of adolescents endorsing at least moderate distress in those two school situations were 90.5 and 87.3 %, respectively. Furthermore, these situations were also frequently avoided. Respectively, 65.1 and 69.8 % reported at least moderate avoidance (Beidel et al. 2007). In all, these two studies conducted with clinical populations show a very high prevalence of fear and avoidance of school-related social situations.

Other studies have investigated the frequency of social fears and/or avoidance in community samples of adolescents. Essau et al. (1999) investigated the frequency of social fears in a large community sample of German adolescents aged 12–17 years. The most commonly feared social situations were performance/test situations and public speaking, reportedly feared by 31.1 and 19.7 % of the sample, respectively. In a second, large sample of 14–24-year-olds, Wittchen et al. (1999) reported a slightly lower prevalence, with 18.2 and 13.2 % of the sample fearing performance/test situations and public speaking, respectively. Ranta et al. (2007) administered the Social Phobia Inventory (SPIN; Connor et al. 2000) in a large Finnish population sample of adolescents aged between 12 and 16 years. Just over 12 % of the sample reported extreme avoidance of speeches (Ranta et al. 2007). The situations investigated in these three studies are not specific to the school setting, and the findings are not related to adolescents' general level of social anxiety. Hence, these studies do not specifically inform about the impact of school-related social situations on socially anxious adolescents.

Gren-Landell et al. (2009) study of a large sample of Swedish adolescents (12–14 years) attending secondary school investigated the fear of specific social situations, including school situations, using a self-report measure. The school situations included in the questionnaire were "speaking in front of the class," "raising your hand during a lesson," "being together with others during breaks," and "eating together with others during lunch break." In the total sample, "speaking in front of the class" was the most feared situation, with 6.2 % endorsing marked fear of this situation. Of the students who fulfilled DSM-IV criteria for SAD ($n=93$), 63.4 % reported marked fear in the situation "speaking in front of the class"; this was the most common fear in this group. In contrast, only 3.6 % of the students who did not fulfill SAD criteria ($n=2{,}035$) reported marked fear in this school situation. For the other three school situations, up to 15 % of adolescents in the SAD group reported marked fear in contrast with 2.3 % of the non-SAD group

(Gren-Landell et al. 2009). In a second study, Ranta et al. (2012) compared a group of adolescents (12–17 years) diagnosed with SAD ($n=22$) with a group without SAD ($n=299$). Based on reports on the SPIN, 64 % of the SAD group reported avoiding speeches at least "very much" versus 31 % of the non-SAD group. Although the latter study did not focus on school situations specifically, the results are consistent with those of Gren-Landell et al. (2009), inasmuch as more than 60 % of clinically socially anxious adolescents reported moderate fear or avoidance of speech situations.

The impact of school-related social situations on adolescents with high levels of social anxiety is well illustrated by findings from the Social Anxiety and Normal Development (SAND) study (Westenberg et al. 2009). This study made use of a sample of adolescents with a wide range of social anxiety levels. The adolescents completed a questionnaire that asked how distressed they felt in 20 different social situations and how frequently they tried to avoid these situations (Sumter et al. 2009). The questionnaire was based on the social phobia module from the ADIS-C (Silverman and Albano 1996). The questionnaire includes situations that are specific to the school context such as answering questions in class, giving a speech in class, and asking the teacher a question or asking for help. The distress and avoidance questions are answered on a 9-point scale. For the present chapter, we compared the socially anxious and non-anxious adolescents, as described below.

A group of high and low socially anxious adolescents was selected (12–18 years), using scores on the Social Anxiety Scale for Adolescents (SAS-A; La Greca and Lopez 1998). Forty high socially anxious adolescents were selected based on their scoring in the top 20 % of their gender-specific distribution. The high socially anxious group had a mean SAS-A score of 56.73, which is above the clinical cutoff recommended by La Greca (1998). Subsequently, an equal number of adolescents were selected with low (but not the lowest) social anxiety scores, SAS-A scores between 10 and 32 % according to the gender-specific distribution. The percentage of adolescents in each social anxiety group (high and low) endorsing a low, moderate, and high degree of distress and avoidance is presented in Table 7.1. The table presents distress and avoidance results for all 20 social situations included in the questionnaire, but for the purposes of this chapter, we now focus our discussion on the social situations that are relevant to the school context.

With regard to experienced distress, significant differences between high and low socially anxious adolescents can be seen, particularly in the following school-related social situations: "answering questions in class," "giving a speech in class," "reading aloud in class," "writing on the board," and "taking tests." For the majority of these five school situations, none of those in the low socially anxious group endorsed high distress, compared to between 6 and 25 % of those in the high socially anxious group. As well as experiencing more distress in school-related social situations, high socially anxious adolescents were more likely to try to avoid these situations relative to low socially anxious adolescents. For the classroom situations "answering questions," "giving a speech," "reading aloud," and "writing on the board," between 20 and 27 % of high socially anxious adolescents indicated high avoidance, compared to 7 % or fewer of low socially anxious adolescents.

Table 7.1 Distress and avoidance per ADIS situation in high (HSA) and low (LSA) socially anxious participants aged 12 years and older

ADIS situation	Distress %							Avoidance %						
	Low (0–2)		Moderate (3–5)		High (6–8)		Mann-Whitney U	Low (0–2)		Moderate (3–5)		High (6–8)		Mann-Whitney U
	LSA	HSA	LSA	HSA	LSA	HSA		LSA	HSA	LSA	HSA	LSA	HSA	
1. Answering questions in class	95.5	72.7	2.3	20.5	2.3	6.8	751.0*	81.8	52.3	15.9	27.3	2.3	20.5	**656.5***
2. Giving a speech in class	79.5	47.7	20.5	27.3	0	25.0	**610.5****	84.1	54.5	9.1	18.2	6.8	27.3	**670.0***
3. Reading aloud in class	95.5	59.1	4.5	29.5	0	11.4	**611.0****	86.4	63.6	11.4	11.4	2.3	25.0	723.0*
4. Asking the teacher a question or for help	95.5	77.3	4.5	18.2	0	4.5	790.0	86.4	70.5	11.4	13.6	2.3	15.9	799.5
5. Taking tests	88.6	65.9	11.4	18.2	0	15.9	730.5*	90.9	84.1	6.8	4.5	2.3	11.4	895.5
6. Writing on the board	100	70.5	0	15.9	0	13.6	**682.0****	90.9	63.6	6.8	13.6	2.3	22.7	**692.0***
7. Working/playing with a group of kids	100	86.4	0	13.6	0	0	836.0	95.5	81.8	4.5	15.9	0	2.3	835.0
8. Gym class	95.5	79.5	2.3	15.9	2.3	4.5	816.5	88.6	86.4	6.8	9.1	4.5	4.5	947.0
9. Walking in the hallways	97.7	77.3	2.3	20.5	0	2.3	769.5*	100	86.4	0	9.1	0	4.5	836.0
10. Starting or joining in on a conversation	97.7	86.4	2.3	9.1	0	4.5	857.0	97.7	77.3	2.3	13.6	0	9.1	**768.0***
11. Using school or public bathrooms	90.9	79.5	9.1	13.6	0	6.8	852.0	75.0	61.4	11.4	20.5	13.6	18.2	843.0
12. Eating in front of others	95.5	70.5	4.5	22.7	0	6.8	**723.0***	97.7	84.1	2.3	6.8	0	9.1	834.0
13. Meetings such as scouts or team	97.7	84.1	0	11.4	2.3	4.5	838.5	93.2	81.8	6.8	13.6	0	4.5	855.0
14. Answering or talking on the telephone	93.2	77.3	6.8	15.9	0	6.8	809.5	86.4	63.6	13.6	25.0	0	11.4	733.0*

Table 7.1 (continued)

ADIS situation	Distress %							Avoidance %						
	Low (0–2)		Moderate (3–5)		High (6–8)		Mann-Whitney U	Low (0–2)		Moderate (3–5)		High (6–8)		Mann-Whitney U
	LSA	HSA	LSA	HSA	LSA	HSA		LSA	HSA	LSA	HSA	LSA	HSA	
15. Musical or athletic performances	90.9	59.1	9.1	20.5	0	20.5	**642.0****	90.9	68.2	6.8	15.9	2.3	15.9	741.0*
16. Inviting a friend to get together	95.5	75.0	4.5	18.2	0	6.8	767.0*	93.2	77.3	6.8	15.9	0	6.8	809.5
17. Speaking to an adult	97.7	79.5	2.3	13.6	0	6.8	790.5*	97.7	72.7	2.3	20.5	0	6.8	**724.5***
18. Talking to persons you don't know well	100	47.7	0	31.8	0	20.5	**462.0****	97.7	54.5	2.3	18.2	0	27.3	**544.0****
19. Attending parties	93.2	79.5	4.5	11.4	2.3	9.1	834.5	90.9	84.1	6.8	9.1	2.3	6.8	899.5
20. Having picture taken	97.7	75.0	2.3	20.5	0	4.5	**747.0***	95.5	77.3	2.3	15.9	2.3	6.8	794.0

$^{**}p<.001$; $^{*}p<.01$; (1-tailed). *P* values in bold <.0025 (Bonferroni correction). HSA=44 (23 boys, 21 girls), LSA=44 (20 boys, 24 girls). HSA-LSA differences tested with Mann-Whitney U

Remarkably, the school-related situations associated with "asking the teacher a question/for help" and "working/playing with a group of kids" (both of which may occur in the classroom but are not limited to the classroom) did not show social anxiety group differences for distress and avoidance. The lack of group differences for these situations may be because students can choose whether to ask a question and when and where to ask it and can choose with whom they work or play. In contrast, the activities causing considerable distress and avoidance for high socially anxious students – "answering questions," "giving a speech," "reading aloud" and "writing on the board" – are all guided by the teacher and therefore offer the student little to no choice.

A consistent finding in the studies reviewed here is that socially anxious adolescents are particularly fearful of, and would like to avoid, *public performance* situations in their own classroom: "giving a speech in class," "reading aloud in class," "raising your hand during lessons," "asking or answering questions in class," and "writing on the board." This is likely to have negative consequences for the socially anxious adolescent and might lead to, for example, decreased participation in school activities and thus lower academic results. In contrast, socially anxious adolescents report less fear and avoidance of other classroom situations (e.g., "asking teacher for help," "working with group of kids"). These situations do not directly expose the adolescent to public scrutiny and might offer more choice with respect to interaction partners. The possibility of choosing one's interaction partner(s) is relevant to socially anxious adolescents because this could provide the opportunity to minimize the likelihood of being negatively treated or victimized (section "Factors explaining social anxiety in the school setting"), thereby reducing fear for, and avoidance of, these types of school situations.

School Refusal

Social Anxiety and School Absenteeism

Because of the inherently social nature of school, it is self-evident that social anxiety would sometimes contribute to school absenteeism. Studies of adults' retrospective reports provide tenuous support for this notion. For example, Davidson et al. (1993) found that a marginally significantly higher proportion of adults with SAD reported that they "played truant at least twice in a year" during schooling relative to adults without SAD (p. 713). In Van Ameringen and colleagues' (2003) study of anxiety-disordered adults, there were 98 subjects who reported that they "thought that they left school prematurely" (p. 565). Of these, the majority (61 %) had a current diagnosis of generalized social phobia (GSP). One hundred and three subjects did not think that they left school early. Only 45 % of this group had a current diagnosis of GSP, and this percentage was significantly less compared with the percentage (61 %) of those who left school prematurely. The problem with adult studies such as these is that they do not establish a concurrent relationship between social anxiety and school absenteeism.

Stronger evidence comes from a number of community-based cross-sectional studies conducted with the youth. In a German study of over 3,000 adolescents and young adults (14–24 years; Wittchen et al. 1999), it was found that 57 % of those with GSP reported that "social fears or avoidance interfered a lot" with work, school, or household management (p. 312). Further, 15 % of those with GSP reported being unable to go to school or work on at least 3 days in the past month as a result of GSP. Among 174 African-American youth (*M* age = 11.7 years), a positive association was found between actual/desired avoidance of situations involving interaction with peers or evaluation in class, on the one hand, and unexcused absences from school on the other hand (Lyon 2010). Presumably the youth's actual or desired avoidance of social or evaluative situations at school was fueled by some degree of social anxiety. No associations were found between unexcused absences and nonsocial factors such as the pursuit of attention from parents. In a survey conducted in the continental United States with over 10,000 adolescents (13–18 years), those diagnosed with SAD were found to report greater impairment in the area of school/work (in the worst month of the past year) relative to shy adolescents and adolescents with no shyness (Burstein et al. 2011). Unfortunately rates of school absenteeism were not reported. Most recently, a study of 865 Norwegian adolescents (16–21 years; *M* age = 17.2 years) involved a comparison between high-anxious youth often absent from school and high-anxious youth attending school regularly (Ingul and Nordahl 2013). Those who were often absent from school had higher social anxiety and fewer close friends. Because absenteeism was analyzed categorically rather than dimensionally, it is premature to conclude that progressively higher levels of social anxiety will be associated with progressively higher levels of absenteeism.

The aforementioned studies conducted with young people predominantly focused on adolescence. This is a developmental period in which the prevalence of SAD increases (Costello et al. 2003) and the prevalence of school attendance problems increases (Heyne 2006; Nakamura et al. 2010). A relationship between social anxiety and school absenteeism may also exist earlier in development, as suggested by the study of Weeks et al. (2009). In their predominantly Caucasian sample of 178 Canadian children (7–8 years; *M* age = 7.6 years), a positive association was found between social anxiety and the desire to avoid school. Perhaps the desire to avoid school during childhood does not translate into school absenteeism as quickly as it does in adolescence. That is, the parents of a socially anxious child may be more willing and able to get their child to attend school than are the parents of a socially anxious adolescent.

Social Anxiety and School Refusal

School refusal is a type of school attendance problem that is often differentiated from truancy (Heyne et al. in press). The term "school refusal" is used to describe a young person's reluctance or refusal to attend school when it is paired with emotional distress (e.g., fearfulness, anxiety, somatic complaints, unhappiness); is not concealed from parents and often involves the young person staying at home; and is not associated with severe antisocial behavior (Berg 1997, 2002; Berg et al. 1969;

Bools et al. 1990). Truancy, on the other hand, is said to occur when a young person is absent from school and the parents do not know about the child's absence (Kearney 2002) or whereabouts (Berg et al. 1985). Moreover, truancy is often associated with severe antisocial behaviors (Vaughn et al. 2013), and it is not commonly associated with anxiety (Heyne et al. in press). Following, we review literature indicating the extent to which the serious problem of school refusal may be associated with social factors, especially social anxiety. We also review the negative impact that social factors seem to have on the short- and longer-term well-being of school-refusing youth.

In an early study of 29 youth (*M* age = 14.9 years) diagnosed with DSM-III-R social phobia, Strauss and Last (1993) found that the most common fear exhibited was "a fear of school" (p. 146). Indeed, almost two-thirds (64 %) of the socially phobic youth exhibited a fear of school. It is worth bearing in mind, however, that a fear of school is not synonymous with the presence of school refusal as defined by Berg and colleagues (Berg 1997, 2002; Berg et al. 1969; Bools et al. 1990). We turn now to studies which were based on samples of school refusers selected according to the comprehensive criteria of Berg and colleagues.

Place et al. (2002) interviewed the families of 17 school refusers (aged 12–15 years). These youth had difficulty with peer relationships, a sense of isolation (most did not belong to a friendship group when they started secondary school), and were bullied and teased at school. It is likely that social anxiety contributed to or stemmed from the social difficulties experienced by these school-refusing youth. Heyne et al. (1998) assessed self-efficacy among 135 children and adolescents (5–15 years; *M* age = 11.4 years) referred for school refusal. Across the sample, youth's perception of their ability to cope was lowest for the social-related situation of answering peers' questions about absences from school and highest for the non-social situation of doing schoolwork. The low level of self-efficacy for the social-related situation may be associated with social anxiety, in line with Rudy et al. (2014) finding that social self-efficacy uniquely contributed to levels of social anxiety among youth. In Buitelaar et al. (1994) follow-up study of 25 school-refusing adolescents (*M* age at referral = 14.8 years), the majority were found to have "unsatisfactory or insufficient social relationships" prior to referral (p. 251). Further, one of the most common diagnoses at initial contact was avoidant disorder of childhood or adolescence (AD), which overlaps extensively with SAD (APA 1994). In another study of school-refusing adolescents (11–17 years; *M* = 14.6 years), SAD was a primary or secondary diagnosis among approximately two-thirds of the sample (65 %; Heyne et al. 2011).

Two additional studies reportedly investigated school refusal even though Berg and colleagues' school refusal criteria were not used to recruit subjects. Bernstein et al. (2001) studied 41 adolescents (*M* age = 15.8 years) who attended school less than 80 % of the time and were diagnosed with both an anxiety disorder and a depressive disorder. About two-thirds (67 %) of these adolescents had a diagnosis of SAD. In the Beidas et al. (2010) study of children and adolescents (7–16 years; *M* = 11.0 years) with "denial to attend school or difficulty remaining in school," it was found that more youth presented with a principal diagnosis of SAD (n = 11) than with generalized anxiety disorder ($n=7$) or separation anxiety disorder ($n=9$) (p. 255).

Results from the aforementioned studies of referred school refusers need to be interpreted cautiously because of a bias that may occur due to referral and intake procedures. In one setting, for example, school refusers may be referred to a school refusal program, and in another setting, they may be referred to a general anxiety team. If school refusers are referred to an anxiety team because of the co-occurrence of anxiety symptoms, and a study is then based on a sample drawn from this population, there may be an inflated association between school refusal and anxiety symptoms. Community-based studies provide a less biased picture of the relationship between social anxiety and school refusal. Recently, Nair et al. (2013) reported on a community sample of 500 adolescents (11–19 years) from rural India. Based on logistic regression, a significant association was found between meeting SAD diagnostic criteria and meeting the criteria for school refusal,[1] even when controlling for comorbid major depressive disorder and dysthymia. The odds ratio statistic indicated an eightfold increase of school refusal among adolescents meeting criteria for SAD. A decade earlier, the largest comprehensive community-based study of school attendance problems was conducted by Egger et al. (2003). These researchers studied school attendance problems according to type, drawing on data from more than 1,400 youth aged 9–16 years from North Carolina in the United States. They found that being shy with peers, having difficulty making friends, and being bullied or teased were significantly associated with anxious school refusal. The same social factors were not associated with truancy. In an uncorrected model, the diagnosis of SAD was significantly associated with school refusal and not with truancy. In a corrected model (i.e., controlling for the effects of comorbid disorders), SAD was not associated with school refusal, probably because SAD was highly predictive of simple phobia and depression, both of which were associated with school refusal in uncorrected models. It may be that many socially anxious youth find it difficult to attend school *because of* the depressive affect they experience when confronted with school, and the school setting may have become a phobic stimulus because of the socially challenging aspects of school.

There is currently no research on the direction of influence between social factors and school refusal. Anecdotally, Buitelaar et al. (1994) referred to "the importance of social relationship factors in the development of school refusal" (p. 252). It is feasible that social anxiety is one of the factors that contributes to the development of school refusal, but also to its maintenance. It is equally feasible that school refusal perpetuates social anxiety. As noted by Albano (1995), continued absence from school severely reduces the quality and number of opportunities for socially anxious school refusers to increase social interactions. Consequently, there are fewer opportunities for interventions such as socially-related exposure tasks and practicing social skills. Longitudinal studies are needed in order to determine the

[1] The authors used the term "school phobia," and adolescents were deemed to have school phobia if their score on the school phobia subscale of the self-report Screen for Child Anxiety Related Emotional Disorders (SCARED) was ≥ 3.

(bi)directionality of the relationship between social anxiety and school refusal and to determine which factors moderate and mediate the relationship.

The relationship between social anxiety and school refusal appears to be age related. Kearney and Albano (2004) examined the function of youths' school refusal, drawing on questionnaire responses from 143 youth (5–17 years; $M = 11.6$) and their parents. Youth who refused school to escape from aversive social and/or evaluative situations were typically older, whereas younger school refusers were more likely to endorse other reasons for refusing to attend. More specifically, the mean age of youth seeking to escape aversive social and/or evaluative situations was 14.4 years ($SD = 1.8$), whereas youth seeking to avoid stimuli that provoke negative affectivity were 11.8 years on average ($SD = 2.7$), youth refusing school for attention were 9.2 years on average ($SD = 2.8$), and youth pursuing tangible reinforcement outside of school were 12.9 years on average ($SD = 2.8$). Although this study did not measure social anxiety per se, the older youth's motivation to escape aversive social and/or evaluative situations is clearly related to social anxiety. Last and Strauss (1990) reported that, at intake, school refusers with SAD were older than school refusers with separation anxiety disorder.

The higher prevalence of social anxiety among older school refusers, as reported by Last and Strauss (1990), may simply be a reflection of the higher prevalence of SAD among older youth relative to younger youth (e.g., Costello et al. 2003). It might also be explained by the increasingly complex and demanding nature of the secondary school environment relative to the primary school environment. Galloway (1985) argued that, as the child grows older, school attendance problems are increasingly under the influence of school-based factors. At secondary school the student is confronted with a larger and more complex social environment involving multiple teachers, moving between classes, and needing to function more autonomously (Steinberg 2005, cited in Holmbeck et al. 2012). These aspects of secondary schooling, combined with the increasing importance of the peer context during adolescence, may lead some vulnerable youth to become overwhelmed and to escape to the security of the home environment.

There is accumulating evidence that social anxiety is associated with poor response to treatment for school refusal. In Bernstein and colleagues' (2001) 1-year follow-up of school-refusing adolescents treated with cognitive-behavioral therapy (CBT) plus imipramine or CBT plus placebo, the retention rate of disorders was higher for SAD (50 % retention) and AD (50 % retention) relative to other disorders. In further analysis of data from the original cohort, Layne et al. (2003) found that the presence of AD was a significant predictor of poorer school attendance at posttreatment.[2] There was no treatment group by diagnosis (AD/no AD) interaction effect, suggesting that the additional use of pharmacotherapy does not change the impact of social avoidance on the outcome of CBT for school refusal. Heyne et al. (2011) reported that school attendance 2 months following treatment was lower for school-refusing adolescents who still met criteria for SAD (18 % of school-time attended) relative to those who had no disorder or a disorder other than SAD following

[2] Social anxiety disorder was not analyzed as a predictor of treatment outcome.

treatment (68 % of school-time attended). Interestingly, adolescent school refusers who still met criteria for SAD at 2-month follow-up less commonly had friends in the same class at pretreatment, relative to adolescents who did not meet criteria for SAD at follow-up (50 % versus 80 %, respectively). McShane et al. (2004) investigated longer-term outcomes for 192 youth who were aged between 12 and 18 years when treated for school refusal. A pretreatment diagnosis of SAD was found to predict poorer functional outcomes (i.e., unemployment or home schooling) 3 years after treatment. More specifically, only 40 % of those with SAD at pretreatment were doing well 3 years after treatment, compared with 79 % of those without SAD.

In all, social anxiety and related social factors (e.g., difficulty with peer relationships) are linked to the difficulty that some young people have with attending school regularly. Among school refusers with SAD, the refusal to attend school may be regarded as the avoidance component of the youths' social anxiety. Studies suggest that SAD among school-refusing adolescents is often treatment resistant and that SAD is associated with poor outcomes well after the end of treatment for school refusal. Suggestions to improve outcomes for school refusers with SAD have included the following: adjunctive interventions such as social skills training and pharmacotherapy (Layne et al. 2003); starting with individual treatment and progressing to group-based treatment (Albano 1995); greater flexibility at school, such as reduced academic demands for adolescents already burdened with the challenge of social anxiety (Heyne et al. 2011); longer and more intensive treatment (Heyne et al. 2011; McShane et al. 2004); and targeting social isolation and promoting participation in prosocial activities (Ingul and Nordahl 2013). According to Place et al. (2000); there is little likelihood of school refusers ever returning to mainstream schooling if peer functioning cannot be improved.

Factors Explaining Social Anxiety in the School Setting

Social Interactions with Classmates

Socially anxious adolescents may encounter all sorts of negative outcomes from their interactions with classmates. The range of negative behaviors that can be experienced in the classroom varies from neglect, and lack of acceptance and support at one end to rejection and direct teasing and physical aggression at the other (see Kingery et al. 2010 for a review). The relation between social anxiety and these forms of victimization appears to be bidirectional (for a review, please see Garcia-Lopez et al. 2011). A meta-analysis of longitudinal studies showed that internalizing problems, including withdrawal and anxiety, predicted an increase in peer victimization and peer victimization, in turn, predicted an increase in internalizing problems (Reijntjes et al. 2010). Socially anxious students seem to be trapped in a vicious cycle of social anxiety and victimization (Ollendick and Hirshfeld-Becker 2002; Siegel et al. 2009). This conclusion is based on studies using self-report measures (e.g., La Greca and Harrison 2005; Ranta et al. 2009; Storch and Masia-Warner 2004) as well as ratings from classmates in sociometric studies (e.g., Erath et al. 2007; Inderbitzen et al. 1997). Furthermore, observations in the school and classroom have substantiated the negative treatment of socially anxious students (Blöte et al. 2007, 2010; Spence et al. 1999).

Some features of the social environment may to some extent protect socially anxious youth against the harmful effects of negative peer treatment. For example, the number and quality of friendships, being a member of a "crowd" (be it a high-status or low-status crowd), and being liked by at least some peers have all been found to predict lower levels of social anxiety (La Greca and Harrison 2005; London et al. 2007) over time. However, there is no evidence that friendship and crowd membership variables play a mediating or moderating role in the link between victimization and social anxiety (La Greca and Harrison 2005). These variables predicted lower levels of social anxiety independent of the degree of victimization.

In the following section, we explore *why* socially anxious adolescents are treated in a negative way by classmates. We firstly address factors in socially anxious students themselves and then factors in the peer group.

Factors in the Socially Anxious Student

Most socially anxious youth are withdrawn, inhibited, or shy in the social situations they fear. They lack social skills or, if they have those skills, do not employ them in feared situations (Kingery et al. 2010). They may show safety behaviors (Clark 2001; Garcia-Lopez 2013; Hodson et al. 2008; Ranta et al. 2014) to keep the social interaction at a minimum (e.g., by avoiding eye contact and keeping quiet, using "shadow friend") and to prevent making a negative impression on others (e.g., by firmly holding an object to keep their trembling under control or keeping their arms close to their body to hide sweat stains). A number of studies have been conducted on the relation between these behavioral features and peer responses, some of the studies in the domain of social anxiety and some in the domain of social withdrawal and inhibition.

At the behavioral level, there is a clear overlap between social anxiety and social withdrawal and inhibition, although not all socially anxious adolescents are inhibited and withdrawn, with some even being risk-seeking and aggressive (Erath et al. 2012; Hanby et al. 2012). At the same time, not all socially withdrawn, inhibited youth will be socially anxious, although in childhood as well as adolescence, social withdrawal is associated with (social) anxiety (Rubin and Coplan 2004). The reason we do not know the extent to which social withdrawal overlaps with social anxiety is that social anxiety studies and social withdrawal studies are conducted in different domains of psychological/psychiatric research, the clinical psychology and developmental psychology domain, respectively (Kingery et al. 2010). Nevertheless, studies on social withdrawal and its consequences for young people's development might be useful in understanding the peer relations of socially anxious youth. For this reason, we review these studies in this chapter.

In the following sections, we address the question of what actually determines whether socially anxious adolescents will be neglected, disliked, rejected, or victimized in their school environment. Is it because of socially anxious students' social withdrawal, their safety behaviors, lack of confidence, and nervousness? Is it perhaps because their anxiety is expressed in their body posture, facial expression, voice, way of verbally communicating, and physical appearance? We also consider how much time it takes before these students are perceived as socially anxious and are treated in a negative way. We therefore discuss studies related to (a) the first impression that socially anxious adolescents make on peers who are not acquainted with them; (b) research on emerging social relations in new peer groups; and (c) socially anxious adolescents' ongoing relations in groups with familiar peers.

First Impressions

Recently, a few studies investigated the impression that socially anxious adolescents make on unfamiliar peers. A study by Miers et al. (2010) addressed peer perceptions of the social performance of socially anxious youth. Participants in this study were adolescents aged between 13 and 17 years, divided into a high and a low socially anxious group based on their anxiety scores on the SAS-A (La Greca and Lopez 1998). These participants gave a speech in front of a prerecorded audience. Video-recorded 2-min fragments of the speeches were observed by whole school classes of unfamiliar peers who individually rated the fragments. Peer observers rated speaker behavior on speech content, facial expressions, posture/body movement, and way of speaking (voice, language). Results showed that high socially anxious speakers were judged as performing more poorly on all four behavioral aspects. After controlling for self-reported depressive symptoms, the differences between the high- and low-anxiety groups were still significant, except for facial expression. So, peer responses to the speakers' behavior could mainly be ascribed to speakers' social anxiety and not their depressed mood. Furthermore, the four aspects of perceived speaker behavior were strongly related, and the authors concluded that because no particular behavior made a unique contribution to predicting which group speakers belonged to (i.e., high or low anxious), there may be a general lack of social skills in socially anxious speakers. An alternative conclusion reached by the authors was that socially anxious speakers exhibit certain behavior that elicits a negative halo effect (a general impression determining the judgment of individual qualities of a person, Thorndike 1920) in other people's judgments.

Another study further supports the proposition that socially anxious adolescents make a general negative impression on unfamiliar peers, and it also presents evidence regarding mediators in the social anxiety – rejection link. Blöte et al. (2015) divided adolescents (13–17 years) into a high socially anxious group and a low socially anxious group. The video-recorded speeches of these adolescents were observed by whole classes of unfamiliar same-aged peers. The peers rated the speeches with respect to the social performance of the speaker and the speaker's likeability (rejection). Each peer rated the speakers on only one of the four behavioral aspects in order to prevent carryover effects that might have caused the high intercorrelations in the Miers et al. (2010) study. Trained adult observers also rated the social performance using the Performance Questionnaire (PQ; Cartwright-Hatton et al. 2005; Miers et al. 2009). The physical attractiveness of the speakers was rated by different peers (i.e., different to those rating social performance and likeability) using photographs (screenshots) of the speakers taken before they started their speech. Results showed that the ratings of the four different aspects of social performance were once again strongly related. That is, the result replicated that of the Miers et al. (2010) study, even when different peers rated different aspects of social performance. The main findings of the study were that socially anxious adolescents were relatively less liked compared to their non-anxious counterparts and that physical attractiveness and social performance equally mediated the link between social anxiety and peer liking. However, the mediation effect was partial, as the direct link between social anxiety and peer liking was still significant after including the mediators in the model. The authors argued that there may be one or more characteristics other than physical appearance and social performance that lead peers to reject socially anxious adolescents who are unfamiliar to them.

A study by Verduin and Kendall (2008) suggests that overt nervousness may be one of these other mediators in the link between social anxiety and likeability. The study investigated the effect of anxiety on peer liking in children and young adolescents (9–13 years). Same-aged unfamiliar peers rated video-recorded speeches of youth with different anxiety disorders, among them a group with social phobia and a control group without any anxiety disorder. Peers rated the state anxiety and likeability of the speakers. Results suggested that peer-rated state anxiety partially mediated the link between social phobia and peer liking. The authors argued that there must be other characteristics in addition to overt nervousness, such as depression or poor social skill, that make socially phobic youth less attractive to unfamiliar others. This conclusion and the conclusion from the Blöte et al. (2015) study suggest that at least three variables mediate the link between social anxiety and peer liking in first impressions, namely, overt nervousness, social performance, and physical appearance.

There is also evidence that high socially anxious adolescents are perceived as "different" by same-aged unfamiliar peers. Blöte et al. (2012) asked the entire classrooms to rate the video-recorded speeches of high and low socially anxious adolescents from the Miers et al. (2010) study. Results showed that high socially anxious speakers were perceived as less similar to the peer raters themselves compared to low socially anxious speakers and that similarity perceptions mediated the link between social anxiety and peer rejection. Notably, not only low, but also high, socially anxious peer raters perceived high socially anxious speakers as different. As suggested by the authors, the similarity rating may have been influenced by wishful thinking, with peers not wishing to be like the high anxious speakers. The perception of dissimilarity may be part of the general negative halo in the judgments of both high and low socially anxious peers.

A recent study helps to shed further light on the question of why high socially anxious adolescents are less effective in social situations relative to nonsocially anxious adolescents. Blöte et al. (in press) aimed to identify explicit differences in behavior between high and low socially anxious youth. The study used naive observers to describe conspicuous features in the video-recorded speech behavior of socially anxious speakers (9–16 years). Based on these descriptions, the Speech Performance Observation Scale for Youth (SPOSY) was developed, including subscales related to expressiveness, confidence, and agitation. Expressiveness as measured with the SPOSY comprises behavioral features such as looking friendly, having a good intonation, using adequate gestures, and showing facial expressions. It also comprises directing attention to the public. It was found that expressiveness and confidence are important features distinguishing between high and low socially anxious youth. Low expressiveness in combination with a lack of confidence may explain the negative peer responses towards socially anxious youth (Blöte et al. in press; Van Beek et al. 2006).

Emerging Relationships

Very few studies have addressed the relation between social anxiety and peer rejection/victimization in the first weeks or months of newly formed groups. One study by Vernberg et al. (1992) investigated peer relations of relocated adolescents (12–14 years) followed over a period of 8 months. Victimization measures were exclusion and direct aggression. It was found that the level of adolescents' social anxiety did not predict self-reported exclusion or direct aggression experiences in the new social group, but it did negatively affect the development of friendships.

A study by Gazelle et al. (2005) examined the effect of anxious solitude on social interactions with familiar and unfamiliar same-aged peers in young preadolescent girls (9-year-olds). Anxious solitary girls and a control group participated in two playgroups, one made up of familiar female classmates and the other made up of unfamiliar girls. In general, anxious solitary girls were perceived by playmates as less socially competent and were less liked and more victimized by playmates compared to the controls. Notably, these effects were larger in the playgroup of familiar classmates relative to the so-called unfamiliar playgroup. Anxious solitary girls showed more whining, complaining, and repetitive behavior in the familiar playgroup than in the unfamiliar playgroup, and the familiar playgroup reacted more negatively towards them than the unfamiliar playgroup. So, the girls were better off in the new group of unfamiliar peers than in the group of familiar classmates. This does not mean that it is generally better for socially anxious youth to be placed in a new social environment. Gazelle et al. (2005) argue that relatively positive peer behavior in unfamiliar groups may become more negative with time. Once a social group starts to agree on the low social status of the anxious solitary youth, exclusion and victimization may start.

Established Relationships

A number of studies have focused on the social interactions of socially anxious students in their school environment. Spence et al. (1999) conducted school-based observations of socially phobic children and adolescents (7–14 years) and found that youth with social phobia were less socially skilled compared to a control group. They were also treated less positively by school peers. Relative to the control group, the socially phobic youth initiated fewer social interactions and had less interactions with their schoolmates. The socially phobic youth were less socially competent, according to parents' perceptions and the perceptions of the youth themselves. The authors argued that the poor social skills of socially phobic youth may result in negative peer responses.

Erath et al. (2007) ascertained whether social skills and withdrawal-disengagement mediated the link between social anxiety and peer acceptance and victimization. Subjects were 6th and 7th graders (11–12 years) divided into a socially anxious group and a control group. The study used a social interaction task with a research assistant to investigate target students' social skills. A peer nomination procedure (on grade level and school level) was used for measuring peer acceptance and victimization. Teachers rated students' withdrawal-disengagement. Social skills during the interaction task were rated by independent observers. The study found relations between social anxiety on the one hand and peer acceptance and victimization on the other. The link between social anxiety and peer acceptance was mediated by target students' expectations about the quality of their performance and their withdrawal-disengagement. However, no significant mediators were found for the link between social anxiety and victimization. The authors suggested that this is probably due to gender differences in the relations between various variables and victimization. For example, the relation between victimization and social anxiety was stronger in boys than in girls. It is argued that gender differences in adolescent peer interactions and in particular the role of withdrawal and aggression in gender groups are important factors in explaining gender-related victimization. Unexpectedly, students' social skills during the conversation were *not* related to their social anxiety level. The authors argued that using adults as interaction partners instead of same-aged peers might explain why socially anxious adolescents did not perform more poorly in the interaction task.

Two studies from our own research group on the link between social anxiety and victimization investigated the behavior of classmates towards socially anxious students (13–16 years) giving an oral presentation in their own classroom (Blöte et al. 2007, 2010). An important question posed in the first study was how class behavior is related to speakers' trait social anxiety and state anxiety as indicated by observations of nervous and communicative behavior (Blöte et al. 2007). An independent observer rated the behavior of the speakers as well as class behavior. Class behavior was also rated by the speakers themselves. Both the independent observer and speakers used the Class Behavior List (CBL) which consists of a selection of items from the Perception of Treatment Lists (PTLs) (Blöte and Westenberg 2007). Furthermore, the independent observer rated the speaker's nervousness and level of interaction with the class. It was found that class behavior as rated by the independent observer was related to speakers' trait social anxiety. Speakers with higher levels of social anxiety were treated more negatively. Class behavior was not related to speakers' overt nervousness during the speech. This is remarkable because socially anxious individuals assume that their nervousness is apparent and negatively influences others' behavior towards them (e.g., Cartwright-Hatton et al. 2005; Rapee and Lim 1992). Given that the level of the speaker's interaction with the class was not related to class behavior either, the question of how trait social anxiety may affect peer behavior could not be answered.

The second study looked more closely at the characteristics of socially anxious adolescent speakers (13–18 years) in order to explain negative responses from classmates (Blöte et al. 2010). For example, what is the importance of social skills, such as looking friendly and speaking in a clear voice, and of overt nervousness, as indicated by blushing or stuttering? And what role does the quality of the speech play? Social skills and nervousness were observed and recorded by an independent observer using an adapted Dutch version of the PQ (Cartwright-Hatton et al. 2005; Miers et al. 2009). To evaluate the speeches, the Speech Content Evaluation Scale was developed. Using the CBL, class behavior was rated by an independent observer, the teacher, and the speakers themselves (Blöte et al. 2007). Results showed that, according to the independent observer, the teacher, and the speakers themselves, socially anxious speakers were treated more negatively by their classmates. Furthermore, class behavior was better predicted by the social skills of the speakers than by their overt nervousness. Surprisingly, with all other variables controlled for, higher-quality speeches elicited more negative class responses (i.e., speeches with the speaker's point of view made clearly, presented systematically, with a logical line of thought). The authors argued that classmates might respond more positively to socially attractive behavior, such as making personal remarks and jokes, than to a well-prepared speech (Blöte et al. 2010).

Peer Group Factors

Studies on specific peer and peer group factors that influence the rejection/victimization of high socially anxious adolescents are few. As far as "first impression" studies are concerned, one would expect that peers who are socially anxious themselves may not immediately reject unfamiliar adolescents who appear anxious. However, the study by Verduin and Kendall (2008) did not support this proposition. Although peer observers with higher levels of social anxiety did rate speakers as more likable, their social anxiety was not a moderator in the link between perceived anxiety and liking of the speakers. That is to say, peers who themselves were socially anxious still liked non-anxious speakers more than anxious speakers. This finding was corroborated by the Blöte et al. (2012) study, which showed that the actual similarity in social anxiety level between speakers and peers was neither related to perceived similarity with the speakers nor to liking of the speakers.

As far as the influence of peer group characteristics on victimization of socially anxious youth in emerging and established relationships is concerned, research has focused on socially withdrawn children. The results of these studies are ambiguous. One study showed that in first-grade classrooms with predominantly withdrawn children, withdrawn boys had a higher social status relative to withdrawn boys in classrooms that had less withdrawn children (Stormshak et al. 1999). Another study, which was longitudinal, found no specific effect of classroom climate on exclusion (Avant et al. 2011). Although solitary anxious students (followed from third through fifth grade) were excluded less during the course of the school year, this was not related to classroom climate. This effect occurred in classrooms with emotionally supportive climates and in classrooms with emotionally unsupportive climates. So, this positive finding is difficult to interpret.

In sum, available research does not clearly identify peer group factors related to social anxiety and peer victimization.

Role of Gender in the Relation Between Social Anxiety and Peer Victimization

Girls and boys differ in their relationships with peers. For example, girls experience more stress in peer relationships and tend to talk more with friends about their problems, possibly making the problems bigger, whereas boys tend to ruminate less, taking problems more lightly (Rose and Rudolph 2006). Therefore, the relation between social anxiety and peer victimization might be different for boys and girls. However, studies on gender as a moderating variable in the relation between social anxiety and peer victimization have yielded mixed results. For example, in a prospective study, Siegel et al. (2009) found that social anxiety predicted an increase in relational victimization (exclusion, friendship withdrawal) in both sexes. In contrast, other prospective studies showed that social anxiety predicted an increase in victimization only for girls (Tillfors et al. 2012) or only for boys (Ranta et al. 2013).

As far as the influence of victimization on social anxiety is concerned, relational victimization predicts an increase in social anxiety in girls (Ranta et al. 2013; Siegel et al. 2009; Vernberg et al. 1992) whereas direct victimization predicts social anxiety in boys (Ranta et al. 2013). In addition, the effect of victimization on social anxiety appears to depend on adolescent males' self-worth. A cross-sectional study on 6th graders (11–13 years) found that boys' self-worth was a moderator in the link between victimization and general anxiety (that included social anxiety; Grills and Ollendick 2002). That is to say, boys with higher self-worth were affected less by victimization. Their self-worth may protect them from becoming anxious. However, girls' self-worth seems to play a different role as it was found to be a mediator between victimization and anxiety. This suggests that victimization negatively affects girls' self-worth and low self-worth then makes them more anxious (Grills and Ollendick 2002).

Conclusion and Discussion of Social Interactions

In sum, for socially anxious adolescents, interactions with classmates are rather difficult. Socially anxious students are more likely than nonsocially anxious students to be victimized, not accepted, and not supported, and these negative outcomes from social interactions in turn increase their social anxiety (Reijntjes et al. 2010). Figure 7.1 presents a schematic overview of the course of peer relationships over time. The figure is partly based on the results of the reviewed studies and partly, where studies were lacking, on extrapolations. Importantly, Fig. 7.1 shows that negative judgments and rejection by peers start in the very first minutes of social contacts. Probably, negative outcomes from social interactions then worsen when students get to know each other more and their low social status in the group has been determined, up to the point where, in their ongoing relationships, a certain negative interaction pattern is firmly established.

The first impression socially anxious students make (relative to their non-anxious counterparts) on unfamiliar age-mates is generally a negative one. They are perceived as anxious (Verduin and Kendall 2008) and socially ineffective (Miers et al. 2010). Socially anxious students are also seen as "different" (Blöte et al. 2012) and as physically less attractive (Blöte et al. 2015). These perceptions seem to play a role in the immediate dislike/rejection by peers towards them. However, we cannot

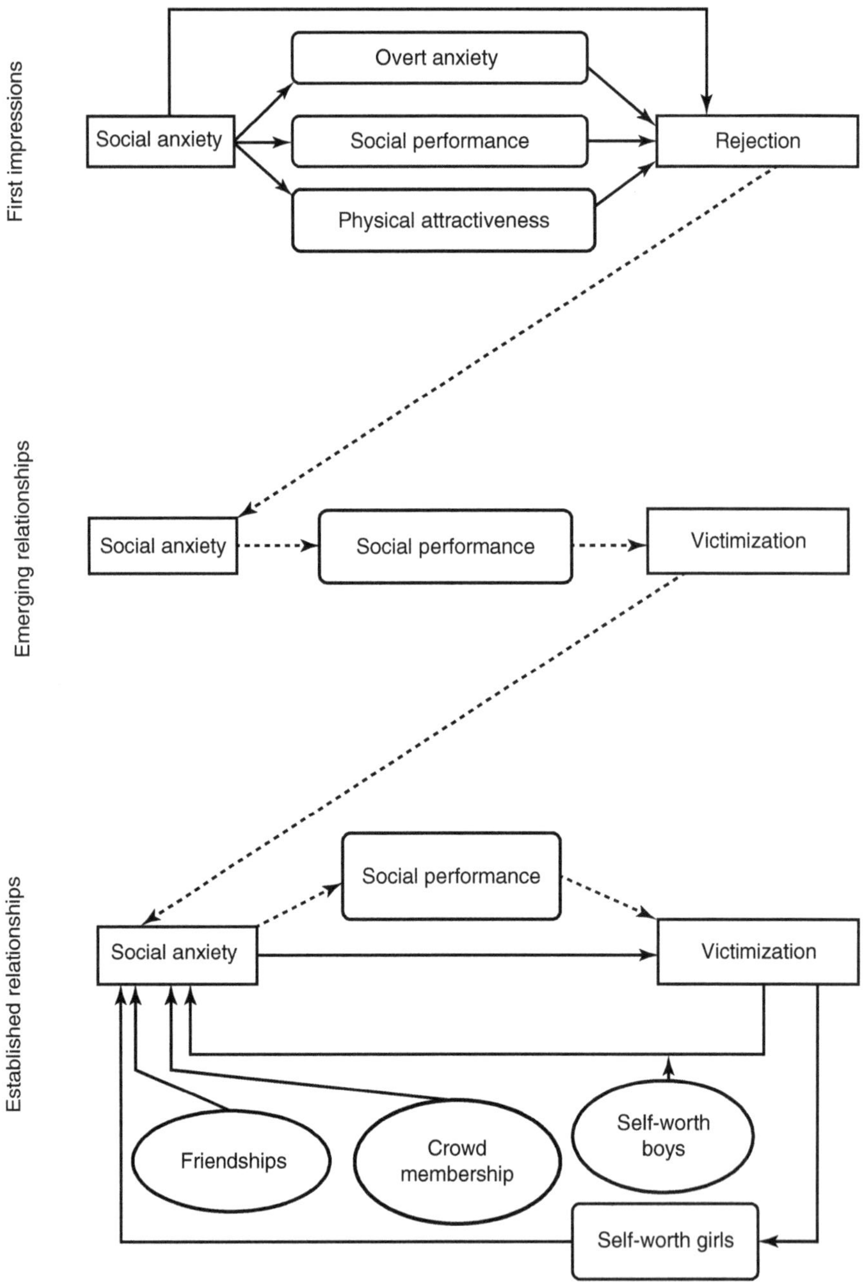

Fig. 7.1 Overview of results of studies reviewed in this chapter regarding the association between social anxiety and rejection/victimization. *Solid lines* tested pathways; *Dotted lines* hypothesized pathways

conclude from the reviewed studies that some aspects in the behavior of socially anxious students are more important than others in eliciting negative peer judgments. The studies seem to suggest that a general negative halo effect (Alden and Taylor 2004; Miers et al. 2010) is at work in peer judgments of high socially anxious adolescents. Future studies are needed to ascertain whether this immediate negative impression is triggered by one or more specific characteristics, which is then carried over to other aspects of the person judged. High socially anxious adolescents may show their anxiety in their behavior and facial/body expression (possibly lacking expressiveness), and peers may not like this, consequently extending their negative opinion to the whole person (Blöte et al. 2015). The finding that socially anxious students are negatively judged and disliked very quickly, in the first minutes of their social performance, is quite disconcerting in view of the possible consequences of this response. Negative self-perceptions of socially anxious students about their social performance seem to be immediately confirmed by peers. This in turn will have consequences for their behavior in subsequent peer interactions.

In light of the negative first impression socially anxious students make on peers, it is not surprising that they encounter negative social outcomes when entering unfamiliar social groups. It is not yet clear which behaviors specifically elicit the negative peer responses in emerging social relationships (just as it was not clear in first impressions), although the Gazelle et al. (2005) study suggests that in girls, "annoying" behaviors like whining and complaining might (partly) mediate the link between anxious solitude and victimization. Furthermore, this study suggested that placing a victimized socially anxious student in a new social group will have some positive effect at first, when the social status of this student is not yet determined by the group. However, this effect is only temporary and victimization may increase over time.

In established relationships, socially anxious students' poor social skills may (partly) explain why they are treated in a negative way by schoolmates (Blöte et al. 2010). Nervous behavior that appears to be a trigger for dislike/rejection at first sight (Verduin and Kendall 2008) does not seem to have this effect among classmates who have known each other for some time (Blöte et al. 2007, 2010). In that situation the social status of individual students has been agreed on and unpopular students are disliked by classmates regardless of whether or not they are nervous during a social performance. However, this explanation needs the necessary caution because of method differences between studies, in particular differences in age and diagnostic status of the participants and in the age of the observers. Verduin and Kendall (2008) studied preadolescents and young adolescents with social phobia and used peer-rated nervousness, whereas Blöte et al. (2007) and (2010) studied a normative sample of older adolescents whose nervousness was judged by an adult observer. Future studies will be needed in order to better understand the role of overt nervousness in peer rejection/victimization.

In view of differences in peer interactions between boys and girls (Rose and Rudolph 2006); it seems likely that the relation between social anxiety and victimization is different between the sexes. Some studies indeed found evidence for the moderating effect of gender (Ranta et al. 2013; Siegel et al. 2009; Tillfors et al. 2012). At the same time, it is difficult to draw conclusions from these studies because of the dissimilar findings. They present an ambiguous picture of the effect of social anxiety on victimization and, in turn, also of victimization on social anxiety for boys and girls. A complicating factor is that different forms of victimization are used in studies, for example, overt/direct victimization (physical or verbal), relational victimization (social exclusion, friendship withdrawal), and reputational victimization (negative interference in other person's relationships). Focusing on these specific kinds of victimization, however, further complicates drawing conclusions as results on the specific kinds of victimization have also been equivocal. More research is needed that pays attention to the different forms that victimization takes for boys and girls. Moreover, the moderators in the relation between victimization and social anxiety might be different for boys and girls. Self-worth has been shown to play a different moderating role between the sexes (Grills and Ollendick 2002), and depression may also play such a role (Ranta et al. 2013).

Very little is known about which peer group factors influence the victimization of socially anxious students in classrooms. This is unfortunate because it means that schools cannot yet be informed about evidence-supported ways to prevent or stop victimization of socially anxious students. Having (good) friends and belonging to a social group may protect socially anxious students (as well as non-anxious students) to some extent from becoming (more) socially anxious (La Greca and Harrison 2005). Furthermore, common sense would say that the presence of more socially anxious students in a group would have a positive effect because these students would be less negative towards each other. However, studies on first contacts show that both socially anxious and non-anxious students do not like their socially anxious counterparts (Blöte et al. 2012; Verduin and Kendall 2008). It is still possible that socially anxious students who are familiar with each other will support and protect each other from the negative effects of victimization in the classrooms. For example, they may make friends or form a "crowd" which may help them to be more assertive or to be less affected by peer victimization. New studies are needed to draw any firm conclusions about this and other classroom effects on socially anxious students.

Cognitive Factors

The previous sections show that there is quite substantial evidence for negative treatment of socially anxious youth by their age peers, both familiar and unfamiliar, as compared to non-anxious youth. That is, socially anxious youth are more likely to be rejected, neglected, and victimized. In contrast, the cognitive theories of SAD (Clark and Wells 1995; Rapee and Heimberg 1997) place more emphasis on the negative perceptions socially anxious individuals have of social situations and their own performance in these situations. Several empirical studies show that socially anxious youth indeed have negative social perceptions. Compared to non-anxious youth, they interpret ambiguous social cues in a negative way (e.g., Blöte et al. 2014; Miers et al. 2008; Vassilopoulos and Banerjee 2008) and engage in negative interpretations or evaluations of their own behavior in social situations (Alfano et al. 2006; Inderbitzen-Nolan et al. 2007; Miers et al. 2009, 2011; Ranta et al. 2014).

One of the main questions to arise out of the cognitive approach is whether the negative perceptions of socially anxious individuals are based on a "kernel of truth" (Norton and Hope 2001) or are biased relative to an objective source of information. Cognitive theories imply that social experiences and feedback from other persons in social situations influence the development of negative perceptions of one's own social performance. Given the evidence reviewed in section "Social interactions with classmates" that socially anxious youth experience more negative social interactions at school, this would suggest that negative social perceptions in socially anxious youth are, at least to some degree, warranted. Indirect evidence for the kernel-of-truth hypothesis was provided in a study on the social perceptions of high socially anxious students and their classmates (8th–10th graders; aged 13–18 years). All pupils in a class were asked to imagine an oral presentation situation in their class where they or their classmates give a presentation (Blöte and Westenberg 2007). They then filled in a questionnaire how they saw themselves treated in such a situation and how hypothetical classmates showing either fearful or relaxed behavior were treated. The socially anxious students reported that they felt negatively treated by classmates when giving a speech. These perceptions seemed warranted as their classmates also perceived that the behavior towards the hypothetical socially anxious (fearful) students in their class was more negative compared to class behavior towards students who were nonsocially anxious (i.e., relaxed) (Blöte and Westenberg 2007).

Direct evidence for the kernel-of-truth hypothesis could be provided by a direct comparison between self-evaluations of high and low socially anxious youth with evaluations of peer observers. If high socially anxious youth would evaluate themselves as poorer with respect to social performance than their low-anxious counterparts while the peer observers would not perceive a difference between these groups, then we could speak of biased self-perceptions (Miers et al. 2009). Alternatively, if the peer observers would also perceive a difference between high- and low-anxious youth, the negative perceptions would be warranted, supporting the "kernel-of-truth" notion.

We are not aware of a study that has compared the self-evaluations of socially anxious youth with evaluations of peer observers. However, some studies have investigated whether socially anxious youth have negatively biased perceptions of their social performance using the performance evaluations of adult observers as a standard. In terms of appearing nervous during a social performance situation, studies consistently show that socially anxious youth perceive themselves as looking more nervous than do adult observers of these socially anxious youth (e.g., Cartwright-Hatton et al. 2005; Inderbitzen-Nolan et al. 2007; Miers et al. 2009). Thus, socially anxious youths' negative perceptions of their nervous behavior seem to be unwarranted.

When comparing self- to observer evaluations of social skills, a negative bias may not apply to all socially anxious youth. Miers et al. (2009) investigated high and low socially anxious youth's (aged 9–17 years) evaluations of social performance during a short speech. The speeches were recorded and shown to independent adult observers who evaluated the performance using the same questionnaire as the participants. When analyzing the whole high socially anxious group, Miers et al. (2009) found that participants and observers were in agreement about the poorer social skills of high socially anxious youth. This suggested that the perceptions of high socially anxious youth were warranted. However, the authors also split the high socially anxious group into two groups using the observers' performance evaluations: those with a good speech performance and those with a poor speech performance. This analysis showed that the negative self-perceptions were justified only for the socially anxious youth who had a poor speech performance. In contrast, for the socially anxious youth whose performance was judged as good, their negative perceptions were unwarranted. Hence, the "kernel-of-truth" hypothesis seems to apply only to socially anxious youth who are indeed less socially skilled (as determined by adult observers).

In sum, with regard to the way they are treated by peers, the negative cognitions of socially anxious adolescents seem partly warranted and partly colored by internal processes. Socially anxious adolescents rightly expect negative responses from others. Based on these expectations, they interpret neutral responses in a negative way. As far as adolescents' self-perceptions of social performance are concerned, they are "incorrect" in thinking that they make a nervous impression (more nervous than others), and some of them are right in evaluating their own social performance as poor. Socially anxious adolescents who perform well may have negatively biased self-perceptions, whereas poor performing socially anxious adolescents may be correct in judging their performance as poor.

It seems important that future studies make a direct comparison between self-evaluations of performance, on the one hand, and performance evaluations by peers (using the same measure) on the other hand. In this way, we can better investigate whether the negative self-perceptions are based on a kernel of truth or are biased.

Implications: How to Break the Vicious Cycle?

The school environment, and more specifically the formal classroom situation, clearly presents a real challenge to socially anxious adolescents. A number of these adolescents experience considerable distress at school and try to avoid distressing classroom situations. In some cases, socially anxious adolescents may show a more severe form of avoidance by refusing to go to school altogether. Moreover, studies indicate that school refusers with AD or SAD have poorer school attendance and that SAD among school-refusing adolescents is often treatment resistant. In all, this chapter sketches a rather bleak picture of the school experiences of socially anxious students.

What makes successful interventions for socially anxious students particularly difficult is that these students not only *think* that they perform poorly in social situations but that some of them actually are less socially skilled, less confident, and less expressive and consequently elicit negative responses from peers. At first glance, peers see them as different and reject them. Later on, when social relationships are being formed, socially anxious students may be victimized. In sum, these students are trapped in a vicious cycle of social anxiety, negative expectations about their social performance and how peers will respond to their performance, actual negative peer responses, and, as a result, increased social anxiety.

It is a complex task to break this vicious cycle, because so many aspects of the socially anxious student and their environment are involved: not only their social skills but also their social cognitions; not only their behavior, but also their physical appearance; and not only these factors on their own, but also the transactions between them. In view of this multiplicity of factors, effective interventions should address a variety of factors, notably negative thinking, poor social skills, as well as physical appearance features. In addition to a change towards less negative thinking, learning more expressive behavior and wearing more attractive clothing and hairstyle may diminish the immediate negative response from peers and create a more positive halo effect. Improved social skills and greater physical attractiveness may also support more positive self-perceptions. Furthermore, the school context would ideally be included in the intervention, since an established pattern of negative social interactions is not easily changed by changes in just one of its participants. Teachers could play an important role by modeling supportive behavior towards socially anxious students and facilitating positive responses from socially anxious students' peers. In order for interventions to have a positive effect, socially anxious students need the opportunity to practice newly learned behavior in their classroom without being bullied or laughed at.

Regarding school refusal, no prospective studies have yet been reported which identify social anxiety as a risk factor for school refusal. Social anxiety should be studied in this respect, together with school- and family-based factors that might exacerbate or mitigate against the development of school refusal among socially anxious youth. To our way of thinking, the apparent link between social anxiety and school refusal calls for indicated prevention interventions for school refusal, targeting youth with social anxiety. Interventions which help improve socially anxious youth's social connection may help prevent school refusal. In indirect support of this, Alfano et al. (2009) found that decreases in loneliness mediated treatment-related improvements in socially anxious children and adolescents. Because of the inherently social nature of schooling and the increased importance of being able to "fit in" with the peer group (Holmbeck et al. 2012); reduced loneliness may be especially important for school-refusing adolescents. A related factor is friendship quality. Baker and Hudson (2013) found that children and young adolescents (aged 7–13 years) who reported higher friendship quality were more likely to be free of anxiety disorder 6 months following CBT for anxiety. The role of friendship quality will be especially important in interventions to prevent or treat school refusal among socially anxious youth. Because bullying and teasing have also been linked with school refusal (Egger et al. 2003); they require specific attention at the individual level (e.g., social skills training addressing assertiveness) and at the school level (i.e., school-based prevention and response to bullying).

Future Studies

As far as research on social anxiety in students is concerned, there is a lack of knowledge about potential moderators and mediators in the link between social anxiety and victimization. We need to know more about the moderating role gender plays in this link. A number of studies found that the effect of victimization on social anxiety and, reversely, of social anxiety on victimization is different for boys and girls. Unfortunately, until now, the findings are ambiguous with regard to how gender affects the link between social anxiety and victimization. There is also a lack of knowledge about which factors give rise to victimization of some socially anxious students but not others and which factors may protect socially anxious students against the harmful effects of victimization.

Finally, it seems important to focus on same-aged peers as observers and judges of socially anxious students' behavior, because (a) students will behave differently in interactions with same-aged peers than with adults, for example, showing social skills during interactions with adults which they do not show during interactions with peers; (b) students' social interactions are mostly with classmates and not adults/teachers; and (c) same-aged peers are likely to have different standards for appropriate behavior and appearance relative to adults. In view of the high degree of socially anxious students' distress and avoidance encountered when they give a speech in class, an oral presentation task may provide a good opportunity to study social anxiety in students.

References

Albano AM (1995) Treatment of social anxiety in adolescents. Cogn Behav Pract 2:271–298

Alden LE, Taylor CT (2004) Interpersonal processes in social phobia. Clin Psychol Rev 24:857–882

Alfano CA, Beidel DC, Turner SM (2006) Cognitive correlates of social phobia among children and adolescents. J Abnorm Child Psychol 34:182–194. doi:10.1007/s10802-005-9012-9

Alfano CA, Pina AA, Villalta IK, Beidel DC, Ammerman RT, Crosby LE (2009) Mediators and moderators of outcome in the behavioral treatment of childhood social phobia. J Am Acad Child Adolesc Psychiatry 48:945–953

Avant T, Gazelle H, Faldowski R (2011) Classroom emotional climate as a moderator of anxious solitary children's longitudinal risk for peer exclusion: a child×environment model. Dev Psychol 47:1711

Baker JR, Hudson JL (2013) Friendship quality predicts treatment outcome in children with anxiety disorders. Behav Res Ther 51:31–36

Beidas RS, Crawley SA, Mychailyszyn MP, Comer JS, Kendall PC (2010) Cognitive-behavioral treatment of anxious youth with comorbid school refusal: clinical presentation and treatment response. Psihologijske teme 19:255–271

Beidel DC, Turner SM, Young BJ, Ammerman RT, Sallee FR, Crosby L (2007) Psychopathology of adolescent social phobia. J Psychopathol Behav Assess 29:46–53

Berg I (1997) School refusal and truancy. Arch Dis Child 76:90–91

Berg I (2002) School avoidance, school phobia, and truancy. In: Lewis M (ed) Child and adolescent psychiatry: a comprehensive textbook, 3rd edn. Lippincott Williams & Wilkins, Sydney, pp 1260–1266

Berg I, Nichols K, Pritchard C (1969) School phobia—its classification and relationship to dependency. J Child Psychol Psychiatry 10:123–141
Berg I, Casswell G, Goodwin A, Hullin R, McGuire R, Tagg G (1985) Classification of severe school attendance problems. Psychol Med 15:157–165
Bernstein GA, Hektner JM, Borchardt CM, McMillan MH (2001) Treatment of school refusal: one-year follow-up. J Am Acad Child Adolesc Psychiatry 40:206–213
Blöte AW, Westenberg PM (2007) Socially anxious adolescents' perception of treatment by classmates. Behav Res Ther 45:189–198. doi:10.1016/j.brat.2006.02.002
Blöte AW, Kint MJW, Westenberg PM (2007) Peer behavior toward socially anxious adolescents: classroom observations. Behav Res Ther 45:2773–2779. doi:10.1016/j.brat.2007.06.011
Blöte AW, Duvekot J, Schalk RDF, Tuinenburg EM, Westenberg PM (2010) Nervousness and performance characteristics as predictors of peer behavior towards socially anxious adolescents. J Youth Adolesc 39:1498–1507. doi:10.1007/s10964-009-9463-3
Blöte AW, Bokhorst CL, Miers AC, Westenberg PM (2012) Why are socially anxious adolescents rejected by peers? The role of subject-group similarity characteristics. J Res Adolesc 22: 123–134. doi:10.1111/j.1532-7795.2011.00768.x
Blöte AW, Miers AC, Heyne DA, Clark DM, Westenberg PM (2014) The relation between social anxiety and audience perception: examining Clark and Wells' (1995) model among adolescents. Behav Cogn Psychother 42:555–567
Blöte AW, Miers AC, Westenberg PM (2015) The role of social performance and physical attractiveness in peer rejection of socially anxious adolescents. J Res Adolesc. doi:10.1111/jora.12107
Blöte AW, Poungjit A, Miers AC, Van Beek Y, Westenberg PM (in press) The Speech Performance Observation Scale (SPOSY): assessing social performance characteristics related to social anxiety (Journal of Experimental Psychopathology)
Bools C, Foster J, Brown I, Berg I (1990) The identification of psychiatric disorders in children who fail to attend school: a cluster analysis of a non-clinical population. Psychol Med 20:171–181
Buitelaar JK, van Andel H, Duyx JHM, van Strien DC (1994) Depressive and anxiety disorders in adolescence: A follow-up of adolescents with school refusal. Acta Paedopsychiatr 56:249–253
Burstein M, He JP, Kattan G, Albano AM, Avenevoli S, Merikangas KR (2011) Social phobia and subtypes in the national comorbidity survey–adolescent supplement: prevalence, correlates, and comorbidity. J Am Acad Child Adolesc Psychiatry 50:870–880, http://dx.doi.org/10.1016/j.jaac.2011.06.005
Cartwright-Hatton S, Tschernitz N, Gomersall H (2005) Social anxiety in children: social skills deficit, or cognitive distortion? Behav Res Ther 43:131–141
Clark DM (2001) A cognitive perspective on social phobia. In: Crozier WR, Alden LE (eds) International handbook of social anxiety. Wiley, Chichester, pp 405–430
Clark DM, Wells A (1995) A cognitive model of social phobia. In: Heimberg RG, Liebowitz MR, Hope DA, Schneier FR (eds) Social phobia: diagnosis, assessment, and treatment. Guilford Press, New York, pp 69–93
Connor KM, Davidson JRT, Churchill LE, Sherwood A, Weisler RH, Foa E (2000) Psychometric properties of the Social Phobia Inventory (SPIN) New self-rating scale. Br J Psychiatry 176:379–386
Costello EJ, Mustillo S, Erkanli A, Keeler G, Angold A (2003) Prevalence and development of psychiatric disorders in childhood and adolescence. Arch Gen Psychiatry 60:837–844
Davidson JRT, Hughes DL, George LK, Blazer DG (1993) The epidemiology of social phobia: findings from the Duke Epidemiological Catchment Area Study. Psychol Med (London) 23:709–718
Eckert P (1989) Jocks and burnouts: social categories and identity in the high school. Teachers College Press, New York
Egger HL, Costello JE, Angold A (2003) School refusal and psychiatric disorders: a community study. J Am Acad Child Adolesc Psychiatry 42:797–807

Erath SA, Flanagan KS, Bierman KL (2007) Social anxiety and peer relations in early adolescence: behavioral and cognitive factors. J Abnorm Child Psychol 35:405–416
Erath SA, Tu KM, El-Sheikh M (2012) Socially anxious and peer-victimized preadolescents: "doubly primed" for distress? J Abnorm Child Psychol 40:837–848
Essau CA, Conradt J, Petermann F (1999) Frequency and comorbidity of social phobia and social fears in adolescents. Behav Res Ther 37:831–843
Galloway D (1985) Schools and persistent absentees. Pergamon Press, Oxford
Garcia-Lopez LJ (2013) Tratando…trastorno de ansiedad social [Treating…social anxiety disorder]. Piramide, Madrid in the References for that chapter.
Garcia-Lopez LJ, Irurtia MJ, Caballo VE, Díaz-Castela MM (2011) Ansiedad social y abuso psicológico [Social anxiety and psychological abuse]. Behav Psycholy 19:223–236
Gazelle H, Putallaz M, Li Y, Grimes CL, Kupersmidt JB, Coie JD (2005) Anxious solitude across contexts: girls' interactions with familiar and unfamiliar peers. Child Dev 76:227–246
Gren-Landell M, Tillfors M, Furmark T, Bohlin G, Andersson G, Svedin CG (2009) Social phobia in Swedish adolescents. Soc Psychiatry Psychiatr Epidemiol 44:1–7
Grills AE, Ollendick TH (2002) Peer victimization, global self-worth, and anxiety in middle school children. J Clin Child Adolesc Psychol 31:59–68
Hanby MSR, Fales J, Nangle DW, Serwik AK, Hedrich UJ (2012) Social anxiety as a predictor of dating aggression. J Interpers Violence 27:1867–1888. doi:10.1177/0886260511431438
Heyne D (2006) School rfeusal. In: Fisher JE, O'Donohue WT (eds) Practitioner's guide to evidence-based psychotherapy. Springer, New York, pp 600-619
Heyne D, King N, Tonge B, Rollings S, Pritchard M, Young D, Myerson N (1998) The self-efficacy questionnaire for school situations: development and psychometric evaluation. Behav Chang 15:31–40
Heyne D, Sauter FM, Van Widenfelt BM, Vermeiren R, Westenberg PM (2011) School refusal and anxiety in adolescence: non-randomized trial of a developmentally sensitive cognitive behavioral therapy. J Anxiety Disord 25:870–878
Heyne D, Sauter FM, Maynard BR (in press) Moderators and mediators of treatments for youth with school refusal or truancy. In: Maric M, Prins PJM, Ollendick TH (eds) Mediators and moderators of youth treatment outcomes. Oxford University Press, New York
Hodson KJ, McManus FV, Clark DM, Doll H (2008) Can Clark and Wells' (1995) cognitive model of social phobia be applied to young people? Behav Cogn Psychother 36:449–461
Holmbeck GN, Devine KA, Wasserman R, Schellinger K, Tuminello E (2012) Guides from developmental psychology for therapy with adolescents. In: Kendall PC (ed) Child and adolescent therapy: cognitive-behavioral procedures. Guilford, New York, pp 429–470
Inderbitzen HM, Walters KS, Bukowski AL (1997) The role of social anxiety in adolescent peer relations: differences among sociometric status groups and rejected subgroups. J Clin Child Psychol 26:338–348
Inderbitzen-Nolan HM, Anderson ER, Johnson HS (2007) Subjective versus objective behavioral ratings following two analogue tasks: a comparison of socially phobic and non-anxious adolescents. J Anxiety Disord 21:76–90
Ingul JM, Nordahl HM (2013) Anxiety as a risk factor for school absenteeism: what differentiates anxious school attenders from non-attenders? Ann Gen Psychiatry 12:25
Kearney CA (2002) Identifying the function of school refusal behavior: a revision of the School Refusal Assessment Scale. J Psychopathol Behav Assess 24:235–245
Kearney CA, Albano AM (2004) The functional profiles of school refusal behavior diagnostic aspects. Behav Modif 28:147–161
Kingery JN, Erdley CA, Marshall KC, Whitaker KG, Reuter TR (2010) Peer experiences of anxious and socially withdrawn youth: an integrative review of the developmental and clinical literature. Clin Child Fam Psychol Rev 13:91–128. doi:10.1007/s10567-009-0063-2
La Greca AM (1998) Social anxiety scales for children and adolescents: manual and instructions for the SASC, SASC-R, SAS-A (adolescents), and parent versions of the scales. University of Miami, Department of Psychology, Miami

La Greca AM, Harrison HM (2005) Adolescent peer relations, friendships, and romantic relationships: do they predict social anxiety and depression? J Clin Child Adolesc Psychol 34:49–61. doi:10.1207/s15374424jccp3401_5
La Greca AM, Lopez N (1998) Social anxiety among adolescents: linkages with peer relations and friendships. J Abnorm Child Psychol 26:83–94
Last CG, Strauss CC (1990) School refusal in anxiety-disordered children and adolescents. J Am Acad Child Adolesc Psychiatry 29:31–35
Layne AE, Bernstein GA, Egan EA, Kushner MG (2003) Predictors of treatment response in anxious-depressed adolescents with school refusal. J Am Acad Child Adolesc Psychiatry 42:319–326
London B, Downey G, Bonica C, Paltin I (2007) Social causes and consequences of rejection sensitivity. J Res Adolesc 17:481–506. doi:10.1111/j.1532-7795.2007.00531.x
Lyon AR (2010) Confirmatory factor analysis of the School Refusal Assessment Scale-Revised in an African American community sample. J Psychoeduc Assess 28:511–523
McShane G, Walter G, Rey JM (2004) Functional outcome of adolescents with school refusal. Clin Child Psychol Psychiatry 9:53–60
Miers AC, Blöte AW, Bögels SM, Westenberg PM (2008) Interpretation bias and social anxiety in adolescents. J Anxiety Disord 22:1462–1471. doi:10.1016/j.janxdis.2008.02.010
Miers AC, Blöte AW, Bokhorst CL, Westenberg PM (2009) Negative self-evaluations and the relation to performance level in socially anxious children and adolescents. Behav Res Ther 47:1043–1049. doi:10.1016/j.brat.2009.07.017
Miers AC, Blöte AW, Westenberg PM (2010) Peer perceptions of social skills in socially anxious and nonanxious adolescents. J Abnorm Child Psychol 38:33–41. doi:10.1007/s10802-009-9345-x
Miers AC, Blöte AW, Westenberg PM (2011) Negative social cognitions in socially anxious youth: distorted reality or a kernel of truth? J Child Fam Stud 20:214–223. doi:10.1007/s10826-010-9423-2
Nair MKC, Russell PSS, Subramaniam VS, Nazeema S, Chembagam N, Russell S, Charles H (2013) School phobia and anxiety disorders among adolescents in a rural community population in India. Indian J Pediatr 80:171–174
Nakamura M, Kondo I, Kubota A, Furukawa I, Suzuki T, Nakamura H, Hayakawa N, Ojima T, Aoki N (2010) School-attendance problems, subjective symptoms and lifestyle factors: the Shizuoka health and lifestyle survey of students [Nihon koshu eisei zasshi]. Jpn J Public Health 57:881–890
Norton PJ, Hope DA (2001) Kernels of truth or distorted perceptions: self and observer ratings of social anxiety and performance. Behav Ther 32:765–786
Ollendick TH, Hirshfeld-Becker DR (2002) The developmental psychopathology of social anxiety disorder. Biol Psychiatry 51:44–58. doi:10.1016/s0006-3223(01)01305-1
Place M, Hulsmeier J, Davis S, Taylor E (2000) School refusal: a changing problem which requires a change of approach? Clin Child Psychol Psychiatry 5:345–355
Place M, Hulsmeier J, Davis S, Taylor E (2002) The coping mechanisms of children with school refusal. J Res Spec 1–10
Ranta K, Kaltiala-Heino R, Koivisto AM, Tuomisto MT, Pelkonen M, Marttunen M (2007) Age and gender differences in social anxiety symptoms during adolescence: the Social Phobia Inventory (SPIN) as a measure. Psychiatry Res 153:261–270, http://dx.doi.org/10.1016/j.psychres.2006.12.006
Ranta K, Kaltiala-Heino R, Pelkonen M, Marttunen M (2009) Associations between peer victimization, self-reported depression and social phobia among adolescents: the role of comorbidity. J Adolesc 32:77–93, http://dx.doi.org/10.1016/j.adolescence.2007.11.005
Ranta K, Kaltiala-Heino R, Rantanen P, Marttunen M (2012) The Mini-Social Phobia Inventory: psychometric properties in an adolescent general population sample. Compr Psychiatry 53:630–637
Ranta K, Kaltiala-Heino R, Fröjd S, Marttunen M (2013) Peer victimization and social phobia: a follow-up study among adolescents. Soc Psychiatry Psychiatr Epidemiol 48:533–544

Ranta K, Tuomisto MT, Kaltiala-Heino R, Rantanen P, Marttunen M (2014) Cognition, imagery and coping among adolescents with social anxiety and phobia: testing the Clark and Wells model in the population. Clin Psychol Psychother 21:252–263. doi:10.1002/cpp.1833

Rao PA, Beidel DC, Turner SM, Ammerman RT, Crosby LE, Sallee FR (2007) Social anxiety disorder in childhood and adolescence: descriptive psychopathology. Behav Res Ther 45: 1181–1191. doi:10.1016/j.brat.2006.07.015

Rapee RM, Heimberg RG (1997) A cognitive-behavioral model of anxiety in social phobia. Behav Res Ther 35:741–756, http://dx.doi.org/10.1016/S0005-7967(97)00022-3

Rapee RM, Lim L (1992) Discrepancy between self-and observer ratings of performance in social phobics. J Abnorm Psychol 101:728

Rapee RM, Spence SH (2004) The etiology of social phobia: empirical evidence and an initial model. Clin Psychol Rev 24:737–767

Reijntjes A, Kamphuis JH, Prinzie P, Telch MJ (2010) Peer victimization and internalizing problems in children: a meta-analysis of longitudinal studies. Child Abuse Negl 34:244–252. doi:10.1016/j.chiabu.2009.07.009

Rose AJ, Rudolph KD (2006) A review of sex differences in peer relationship processes: potential trade-offs for the emotional and behavioral development of girls and boys. Psychol Bull 132:98

Rubin KH, Coplan RJ (2004) Paying attention to and not neglecting social withdrawal and social isolation. Merrill-Palmer Q 50:506–534

Rudy BM, Davis TE, Matthews RA (2014) Cognitive indicators of social anxiety in youth: a structural equation analysis. Behav Ther 45:116–125

Siegel RS, La Greca AM, Harrison HM (2009) Peer victimization and social anxiety in adolescents: prospective and reciprocal relationships. J Youth Adolesc 38:1096–1109

Silverman and Albano (1996) is: Silverman, W. K., & Albano, A. M. (1996). The anxiety disorders interview schedule for DSM-IV—Child and parent versions. San Antonio, TX: Psychological Corporation.

Spence SH, Donovan C, Brechman-Toussaint M (1999) Social skills, social outcomes, and cognitive features of childhood social phobia. J Abnorm Psychol 108:211

Storch EA, Masia-Warner C (2004) The relationship of peer victimization to social anxiety and loneliness in adolescent females. J Adolesc 27:351–362, http://dx.doi.org/10.1016/j.adolescence.2004.03.003

Stormshak EA, Bierman KL, Bruschi C, Dodge KA, Coie JD (1999) The relation between behavior problems and peer preference in different classroom contexts. Child Dev 70:169–182

Strauss CC, Last CG (1993) Social and simple phobias in children. J Anxiety Disord 7:141–152

Sumter SR, Bokhorst CL, Westenberg PM (2009) Social fears during adolescence: is there an increase in distress and avoidance? J Anxiety Disord 23:897–903

Thorndike EL (1920) A constant error in psychological ratings. J Appl Psychol 4:25–29

Tillfors M, Persson S, Willén M, Burk WJ (2012) Prospective links between social anxiety and adolescent peer relations. J Adolesc 35:1255–1263

Van Ameringen M, Mancini C, Farvolden P (2003) The impact of anxiety disorders on educational achievement. J Anxiety Disord 17:561–571

Van Beek Y, Van Dolderen MSM, Demon Dubas JJS (2006) Gender-specific development of nonverbal behaviours and mild depression in adolescence. J Child Psychol Psychiatry 47:1272–1283

Van den Bos E, De Rooij M, Miers AC, Bokhorst CL, Westenberg PM (2014) Adolescents' increasing stress response to social evaluation: pubertal effects on cortisol and alpha-amylase during public speaking. Child Dev 85:220–236. doi:10.1111/cdev.12118

Vassilopoulos SP, Banerjee R (2008) Interpretations and judgments regarding positive and negative social scenarios in childhood social anxiety. Behav Res Ther 46:870–876

Vaughn MG, Maynard BR, Salas-Wright CP, Perron BE, Abdon A (2013) Prevalence and correlates of truancy in the US: results from a national sample. J Adolesc 36:767–776

Verduin TL, Kendall PC (2008) Peer perceptions and liking of children with anxiety disorders. J Abnorm Child Psychol 36:459–469

Vernberg EM, Abwender DA, Ewell KK, Beery SH (1992) Social anxiety and peer relationships in early adolescence: a prospective analysis. J Clin Child Psychol 21:189–196

Weeks M, Coplan RJ, Kingsbury A (2009) The correlates and consequences of early appearing social anxiety in young children. J Anxiety Disord 23:965–972

Westenberg PM, Drewes MJ, Goedhart AW, Siebelink BM, Treffers PDA (2004) A developmental analysis of self-reported fears in late childhood through mid-adolescence: social-evaluative fears on the rise? J Child Psychol Psychiatry 45:481–495

Westenberg PM, Bokhorst CL, Miers AC, Sumter SR, Kallen VL, van Pelt J, Blote AW (2009) A prepared speech in front of a pre-recorded audience: subjective, physiological, and neuroendocrine responses to the Leiden Public Speaking Task. Biol Psychol 82:116–124. doi:10.1016/j.biopsycho.2009.06.005

Wittchen HU, Stein MB, Kessler RC (1999) Social fears and social phobia in a community sample of adolescents and young adults: prevalence, risk factors and co-morbidity. Psychol Med 29:309–323. doi:10.1017/s0033291798008174

Social Anxiety and Romantic Relationships

8

Lisa R. Starr and Joanne Davila

Social Anxiety and Romantic Relationships

One of the most dramatic developments in adolescence is the onset of romance. The emergence of romantic relationships introduces adolescents to a key interpersonal context that will continue throughout the life span to be an important, often central, component of social well-being. Little research has explicitly examined how social anxiety—a prevalent problem in adolescence—influences the development of romantic behaviors in adolescence, but existing studies strongly suggest that it is linked to impairments in both romantic behaviors and the interpersonal environment in which they emerge. We begin by describing the nature and developmental significance of adolescent romantic relationships and then discuss how social anxiety affects, and is affected by, them.

Nature of Romantic Relationships in Adolescence

Romantic relationships in adolescence are a normative aspect of development, whose prevalence in the USA rises with age. By age 13, over one-third of adolescents have had a romantic relationship, and by age 17, over 70 % have done so (Carver et al. 2003). Although relationships tend to be short-lived in early adolescence, they increase in length over time (Carver et al. 2003), as well as in depth. In early adolescence, relationships are characterized by affiliation and companionship rather than intimacy (Shulman and Scharf 2000). As adolescence

L.R. Starr, PhD (✉)
Department of Clinical and Social Sciences in Psychology,
University of Rochester, Rochester, NY, USA

J. Davila, PhD
Department of Psychology, Stony Brook University, Stony Brook, NY, USA
e-mail: joanne.davila@stonybrook.edu

K. Ranta et al. (eds.), *Social Anxiety and Phobia in Adolescents: Development, Manifestation and Intervention Strategies*, DOI 10.1007/978-3-319-16703-9_8

progresses, teens are more likely to engage in dyadic dating that involves higher levels of intimacy and closeness, deeper mutual feelings, and more extensive sexual activity (Connolly and Goldberg 1999; Shulman and Scharf 2000). By late adolescence, teens' romantic relationships also include caretaking and caregiving functions and begin to resemble what we typically think of as adult dyadic relationships (Furman and Wehner 1994). In addition, over time, youth spend more time with romantic partners and, by late adolescence, report greater closeness with their romantic partners than with their best friends or their parents (Kuttler and La Greca 2004; Laursen 1996).

The rates of engagement in sexual intercourse among never-married US adolescents show a similar developmental progression to romantic relationships. Approximately 15 % of youth have engaged in sexual intercourse before age 15 years, and rates rise to nearly 70 % by age 19 (Abma et al. 2004). Not surprisingly for most adolescents, dating activities and romantic relationships provide the context for engaging in sexual activities (Kuttler and La Greca 2004).

Adolescent romantic relationships are adaptive in numerous ways that may benefit development and emotional functioning, particularly with regard to identity development and the capacity for intimacy (see Collins 2003; Furman and Shaffer 2003). For instance, high-quality romantic relationships are associated with positive affect, positive self-worth, and a sense of social competence (Connolly and Konarski 1994; Harter 1999; Larson and Richards 1998; Masten et al. 1995; Zimmer-Gembeck et al. 2001, 2004). In addition, affectionate intimate behaviors (e.g., kissing, hugging, holding hands) are associated with positive family relationships, romantic relationship satisfaction, and commitment (e.g., Welsh et al. 2005; Williams et al. 2008).

Adolescent romantic relationships also provide learning experiences that can set the stage for romantic functioning in adulthood. For example, lower romantic competence is associated with early adolescent girls making stronger predictions that they will be unlikely to marry and also with greater engagement in potentially risky sexual activity (Davila et al. 2009a). In addition, higher-quality romantic relationships in adolescence are associated with positive relationships and commitment in early adult relationships (Seiffge-Krenke and Lang 2002), as well as with more adaptive relationship processes (e.g., better conflict resolution and caregiving) in young adulthood (Madsen and Collins 2011).

Adolescent romantic relationships can, however, be a significant challenge or stressor that contributes to psychosocial distress. Romantic relationships are associated with strong negative emotions (e.g., anxiety, anger, jealousy, and depression) among high school youth (Larson et al. 1999). In addition, most adolescents will face specific relationship stressors, including breakups, and interactions with a romantic partner that may involve criticism, conflict, and pressure. Some adolescents will engage in risky sexual activity (e.g., failure to use condoms, multiple sexual partners) that results in negative outcomes (e.g., unplanned pregnancy, sexually transmitted infections), and they will face or engage in relationship aggression. Romantic experiences also can teach young people dysfunctional beliefs about relationships and maladaptive interpersonal behaviors, which they may repeat over time (Waldinger et al. 2002). Not surprisingly then, adolescent romantic relationships and what happens in them are associated with numerous types of psychopathology, including externalizing problems, depression, and anxiety disorders (for a review, see Davila et al. in press).

Adolescent Romantic Relationships and Social Anxiety

Research on associations between social anxiety and romantic processes in adolescence is strikingly limited. This represents a significant shortcoming of the literature, as there are strong empirical and conceptual reasons to believe that social anxiety would influence the development of romantic behaviors. Social anxiety is fundamentally an interpersonal problem, and romantic relationships become an increasingly salient interpersonal context during adolescence. Fear of negative evaluation is a core aspect of social anxiety disorder, and beginning to date inherently exposes youth to interpersonal scrutiny. Thus, the emergence of dating may activate socially anxious youth' fears. In turn, social anxiety may impair the acquisition of romantic skills. We begin with a discussion of how social anxiety impairs a key context in which romantic relationships emerge—peer relationships.

Peer Dysfunction and Implications for the Emergence of Romantic Relationships

Although research explicitly examining the link between social anxiety and adolescent romantic functioning has been fairly limited, studies have clearly tied social anxiety to a variety of impairments in peer relations during adolescence (see Biggs et al. 2011; Davila et al. 2010; Starr et al. 2011), and these may in turn have implications for romantic relationships. Social anxiety is related to peer rejection (Inderbitzen et al. 1997; Vernberg et al. 1992). Peer victimization and exclusion predict social anxiety both cross-sectionally and longitudinally (La Greca and Harrison 2005; Ranta el al. 2009, 2013; Siegel et al. 2009; Storch and Masia-Warner 2004; Vernberg et al. 1992), and socially anxious youth may be more likely to be targeted with peer victimization (although evidence for the latter is somewhat mixed; Siegel et al. 2009; Storch et al. 2005; Vernberg et al. 1992). Socially anxious adolescents are also less likely to belong to high-status peer crowds (La Greca and Harrison 2005). Furthermore, adolescents with social anxiety also report fewer close friends, including friends of the opposite sex (La Greca and Lopez 1998; La Greca and Mackey 2007; Starr and Davila 2008a). Within existing peer relationships and friendships, social anxiety predicts lower perceived support, intimacy, communication, and trust, and fewer positive and more negative interactions (La Greca and Harrison 2005; La Greca and Lopez 1998; Starr and Davila 2008a). In addition, compared to non-anxious youth, socially anxious youth perceive themselves as less interpersonally competent (Starr and Davila 2008a). Disruptions in peer functioning are maintained when controlling for concurrent depressive symptoms (Starr and Davila 2008a), suggesting that they are relatively specific to social anxiety. In sum, adolescents who are socially anxious often find themselves with fewer friends, lower quality friendships, fewer interpersonal skills, and more negative peer experiences.

These impairments in peer relations are likely to generalize to romantic contexts. Romantic relationships rely on many of the same competencies that are important to friendships (e.g., conflict management, emotion regulation, capacity for intimacy, support provision), so to the extent that socially anxious youth lack these skills, they may have difficulty navigating romantic activities. Moreover, early romantic experiences often take place directly within peer contexts. Partners are typically drawn from within social cliques, early dating activities frequently occur in mixed-sex group settings, and friends are often key sources of social support (Brown 1999; Connolly and Goldberg 1999). Thus, if socially anxious youth have fewer friendships, they may have a more difficult time finding a partner in the first place and fewer available social resources for managing the relationships that they are able to establish. Friendships also provide a setting in which interpersonal skills needed for relationships can be modeled, practiced, and mastered; in particular, other-sex friendships provide opportunities to learn how to interact with and relate to other-sex peers (Collins et al. 2009; Connolly et al. 2004; Connolly and Goldberg 1999; Zimmer-Gembeck 2002). Consequently, if social anxiety impedes the development of strong friendships (including heterosocial friendships), it may also leave the youth less developmentally prepared for the relational demands of romantic involvement. Finally, adolescents who are sensitive to stressful peer experiences, such as peer victimization and rejection, may also struggle with romantic activities, which often expose the youth to potentially anxiety-provoking circumstances. In direct support of the idea that the effects of social anxiety on platonic peer relationships generalize to romantic experiences, Hebert et al. (2013) found cross-sectional support for a mediation model in which social anxiety indirectly influenced romantic functioning via disruptions in same-sex friendships, which then predicted impairments in other-sex friendships, which was in turn associated with romantic relationship functioning.

Dating Anxiety

Among some adolescents, social fears and avoidance are relatively specific to romantic situations. *Dating anxiety* refers to worries and inhibition in mixed-sex social situations involving interaction with romantic partners or potential partners, including concerns about negative romantic evaluations (Chorney and Morris 2008; Glickman and La Greca 2004). The construct of dating anxiety is conceptually rooted in social anxiety, and social anxiety is highly correlated with but empirically distinct from dating anxiety (Glickman and La Greca 2004). For example, dating anxiety predicts dating activities beyond the contributions of social anxiety (Glickman and La Greca 2004), predicting lower engagement in dating and hetero-social friendships and fewer positive and more negative qualities within existing romantic relationships (Glickman and La Greca 2004; La Greca and Mackey 2007). Fortunately, dating anxiety appears to decline with age (Glickman and La Greca 2004; Nieder and Seiffge-Krenke 2001), perhaps decreasing as familiarity with dating situations increases and relational skills are acquired.

Romantic Behaviors of Socially Anxious Youth

Social anxiety creates numerous barriers to the formation of romantic relationships. Avoidance of social situations, particularly those that present opportunities for negative evaluation by others (such as asking someone out or going on a date), is a core feature of social anxiety disorder. Social anxiety is also tied to difficulties with key relationship formation mechanisms, such as self-disclosure (Alden and Taylor 2004; Meleshko and Alden 1993; Papsdorf and Alden 1998), meaning that socially anxious youth who attempt to build relationships may often have trouble doing so. Finally, socially anxious individuals are often interpersonally awkward, frequently displaying self-preserving micro-behaviors that provoke rejection by others (Alden and Taylor 2004). As a consequence, they may be less sought after as romantic partners, particularly in adolescence, when the social desirability of one's dating partner has a particularly strong influence on social status and popularity (Brown 1999).

It is therefore not surprising that socially anxious adolescents report lower rates of engagement in romantic relationships and in the heterosocial situations in which they often emerge (Glickman and La Greca 2004; La Greca et al. 2011; La Greca and Harrison 2005; La Greca and Mackey 2007). This pattern is not unique to adolescence. Adults with social anxiety disorder are more likely to report never having been married (Lampe et al. 2003; Schneier et al. 1992; Wittchen et al. 1999), especially those with more severe symptoms (Hart et al. 1999). Social inhibition in childhood prospectively predicts delayed marriage (Caspi et al. 1988), and socially anxious college students report fewer interactions with the opposite sex and less sexual activity (Dodge et al. 1988; Leary and Dobbins 1983). However, the link between social anxiety and adolescent romantic involvement may be particularly important for two reasons. First, romantic interactions may be particularly triggering to socially anxious youth during adolescence simply because they are new and unfamiliar. Second, given the developmental significance of dating and other heterosocial activities during adolescence, inability or unwillingness to pursue these relationships may prevent the acquisition of important developmental skills that contribute to relational functioning throughout the life span. Cross-sectional research has already suggested that social impairments related to adolescent social anxiety seep across different types of interpersonal relationships (Hebert et al. 2013), and an important next step will be to evaluate cascading effects of interpersonal difficulties across developmental stages. For example, it would be interesting to prospectively explore whether socially anxious youth who withdraw from dating during adolescence show greater problems in their relationships later in life.

Less is known about the specific characteristics of the romantic relationships that socially anxious adolescents do manage to establish. However, evidence from the adult literature tentatively suggests that social anxiety predicts a range of problems with romantic functioning. Social anxiety is associated with poorer marital adjustment (Filsinger and Wilson 1983; Whisman 2007). Compared to non-anxious controls, romantically involved adults with social anxiety report lower intimacy, self-disclosure, and emotional expression and are more likely to attribute blame for conflicts to stable partner characteristics (Sparrevohn and Rapee 2009; Wenzel 2002). In one small study, Wenzel et al. (2005) coded videotaped conversations between socially anxious individuals and their romantic partners and found that compared to non-anxious controls, partners with social anxiety displayed more "very negative" behaviors (e.g., character assassination, kitchen sinking, "yes, but" statements; Floyd and Markman 1984) and showed overall poorer social skills. Socially anxious adults also generally display maladaptive interpersonal styles within their close relationships, including problems with assertion, self-disclosure, conflict avoidance, and avoidance of expressing emotion (Cuming and Rapee 2010; Davila and Beck 2002; Grant et al. 2007).

Although social anxiety is typically associated with interpersonal avoidance, among anxious youth who are able to establish satisfying romantic relationships, patterns of interpersonal dependence may sometimes emerge (Darcy et al. 2005). Imagine a socially anxious teen has overcome her social fears to pursue and establish a romantic relationship. She has likely had to battle her fears of negative evaluation at every step of the relationship building process, from initiating contact with her partner to establishing and fostering intimacy. She may not have many other individuals in her life who provide support and companionship and may perceive her chances of attracting another partner as limited. All together, she has invested significant effort in the relationship, relies heavily upon her partner for emotional support and companionship, and lacks confidence in her ability to initiate another relationship. These forces could easily accumulate into a powerful motivation to keep her current relationship intact, resulting in dependent behaviors. Supporting this notion, Darcy et al. (2005) provided evidence that social anxiety is associated with interpersonal dependence in romantic relationships among college students.

More research is needed to establish whether social anxiety also predicts interpersonal dependence on romantic partners at earlier ages. To the extent that it does, however, it may have implications for important relationship processes. Socially anxious teens may be more likely to self-silence in romantic relationships, withholding their opinions and thoughts to maintain the relationship, and this tendency has been linked to depression and relationship problems (Harper et al. 2006; Harper and Welsh 2007). Socially anxious teens may also have difficulty asserting themselves in sexual situations and may make risky sexual choices to preserve their relationships and avoid embarrassment (Bell 2009; Kashdan et al. 2006). Thus, although social anxiety is associated with lower levels of sexual experience overall (Leary and Dobbins 1983), it is possible that among sexually active youth, social anxiety predicts risky sex and problematic outcomes, such as unwanted pregnancy and sexually transmitted infections.

While some socially anxious teens may engage in self-silencing and other relationship-preserving behaviors, others may perceive their romantic relationships as safe places for them to express negative emotions that they normally keep concealed. Supporting this idea, Beck et al. (2006) found that when faced with a social threat task, socially anxious women in more satisfying relationships displayed more negative relationship behaviors. The authors suggested that for socially anxious women, satisfying relationships could function as a secure base where they can feel comfortable expressing negative feelings without fears of rejection. Unfortunately, this tendency may backfire, as another study suggested that uninhibited expression of negative emotions, although beneficial to the romantic relationships of nonsocially anxious individuals, prospectively predicts deteriorating closeness ratings among those with high social anxiety (Kashdan et al. 2007). These studies may suggest a sad irony: once socially anxious individuals finally overcome their social fears to establish closeness and security with romantic partners, they may over-rely on their partners as an outlet for their negative emotions, and this may become burdensome to their partners, ultimately provoking rejection and confirming fears of negative evaluation (not unlike the excessive reassurance-seeking model in depression; Joiner et al. 1999; Starr and Davila 2008b).

Potential Impact of Romantic Involvement on Social Anxiety

Little research has evaluated whether dating has an impact on social anxiety symptoms. On one hand, romantic relationships during early or mid-adolescence longitudinally predict depression and other maladaptive outcomes (see Davila 2008; Davila et al. in press), perhaps because they introduce challenges that young people are developmentally unprepared to manage. As anxiety and depression share core internalizing pathology (Krueger 1999), it is possible that among adolescents predisposed to anxiety, romantic stressors would lead to anxiety symptoms in addition to depression, particularly when youth make helpless attributions about the romantic events. Supporting this idea, in a 1-year follow-up of early adolescent girls, dating activities predicted significant increases in anxiety disorder symptoms (including but not limited to social phobia symptoms), controlling for comorbid disorders (Starr et al. 2012).

On the other hand, romantic relationships may offer corrective experiences to many anxious youth. Romantic activities may serve as a context in which socially anxious adolescents can confront and habituate to feared social situations, practice interpersonal skills, build self-confidence, reduce avoidance, and modify maladaptive schemas. Romantic partners can offer support and encouragement, reducing negative self-concepts and rejection fears. Indeed, in one study, socially anxious college students perceived their romantic relationships as beneficial to their psychological health (Gordon et al. 2012). Of course, negative romantic experiences may have the reverse effect, confirming rejection fears and increasing social anxiety, so the quality of the romantic relationship may be a key moderator of outcomes. However, simple exposure to romantic situations—whether or not they are overwhelmingly positive experiences—would at the very least strip them of their unfamiliarity, and that alone may make them less threatening. Consistent with this idea, Nieder and Seiffge-Krenke (2001) followed adolescents prospectively between ages 14 and 17 and found that self-reported stress related to romantic situations declined over time, suggesting that comfort with dating activities increases along with increased exposure to romantic situations.

Social Anxiety and Same-Sex Relationships

If we know little about how social anxiety affects and is affected by adolescent heterosexual romantic relationships, we barely know anything about its implications for same-sex relationships. Sexual minorities show elevated rates of social phobia, sometimes related to (often accurate) expectations of rejection and victimization based on their sexual orientation (Gilman et al. 2001; Pachankis and Goldfried 2006; Roberts et al. 2011). Social anxiety may inhibit the romantic pursuits of lesbian, gay, and bisexual youth even more that it does for heterosexual teens, given the significant stigma surrounding the formation of same-sex relationships. Many teens may not feel prepared to disclose their sexual minority status to potential partners, and many will avoid that situation by choosing to date other-sex partners (Diamond et al. 1999). Even openly gay youth may feel scrutinized as they pursue developmentally normative dating activities with same-sex partners in public arenas (especially in less tolerant communities). Some evidence suggests that social anxiety leads to sexual risk-taking among gay adolescents. Hart and Heimberg (2005) found that social anxiety predicted unprotected sex among gay male late adolescents, perhaps because socially anxious boys were focused on performance rather than safety or because they were too embarrassed to discuss condom use. More research is needed to understand how social anxiety (including stigma-related fears) interferes with the development of healthy romantic functioning among sexual minority youth.

Future Research Directions

As we have previously emphasized, research examining social anxiety within the context of adolescent romantic experiences is remarkably limited. Researchers are increasingly taking an interest in the ties between the emergence of romantic relationships and psychopathology (Davila et al. in press), and it is surprising that social anxiety, which by definition influences social processes, has been relatively neglected. This is a research area clearly ripe for exploration, with an abundance of intriguing, unanswered questions.

Social Anxiety and Basic Romantic Relationship Processes in Adolescence

One important topic that has been unaddressed in the literature is how social anxiety influences basic relationship processes and romantic milestones in adolescents. For example, an initial stage of romantic contact is infatuation, where adolescents harbor "crushes" on potential partners (Connolly and Goldberg 1999). Many adolescents experience intense emotions and embarrassment during the infatuation stage (especially when interacting with their "crush"), and difficult emotions are often mitigated by friend support. How might these emotions interplay with social anxiety, especially for those with little peer support? In addition, do socially inhibited teens follow typical developmental trajectories in their romantic interactions (i.e., progressing from same-sex friendships to affiliative heterosocial socialization to dyadic dating and adultlike partnerships, with partners becoming an increasingly important source of support over time; Collins et al. 2009; Connolly and Goldberg 1999)? If trajectories are delayed, most of their peers may have moved forward to other stages, leaving socially anxious teens with less peer support. Or, if social anxiety prevents some adolescents from participating in early stages of dating at normative ages, do they progress immediately to dyadic dating to catch up with their peers, and if so, does the lack of exposure to the activities that set the stage for romantic involvement leave them less prepared for the relational demands of dyadic dating (see Hebert et al. 2013)? On an encouraging note, research tentatively suggests that most "late bloomers" do progress through typical stages and, unlike early daters, are not at elevated risk for internalizing disorders (Connolly et al. 2013); however, research on late-starting daters is very limited and has not specifically focused on socially anxious populations.

Moderators and Partner Factors

Another important next step will be to identify moderating variables that intensify or attenuate the association between social anxiety and romantic dysfunction. In the parallel literature on depression, several moderators have been shown to increase the link between depressive symptoms and adolescent romantic activities, including family factors (Davila et al. 2009b; Doyle et al. 2003; Steinberg and Davila 2008), attachment style (Davila et al. 2004), co-rumination (Starr and Davila 2009), pubertal timing (Stroud and Davila 2008), classroom context (Hou et al. 2013), genetic vulnerability (Starr et al. 2014), and female gender (Joyner and Udry 2000; Starr and Davila 2008c).

We expect that several factors also influence social anxiety's relationship to romantic experiences. In line with the adult literature (Hart et al. 1999), we would naturally expect the nature and severity of the social anxiety symptoms to make a difference; for example, we would not anticipate situation-bound social phobia (such as public speaking anxiety) to play a significant role in romantic functioning. Furthermore, the quality of the adolescent's non-romantic relationships likely contributes to romantic impairments. Adolescents who are able to establish at least one high-quality friendship or who have strong, communicative relationships with their family members would have a context to develop interpersonal skills and close relationship models even in the absence of romantic activities. Among romantically involved socially anxious adolescents, those with strong external relationships that provide support and companionship may be less likely to become dependent on their romantic partners and may have better support when relationships turn sour.

Romantic relationships are a two-way street, and an important and often overlooked factor is partner selection. Some youth will respond to their partner's distress with support and patience, and others will lack the capacity, maturity, or inclination to do so. It stands to reason that a more supportive partner could provide a corrective learning experience, whereas a more rejecting partner could confirm social fears and aggravate symptoms. An interesting related question is whether socially anxious youth selectively gravitate toward partners with particular characteristics. Researchers have long observed patterns of assortative mating related to psychiatric disorder and personality traits (Merikangas 1982; Merikangas and Spiker 1982), although less research has directly examined this phenomenon in socially anxious populations. If socially anxious youth are more likely to select partners who are also interpersonally withdrawn, for example, it could have multiple effects; partners may be more able to provide empathetic support and understanding for each other's fears, but they may also end up reinforcing each other's social avoidance.

Effects of Internet-Based Social Networking and Other New Technologies

Modern forms of communication and social networking provide a whole new venue for romantic contact, and these may have ups and downs for socially anxious youth. Communicating with peers, including love interests, via a computer screen or text message strips social interactions of many of their anxiety-inducing elements, potentially reducing the inhibitions of socially anxious youth. This could conceivably have numerous benefits for socially anxious adolescents, including providing more opportunities to initiate romantic contact and obtain social support (e.g., Indian and Grieve 2014; Valkenburg and Peter 2009).

Research in this area is new, and it is too early to say whether the developmental skills practiced in online interactions generalize to face-to-face relationships, but existing evidence suggests that online communication enhances adolescents' relationships, social connectedness, and general well-being (Indian and Grieve 2014; Valkenburg and Peter 2009), as well as romantic relationship qualities (Blais et al. 2008). That said, new technologies may also introduce risky or stressful experiences. For example, negative social networking experiences have been associated with adolescents' reports of social anxiety (Landoll et al. 2013). In addition, one might speculate that socially anxious teens (being eager to please) might be more susceptible to high-risk online romantic interactions (e.g., linking up with high-risk or predatory partners online, "sexting," etc.). As these technologies are new, research investigating them is correspondingly nascent; so far more studies are needed before we can understand the trade-offs of digital social networking for the romantic functioning of socially anxious youth.

Implications for Prevention and Intervention

Given the developmental salience of romantic relationships in adolescence, it is important for therapists treating socially anxious youth to assess romantic behaviors and competencies and determine how these may be influenced by anxiety pathology. Deficits or dating-specific fears may be addressed in treatment using a variety of approaches that have been developed to target general social fears and interpersonal effectiveness, including behavioral rehearsal, imaginal or in vivo exposure to feared situations, cognitive restructuring, assertiveness training, and mindfulness techniques (e.g., Albano et al. 1995; Albano and DiBartolo 2007; Beidel et al. 2000; Garcia-Lopez 2000, 2007, 2013, Garcia-Lopez et al. 2002, 2006, 2009, 2014; Hayward et al. 2000; Masia et al. 2001, 2005, 2007; Roemer and Orsillo 2010). For more details, please see Chap. 8, 12 and 13. In addition, interpersonal psychotherapy may be well suited for anxious adolescents with dating-related concerns, as this therapeutic approach acknowledges the interconnection between relationship problems and emotional functioning and directly targets interpersonal deficits and has been adapted for adolescents and for socially anxious populations (see Mufson et al. this volume, Chap. 11).

Although numerous treatment and prevention programs targeting social anxiety in adolescent populations have garnered empirical support, none of them have incorporated components specifically aimed at improving romantic relationships, and treatment development researchers should consider doing so (see Davila et al. in press). In the 1970s, researchers developed intervention protocols specifically targeting dating anxiety, using methods such as systematic desensitization, social skills training, and other behavioral techniques, and demonstrated preliminary support for their effectiveness, largely in college samples (e.g., Bander et al. 1975; Curran 1975, 1977). However, this research mostly petered out, and to our knowledge, there have been no recent attempts to update these treatments to incorporate more newly developed psychotherapeutic techniques and tailor approaches to modern audiences, nor have there been any dating anxiety interventions specifically developed for adolescents. As dating-specific anxiety is pervasive among early adolescents, prevention-based psychoeducational programs teaching romantic skills and anxiety management at a community level may help instill core romantic competencies and prevent future anxiety-related distress and impairment.

In conclusion, although they have long been marginalized in the psychological literature, researchers are increasingly recognizing the developmental significance of romantic relationships in adolescence. Social anxiety is a widespread problem during adolescence, with dramatic implications for peer functioning. Far more research is needed to understand how this key peer context—romantic relationships—influences and is influenced by the prevalent and socially impairing psychological condition of social anxiety. Better understanding of these associations may have long-term consequences for the amelioration of social anxiety symptoms and the enrichment of romantic functioning among youth.

References

Abma JC, Martinez GM, Mosher WD, Dawson BS (2004) Teenagers in the United States: sexual activity, contraceptive use, and childbearing, 2002, Vital and Health Statistics 23(24), Vital and health statistics. Hyattsville: National Center for Health Statistics

Albano AM, Marten PA, Holt CS, Heimberg RG, Barlow DH (1995) Cognitive behavioral group treatment for social phobia in adolescents: a preliminary study. J Nerv Ment Dis 183:685–692

Albano AM, DiBartolo PM (2007) Cognitive-behavioral therapy for social phobia in adolescence. Oxford University Press, Oxford

Alden LE, Taylor CT (2004) Interpersonal processes in social phobia. Clin Psychol Rev 24: 857–882. doi:10.1016/j.cpr.2004.07.006

Bander KW, Steinke GV, Allen GJ, Mosher DL (1975) Evaluation of three dating-specific treatment approaches for heterosexual dating anxiety. J Consult Clin Psychol 43:259–265. doi:10.1037/h0076528

Beck JG, Davila J, Farrow S, Grant D (2006) When the heat is on: romantic partner responses influence distress in socially anxious women. Behav Res Ther 44:737–748. doi:http://dx.doi.org/10.1016/j.brat.2005.05.004

Beidel DC, Turner SM, Morris TL (2000) Behavioral treatment of childhood social phobia. J Consult Clin Psychol 68:1072–1080

Bell J (2009) Why embarrassment inhibits the acquisition and use of condoms: a qualitative approach to understanding risky sexual behaviour. J Adolesc 32:379–391. doi:http://dx.doi.org/10.1016/j.adolescence.2008.01.002

Biggs BK, Sampilo ML, McFadden MM (2011) Peer relations and victimization in adolescents with social anxiety disorder. In: Alfano CA, Beidel DC (eds) Social anxiety in adolescents and young adults: translating developmental science into practice. American Psychological Association, Washington, DC, pp 143–160

Blais J, Craig W, Pepler D, Connolly J (2008) Adolescents online: the importance of internet activity choices to salient relationships. J Youth Adolesc 37:522–536. doi:10.1007/s10964-007-9262-7

Brown BB (1999) 'You're going out with who?' Peer group influences on adolescent romantic relationships. In: Furman W, Brown BB, Feiring C (eds) The development of romantic relationships in adolescence. Cambridge University Press, New York, pp 291–329

Carver K, Joyner K, Udry JR (2003) National estimates of adolescent romantic relationships. In: Florsheim P (ed) Adolescent romantic relations and sexual behavior: theory, research, and practical implications. Lawrence Erlbaum, Mahwah, pp 23–56

Caspi A, Elder GH, Bem DJ (1988) Moving away from the world: life-course patterns of shy children. Dev Psychol 24:824–831. doi:10.1037/0012-1649.24.6.824

Chorney DB, Morris TL (2008) The changing face of dating anxiety: issues in assessment with special populations. Clin Psychol Sci Pract 15:224–238. doi:10.1111/j.1468-2850.2008.00132.x

Collins W (2003) More than myth: the developmental significance of romantic relationships during adolescence. J Res Adolesc 13:1–24. doi:10.1111/1532-7795.1301001

Collins WA, Welsh DP, Furman W (2009) Adolescent romantic relationships. Annu Rev Psychol 60:631–652. doi:10.1146/annurev.psych.60.110707.163459

Connolly JA, Goldberg A (1999) Romantic relationships in adolescence: the role of friends and peers in their emergence and development. In: Furman W, Brown BB, Feiring C (eds) The development of romantic relationships in adolescence. Cambridge University Press, Cambridge, pp 266–290

Connolly JA, Konarski R (1994) Peer self-concept in adolescence: analysis of factor structure and of associations with peer experience. J Res Adolesc 4:385–403. doi:10.1207/s15327795jra0403_3

Connolly JA, Craig W, Goldberg A, Pepler D (2004) Mixed-gender groups, dating, and romantic relationships in early adolescence. J Res Adolesc 14:185–207. doi:10.1111/j.1532-7795.2004.01402003.x

Connolly JA, Nguyen HNT, Pepler D, Craig W, Jiang D (2013) Developmental trajectories of romantic stages and associations with problem behaviours during adolescence. J Adolesc 36:1013–1024. doi:http://dx.doi.org/10.1016/j.adolescence.2013.08.006
Cuming S, Rapee RM (2010) Social anxiety and self-protective communication style in close relationships. Behav Res Ther 48:87–96. doi:http://dx.doi.org/10.1016/j.brat.2009.09.010
Curran JP (1975) Social skills training and systematic desensitization in reducing dating anxiety. Behav Res Ther 13:65–68
Curran JP (1977) Skills training as an approach to the treatment of heterosexual-social anxiety: a review. Psychol Bull 84:140
Darcy K, Davila J, Beck JG (2005) Is social anxiety associated with both interpersonal avoidance and interpersonal dependence? Cognit Ther Res 29:171–186
Davila J (2008) Depressive symptoms and adolescent romance: theory, research, and implications. Child Dev Perspect 2:26–31
Davila J, Beck JG (2002) Is social anxiety associated with impairment in close relationships? A preliminary investigation. Behav Ther 33:427–446
Davila J, Steinberg SJ, Kachadourian L, Cobb R, Fincham F (2004) Romantic involvement and depressive symptoms in early and late adolescence: the role of a preoccupied relational style. Pers Relat 11:161–178
Davila J, Steinberg SJ, Ramsay M, Stroud CB, Starr L, Yoneda A (2009a) Assessing romantic competence in adolescence: the romantic competence interview. J Adolesc 32:55–75. doi:10.1016/j.adolescence.2007.12.001
Davila J, Stroud CB, Starr LR, Miller MR, Yoneda A, Hershenberg R (2009b) Romantic and sexual activities, parent-adolescent stress, and depressive symptoms among early adolescent girls. J Adolesc 32:909–924. doi:10.1016/j.adolescence.2008.10.004
Davila J, La Greca AM, Starr LR, Landoll R (2010) Anxiety disorders in adolescence. In: Beck JG (ed) Interpersonal processes in anxiety disorders. American Psychological Association, Washington, DC, pp 97–124
Davila J, Capaldi DM, La Greca A (in press) Adolescent/young adult romantic relationships and psychopathology. In: Cicchetti D (ed) Developmental psychopathology, 3rd edn. Wiley, New York
Diamond LM, Savin-Williams RC, Dubé EM (1999) Sex, dating, passionate friendships, and romance: intimate peer relations among lesbian, gay, and bisexual adolescents. In: Furman W, Brown BB, Feiring C (eds) The development of romantic relationships in adolescence. Cambridge University Press, Cambridge, pp 175–210
Dodge CS, Heimberg RG, Nyman D, O'Rien GT (1988) Daily heterosocial interactions of high and low socially anxious college students: a diary study. Behav Ther 18:90–96
Doyle AB, Brendgen M, Markiewicz D, Kamkar K (2003) Family relationships as moderators of the association between romantic relationships and adjustment in early adolescence. J Early Adolesc 23:316–340. doi:10.1177/0272431603254238
Filsinger EE, Wilson MR (1983) Social anxiety and marital adjustment. Fam Relat J Appl Fam Child Stud 32:513–519
Floyd FJ, Markman HJ (1984) An economical observational measure of couples' communication skill. J Consult Clin Psychol 52:97–103. doi:10.1037/0022-006X.52.1.97
Furman W, Shaffer L (2003) The role of romantic relationships in adolescent development. In: Florsheim P (ed) Adolescent romantic relations and sexual behavior: theory, research, and practical implications. Lawrence Erlbaum, Mahwah, pp 3–22
Furman W, Wehner EA (1994) Romantic views: toward a theory of adolescent romantic relationships. In: Montmayer R, Adams GR, Gullota GP (eds) Advances in adolescent development: personal relationships during adolescence, vol 6. Sage, Thousand Oaks, pp 168–175
Garcia-Lopez LJ (2000, 2007) Examining the efficacy of three cognitive-behavioural treatments aimed at overcoming social anxiety in adolescents. University of Murcia: Publication Service
Garcia-Lopez LJ (2013) Tratando…trastorno de ansiedad social [Treating…social anxiety disorder]. Piramide, Madrid

Garcia-Lopez LJ, Olivares J, Turner SM, Beidel DC, Albano AM, Sánchez-Meca J (2002) Results at long-term among three psychological treatments for adolescents with generalized social phobia (II): clinical significance and effect size. Psicologia Conductual [Behav Psychol] 10:165–179

Garcia-Lopez L-J, Olivares J, Beidel D, Albano A, Turner S, Rosa AI (2006) Efficacy of three treatment protocols for adolescents with social anxiety disorder: a 5-year follow-up assessment. J Anxiety Disord 20:175–191. doi:10.1016/j.janxdis.2005.01.003

Garcia-Lopez LJ, Muela JA, Espinosa-Fernández L, Diaz-Castela MM (2009) Exploring the relevance of expressed emotion to the treatment of social anxiety disorder in adolescence. J Adolesc 32:1371–1376. doi:10.1016/j.adolescence.2009.08.001

Garcia-Lopez LJ, Diaz-Castela MM, Muela-Martinez JA, Espinosa-Fernandez L (2014) Can parent training for parents with high levels of expressed emotion have a positive effect on their child's social anxiety improvement? J Anxiety Disord 28:812–822. doi:10.1016/j.janxdis.2014.09.001

Gilman SE, Cochran SD, Mays VM, Hughes M, Ostrow D, Kessler RC (2001) Risk of psychiatric disorders among individuals reporting same-sex sexual partners in the National Comorbidity Survey. Am J Public Health 91:933–939. doi:10.2105/AJPH.91.6.933

Glickman AR, La Greca AM (2004) The dating anxiety scale for adolescents: scale development and associations with adolescent functioning. J Clin Child Adolesc Psychol 33:566–578

Gordon EA, Heimberg RG, Montesi JL, Fauber RL (2012) Romantic relationships: do socially anxious individuals benefit? Cogn Behav Ther 41:140–151. doi:10.1080/16506073.2012.656275

Grant DM, Beck JG, Farrow SM, Davila J (2007) Do interpersonal features of social anxiety influence the development of depressive symptoms? Cognit Emotion 21:646–663

Harper MS, Welsh DP (2007) Keeping quiet: self-silencing and its association with relational and individual functioning among adolescent romantic couples. J Soc Pers Relat 24:99–116. doi:10.1177/0265407507072601

Harper MS, Dickson JW, Welsh DP (2006) Self-silencing and rejection sensitivity in adolescent romantic relationships. J Youth Adolesc 35:435–443. doi:10.1007/s10964-006-9048-3

Hart TA, Heimberg RG (2005) Social anxiety as a risk factor for unprotected intercourse among gay and bisexual male youth. AIDS Behav 9:505–512. doi:10.1007/s10461-005-9021-2

Hart TA, Turk CL, Heimberg RG, Liebowitz MR (1999) Relation of marital status to social phobia severity. Depress Anxiety 10:28–32

Harter S (1999) The construction of the self: a developmental perspective. Guilford Press, New York

Hayward C, Varady S, Albano AM, Thienemann M, Henderson L, Schatzberg AF (2000) Cognitive-behavioral group therapy for social phobia in female adolescents: results of a pilot study. J Am Acad Child Adolesc Psychiatry 39:721–726

Hebert KR, Fales J, Nangle DW, Papadakis AA, Grover RL (2013) Linking social anxiety and adolescent romantic relationship functioning: indirect effects and importance of peers. J Youth Adolesc 42:1708–1720. doi:10.1007/s10964-012-9878-0

Hou J, Natsuaki MN, Zhang J, Guo F, Huang Z, Wang M, Chen Z (2013) Romantic relationships and adjustment problems in China: the moderating effect of classroom romantic context. J Adolesc 36:171–180. doi:http://dx.doi.org/10.1016/j.adolescence.2012.10.008

Inderbitzen HM, Walters KS, Bukowski AL (1997) The role of social anxiety in adolescent peer relations: differences among sociometric status groups and rejected subgroups. J Clin Child Psychol 26:338–348. doi:10.1207/s15374424jccp2604_2

Indian M, Grieve R (2014) When Facebook is easier than face-to-face: social support derived from Facebook in socially anxious individuals. Pers Indiv Differ 59:102–106. doi:http://dx.doi.org/10.1016/j.paid.2013.11.016

Joiner TE Jr, Metalsky GI, Katz J, Beach SRH (1999) Depression and excessive reassurance-seeking. Psychol Inq 10:269–278

Joyner K, Udry JR (2000) You don't bring me anything but down: adolescent romance and depression. J Health Soc Behav 41:369–391

Kashdan TB, Collins RL, Elhai J (2006) Social anxiety and positive outcome expectancies on risk-taking behaviors. Cognit Ther Res 30:749–761. doi:10.1007/s10608-006-9017-x

Kashdan TB, Volkmann JR, Breen WE, Han S (2007) Social anxiety and romantic relationships: the costs and benefits of negative emotion expression are context-dependent. J Anxiety Dis 21:475–492. doi:http://dx.doi.org/10.1016/j.janxdis.2006.08.007

Krueger RF (1999) The structure of common mental disorders. Arch Gen Psychiatry 56:921–926. doi:10.1001/archpsyc.56.10.921

Kuttler A, La Greca AM (2004) Linkages among adolescent girls' romantic relationships, best friendships, and peer networks. J Adolesc 27:395–414. doi:10.1016/j.adolescence.2004.05.002

La Greca AM, Harrison HM (2005) Adolescent peer relations, friendships, and romantic relationships: do they predict social anxiety and depression? J Clin Child Adolesc Psychol 34:49–61

La Greca AM, Lopez N (1998) Social anxiety among adolescents: linkages with peer relations and friendships. J Abnorm Child Psychol 26:83–94

La Greca AM, Mackey ER (2007) Adolescents' anxiety in dating situations: the potential role of friends and romantic partners. J Clin Child Adolesc Psychol 36:522–533. doi:10.1080/15374410701662097

La Greca AM, Davila J, Landoll R, Siegel R (2011) Dating, romantic relationships, and social anxiety in young people. In: Alfano CA, Beidel DC (eds) Social anxiety in adolescence: translating developmental science into practice. American Psychological Association, Washington, DC, pp 93–105

Lampe L, Slade T, Issakidis C, Andrews G (2003) Social phobia in the Australian national survey of mental health and well-being (NSMHWB). Psychol Med 33:637–646

Landoll RR, La Greca AM, Lai B (2013) Aversive peer experiences on social networking sites: development of the social networking-peer experiences questionnaire. J Res Adolesc 23:695–705. doi:10.1111/jora.12022

Larson RW, Richards MH (1998) Waiting for the weekend: friday and saturday nights as the emotional climax of the week. In: Crouter AC, Larson RW (eds) Temporal rhythms in adolescence: clocks, calendars, and the coordination of daily life, vol 82, New directions for child development. Jossey-Bass, San Francisco, pp 37–51

Larson RW, Clore GL, Wood GA (1999) The emotions of romantic relationships: do they wreak havoc on adolescents? In: Furman W, Brown B, Feiring C (eds) The development of romantic relationships in adolescence. Cambridge Press, New York, pp 19–49

Laursen B (1996) Closeness and conflict in adolescent peer relationships: interdependence with friends and romantic partners. In: Bukowski WM, Newcomb AF, Hartup WW (eds) The company they keep: friendships in childhood and adolescence. Cambridge University Press, New York, pp 186–210

Leary MR, Dobbins SE (1983) Social anxiety, sexual behavior, and contraceptive use. J Pers Soc Psychol 45:1347–1354. doi:10.1037/0022-3514.45.6.1347

Madsen SD, Collins W (2011) The salience of adolescent romantic experiences for romantic relationship qualities in young adulthood. J Res Adolesc 21:789–801. doi:10.1111/j.1532-7795.2011.00737.x

Masten AS, Coatsworth JD, Neemann J, Gest SD (1995) The structure and coherence of competence from childhood through adolescence. Child Dev 66:1635–1659. doi:10.2307/1131901

Masia CL, Klein RG, Storch E, Corda B (2001) School-based behavioral treatment for social anxiety disorder in adolescents: results of a pilot study. J Am Acad Child Adolesc Psychiatry 40:780–786

Masia-Warner C, Klein RG, Dent HC, Fisher PH, Alvir J, Albano AM, Guardino M (2005) Schoolbased Intervention for adolescents with social anxiety disorder: results of a controlled study. J Abnorm Child Psychol 33:707–722

Masia-Warner C, Fisher PH, Shrout PE, Rathor S, Klein RG (2007) Treating adolescents with social anxiety disorder in school: an attention control trial. J Child Psychol Psychiatry 48:676–68 doi:10.1111/j.1469-7610.2007.01737.x

Meleshko KG, Alden LE (1993) Anxiety and self-disclosure: toward a motivational model. J Pers Soc Psychol 64:1000–1009

Merikangas KR (1982) Assortative mating for psychiatric disorders and psychological traits. Arch Gen Psychiatry 39:1173–1180

Merikangas KR, Spiker DG (1982) Assortative mating among in-patients with primary affective disorder. Psychol Med 12:753–764. doi:10.1017/S0033291700049059

Nieder T, Seiffge-Krenke I (2001) Coping with stress in different phases of romantic development. J Adolesc 24:297–311. doi:http://dx.doi.org/10.1006/jado.2001.0407

Pachankis JE, Goldfried MR (2006) Social anxiety in young gay men. J Anxiety Dis 20:996–1015. doi:http://dx.doi.org/10.1016/j.janxdis.2006.01.001

Papsdorf M, Alden LE (1998) Mediators of social rejection in social anxiety: similarity, self-disclosure, and overt signs of anxiety. J Res Pers 32:351–369

Ranta K, Kaltiala-Heino R, Pelkonen M, Marttunen M (2009) Associations between peer victimization, self-reported depression and social phobia among adolescents: the role of comorbidity. J Adolesc 32:77–93

Ranta K, Kaltiala-Heino R, Fröjd S, Marttunen M (2013) Peer victimization and social phobia: a follow-up study among adolescents. Soc Psychiatry Psychiatr Epidemiol 48:533–544

Roberts KE, Schwartz D, Hart TA (2011) Social anxiety among lesbian, gay, bisexual, and transgender adolescents and young adults. In: Alfano CA, Beidel DC (eds) Social anxiety in adolescents and young adults: translating developmental science into practice. American Psychological Association, Washington, DC, pp 161–181

Roemer L, Orsillo SM (2010) Mindfulness- and acceptance-based behavioral therapies in practice. Guilford, New York

Schneier FR, Johnson J, Hornig CD, Liebowitz MR, Weissman MM (1992) Social phobia: comorbidity and morbidity in an epidemiologic sample. Arch Gen Psychiatry 49:282–288. doi:10.1001/archpsyc.1992.01820040034004

Seiffge-Krenke I, Lang J (2002) Forming and maintaining romantic relations from early adolescence to young adulthood: evidence of a developmental sequence. In: Shulman S, Seiffge-Krenke I (co-chairs) Antecedents of the quality and stability of adolescent romantic relationships. Symposium at the conference of the society for research on adolescence, New Orleans, April 2002

Shulman S, Scharf M (2000) Adolescent romantic behaviors and perceptions: age- and gender-related differences, and links with family and peer relationships. J Res Adolesc 10:99–118. doi:10.1207/SJRA1001_5

Siegel R, Greca A, Harrison H (2009) Peer victimization and social anxiety in adolescents: prospective and reciprocal relationships. J Youth Adolesc 38:1096–1109. doi:10.1007/s10964-009-9392-1

Sparrevohn RM, Rapee RM (2009) Self-disclosure, emotional expression and intimacy within romantic relationships of people with social phobia. Behav Res Ther 47:1074–1078. doi:http://dx.doi.org/10.1016/j.brat.2009.07.016

Starr LR, Davila J (2008a) Differentiating interpersonal correlates of depressive symptoms and social anxiety in adolescence: implications for models of comorbidity. J Clin Child Adolesc Psychol 37:337–349. doi:10.1080/15374410801955854

Starr LR, Davila J (2008b) Excessive reassurance seeking, depression, and interpersonal rejection: a meta-analytic review. J Abnorm Psychol 117:762–775

Starr LR, Davila J (2008c) Gender differences in adolescent romantic experiences and their relationship to depressive symptoms. Paper presented at the association for behavioral and cognitive therapies, Orlando

Starr LR, Davila J (2009) Clarifying co-rumination: associations with internalizing symptoms and romantic involvement among adolescent girls. J Adolesc 32:19–37

Starr LR, Davila J, La Greca AM, Landoll R (2011) Social anxiety and depression: the teenage and early adult years. In: Alfano CA, Beidel DC (eds) Social anxiety in adolescents and young adults: translating developmental science into practice. American Psychological Association, Washington, DC, pp 75–91

Starr LR, Davila J, Stroud CB, Li PCC, Yoneda A, Hershenberg R, Miller MR (2012) Love hurts (in more ways than one): specificity of psychological symptoms as predictors and consequences of romantic activity among early adolescent girls. J Clin Psychol 68:403–420. doi:10.1002/jclp.20862

Starr LR, Hammen C (2015). Genetic moderation of the association between adolescent romantic involvement and depression: contributions of 5-HTTLPR genotype, chronic stress, and family discord. [Manuscript under review]

Steinberg SJ, Davila J (2008) Romantic functioning and depressive symptoms among early ado lescent girls: the moderating role of parental emotional availability. J Clin Child Adolesc Psychol 37:350–362

Storch EA, Masia-Warner C (2004) The relationship of peer victimization to social anxiety and loneliness in adolescent females. J Adolesc 27:351–362

Storch EA, Masia-Warner C, Crisp H, Klein RG (2005) Peer victimization and social anxiety in adolescence: a prospective study. Aggress Behav 31:437–452. doi:10.1002/ab.20093

Stroud CB, Davila J (2008) Pubertal timing and depressive symptoms in early adolescents: the roles of romantic competence and romantic experiences. J Youth Adolesc 37:953–966

Valkenburg PM, Peter J (2009) Social consequences of the internet for adolescents: a decade of research. Curr Dir Psychol Sci 18:1–5. doi:10.1111/j.1467-8721.2009.01595.x

Vernberg EM, Abwender DA, Ewell KK, Beery SH (1992) Social anxiety and peer relationships in early adolescence: a prospective analysis. J Clin Child Psychol 21:189–196

Waldinger RJ, Diguer L, Guastella F, Lefebvre R, Allen JP, Luborsky L, Hauser ST (2002) The same old song?–Stability and change in relationship schemas from adolescence to young adulthood. J Youth Adolesc 31:17–29. doi:10.1023/A:1014080915602

Welsh DP, Haugen PT, Widman L, Darling N, Grello CM (2005) Kissing is good: a developmental investigation of sexuality in adolescent romantic couples. Sex Res Soc Policy 2(4):32–41. doi:10.1525/srsp.2005.2.4.32

Wenzel A (2002) Characteristics of close relationships in individuals with social phobia: a preliminary comparison with nonanxious individuals. In: A clinician's guide to maintaining and enhancing close relationships. Lawrence Erlbaum, Mahwah, NJ, pp 199–213

Wenzel A, Graff-Dolezal J, Macho M, Brendle JR (2005) Communication and social skills in socially anxious and nonanxious individuals in the context of romantic relationships. Behav Res Ther 43:505–519

Whisman MA (2007) Marital distress and DSM-IV psychiatric disorders in a population-based national survey. J Abnorm Psychol 116:638–643

Williams T, Connolly J, Cribbie R (2008) Light and heavy heterosexual activities of young Canadian adolescents: normative patterns and differential predictors. J Res Adolesc 18: 145–172. doi:10.1111/j.1532-7795.2008.00554.x

Wittchen H-U, Fuetsch M, Sonntag H, Müller N, Liebowitz M (1999) Disability and quality of life in pure and comorbid social phobia: findings from a controlled study. Eur Psychiatry 14:118–131

Zimmer-Gembeck MJ (2002) The development of romantic relationships and adaptations in the system of peer relationships. J Adolesc Health 31:216–225. doi:http://dx.doi.org/10.1016/S1054-139X(02)00504-9

Zimmer-Gembeck MJ, Siebenbruner J, Collins WA (2001) Diverse aspects of dating: associations with psychosocial functioning from early to middle adolescence. J Adolesc 24:313–336. doi:10.1006/jado.2001.0410

Zimmer-Gembeck MJ, Siebenbruner J, Collins WA (2004) A prospective study of intraindividual and peer influences. Arch Sex Behav 33:381–394. doi:10.1023/B:ASEB.0000028891.16654.2c

Adolescent Social Phobia in Clinical Services

9

John D. Guerry, James Hambrick, and Anne Marie Albano

Introduction

Whether a child presenting for treatment for the first time, or an adult recalling when they first began to struggle with excessive fear in social performance situations, the teenage years have been identified repeatedly as a key time for social anxiety disorder (SAD) to take root and flourish in ways that can be determinant for the entire course of the person's life. For this reason, study of SAD during the adolescent years provides both fruitful insight into the origins and course of the disorder and may also offer a crucial context for intervention.

Among anxiety disorders, SAD has one of the earliest onset and, without intervention, tends to follow a chronic course (Brown et al. 2001; Burstein et al. 2011; Juster and Heimberg 1995; Reich et al. 1994; Rosellini et al. 2013; Stein and Stein 2008). In fact, the median age of onset of SAD appears to be more accurately described as bimodal; in one large sample of individuals presenting for treatment, 21 % reported an age of onset before the age of 10, and 47.6 % reported an age of onset during adolescence/early adulthood (14–22) (Rosellini et al. 2013). Age of

J.D. Guerry, PhD
Department of Child and Adolescent Psychiatry and Behavioral Sciences, The Children's Hospital of Philadelphia, Philadelphia, PA, USA
e-mail: guerryj@email.chop.edu

J. Hambrick, PhD • A.M. Albano, PhD, ABPP (✉)
Child and Adolescent Psychiatry, Columbia University Clinic for Anxiety and Related Disorders, New York Presbyterian Hospital/Columbia University Medical Center, New York, NY, USA
e-mail: hambricj@nyspi.columbia.edu; AlbanoA@nyspi.columbia.edu

K. Ranta et al. (eds.), *Social Anxiety and Phobia in Adolescents: Development, Manifestation and Intervention Strategies*, DOI 10.1007/978-3-319-16703-9_9

onset in the middle childhood years (10–14) or adult years (over 23)[1] is relatively rare (Rosellini et al. 2013; Wittchen and Fehm 2003[2]). For more details, please see Chap. 3. A 3-year longitudinal study found that whereas depression typically followed an episodic course, anxiety and symptoms of social anxiety, in particular, tended to operate with trait stability akin to personality attributes (Prenoveau et al. 2011). The early developmental stages of psychopathology (EDSP) study, a prospective, longitudinal study of 3,021 community participants reported that generally by the age of 19, the individual's SAD stabilized or began a progressive worsening that persisted into adulthood (Wittchen and Fehm 2003).

When one looks at the particular challenges of the developmental stage, it is perhaps no surprise that adolescence is such a fertile ground in which SAD can take root. Traditionally, the period between 13 and 18 years old is viewed as one of tumultuous change. Almost immediately after adolescence emerged as a distinct developmental phase, it was famously characterized as a period of "storm and stress" (Hall 1904), during which questions of identity become paramount (Erikson 1959). Of course, the major change that comes to mind for many is the development of sexual maturity through puberty; however, of late the organizational changes within the brain are now thought to be equally epochal. Through the process of synaptic pruning, massive numbers of neuronal connections die off as the brain shifts from a sponge seeking maximal input to a powerfully efficient processing machine (Compas 2004). Adolescents' abilities to represent information symbolically and to reason abstractly significantly mature. Of course, this ultimately positive reorganization has a few short-term costs; the attrition of neuronal connections between the frontal lobes and limbic structures has been implicated in the higher propensity to risky behavior often observed in teens (Steinberg 2004).

In tandem with these improvements in functioning, everyday tasks of living become more difficult during adolescence. Expectations at school and home tend to increase dramatically, as adolescents are expected to function more independently (although often without commensurate increases in freedom). Adolescents at school take on not just more work, but more complicated and academically challenging work. "Multitasking" is expected with greater frequency and flawlessness. Expectations at home can shift to include more responsibility (e.g., more chores or more work) and increased self-direction (e.g., waking oneself up, initiating homework with less monitoring).

[1]One will note that the age-group labels differ somewhat from conventional labels (including, indeed, other chapters in this volume). For the purposes of accurate reporting, we have chosen to conform to the labels used in the research reviewed in this study. We will address this labeling concern in more detail in the conclusion of this chapter.

[2]In fact, the earlier Wittchen and Fehm article reported that epidemiological samples find a unimodal peak onset during childhood and adolescence, between the ages of 10 and 16, while clinical samples report evidence for somewhat lower age of onset of the generalized subtype as compared with the nongeneralized subtype. The nature of these subtypes, as well as their continued redefinition, has been debated as recently as the latest edition of the *Diagnostic and Statistical Manual* (*DSM-5*; APA 2013).

Relationships with parents can become more complicated as well, although not necessarily in the expected way. Relationship patterns change dramatically within the stage of adolescence. For example, in a sample of 495 Slovenian teens between the ages of 13 and 19, Puklek Levpušček (2006) reported that support seeking from and idealization of parents decreased significantly during early and late adolescence; mid-adolescence (during eighth grade) appeared to be a particularly critical point, during which children were most likely to report high self-sufficiency and defensiveness around need for parental support, before developing a more balanced view of self in relation to family during late adolescence. Parents often view their relationships with teens as suddenly more fraught and difficult, as they find their child questioning their authority and values more and more frequently. Infuriatingly, they see their teens walk away from pitched battles over house standards and rules relatively unscathed, viewing the conflict less as a death match over the future and more as an exchange of opinion (Smetana 1997; Steinberg 2001).

Peer relationships become substantially more salient and charged. With the rise of the "invisible audience" and increasing questions about identity and one's future (presumably offshoots of the improved ability to reason symbolically), adolescents become more aware that their own views of self may differ substantially from their peers' opinions, and even the uncertainty over what others' opinions might be can be threatening and worrisome (Elkind 1967). At the same time, the importance of peers becomes paramount as adolescents step into taking charge of their friendships, and the first tentative first steps toward establishing their sexual identity (Buote et al. 2007; LaGreca and Prinstein 1999), just at a moment where their brains and bodies may be least equipped to manage all the input. For more details, please see Chap. 3, 5 and 8.

All this change and much more happen just in the course of normal development. Successful transition through adolescence depends on meeting these new challenges with a strong foundation of early experience. Compounding their significance, the manner and degree to which adolescents are able to meet these challenges may variably confer risk and resilience as they navigate through subsequent developmental transitions during later adulthood. The ways in which SAD further complicates these developmental transitions are myriad and pervasive. For example, symptoms of social anxiety can interfere with the process of differentiating from parents and adopting a more independent role, contribute to avoidance of peers at exactly the moment when peers are meant to become major influences in the development of one's proto-adult identity, and as a result often inhibit or even bring the transition into adulthood to an effective halt. In addressing SAD clinically, therefore, clinicians must take into account all of the vulnerabilities and developmental challenges present in this period and respond in a comprehensive and inclusive way.

This recognition and the recognition that adolescents face specific challenges that are qualitatively distinct from other age groups led Albano and colleagues (1991) to develop cognitive-behavioral group treatment for adolescents (CBGT-A). CBGT-A, a developmental adaptation of Heimberg's successful protocol for treating adults with SAD (Heimberg et al. 1985, 1990; Hope and Heimberg 1993), is designed to be delivered by co-therapists for groups of adolescents between the ages of 13 and 17 years. CBGT-A consists of 16 to 20 90-min group therapy sessions with adolescents scheduled over a 3- to 4-month time period and adds meetings with parents at four strategically placed sessions during the program. The multicomponent protocol is divided into two phases, with the first phase of treatment (i.e., sessions 1 through 8) focusing on psychoeducation and skill building in such areas as social problem-solving, assertiveness, and cognitive restructuring; and the second phase (i.e., sessions 9 through 14) emphasizing within-session behavioral exposure and homework exposure assignments. Session 15 involves exposure tasks performed in front of an audience of parents, and session 16 focuses on final exposures and termination (Albano and Barlow 1996). Empirical research, though limited somewhat in scope, has supported the efficacy of this approach (Albano et al. 1995; Garcia-Lopez et al. 2002, 2006; Hayward et al 2000; Olivares et al. 2002).

This multifaceted approach was an early recognition of the fact that adapting group (or, for that matter, individual) treatment for adolescents requires careful attention not just to the course and challenges in normal development, but also to the early risk factors that render the child vulnerable to anxiety and the conditioning factors and challenges that occur during adolescence which exploit this vulnerability. We will now consider the specific developmental challenges that predict SAD and the types of interventions that can target those challenges. As we will see, effective evidence-based interventions for SAD in adolescents have consistently emphasized a multifaceted approach, consistent with the complex interplay of factors that leads to the onset of SAD.

Anxiety disorders do not typically appear sui generis; they are frequently the product of distal developmental influences, so that an anxiety problem that arises at 14 or 23 can still be influenced by factors that were present at (or even before) birth. Developmental psychologists (and increasingly clinical psychologists) place a premium on developmental pathways, highlighting the various vulnerabilities, conditioning events, and maintaining factors underlying a disorder (Higa-McMillan and Ebesutani 2011; Vasey and Dadds 2001). Although age of onset during adolescence appears to be more strongly related to the presence of some acute stressor or stressors around the time the SAD developed, most researchers believe the individual's response to these stressors is strongly influenced by a variety of vulnerabilities produced by exposure to any number of risk factors (Rosellini et al. 2013). It is also worth considering early factors in the onset of SAD because earlier age of onset predicts increases in symptom severity, autonomic arousal, depression, higher levels of neurotic temperament, and functional impairment (Rosellini et al. 2013: see Knappe et al. Chap. 3, this volume). Failing to consider the early factors that predict SAD in adolescence would therefore mean that not only would we miss the key predictors of why SAD develops in adolescence, but that we would also neglect the most severely afflicted, those who may experience exponentially exacerbated difficulties during their teenage years.

Biological Risk Factors

As with so many mental and emotional disorders, the road toward adolescent SAD can begin before the child is even born. A broad scientific consensus has gathered in support of the heritability of SAD (e.g., Fyer et al. 1993, 1995; Hughes et al. 2009; Kendler et al. 1992; Mannuzza et al. 1995; Reich and Yates 1988). First-degree relatives of adults with SAD are three times more likely to be afflicted with SAD (compared with first-degree relatives of control participants) (Fyer et al. 1993, 1995; Mannuzza et al. 1995; Reich and Yates 1988). Twin studies have yielded heritability estimates of 30–65 % (Kendler et al. 1992; Beatty et al. 2002). These estimates are more pronounced as a function of subtype of SAD. For example, Stein and colleagues (1998) found that first-degree relatives of adults with generalized SAD were ten times more at risk for generalized SAD; no enhanced risk was found for the nongeneralized subtype.

It should be noted that the heritability estimates reported here are not necessarily specific risk for SAD. Whereas both of the Fyer et al. (1993, 1995) and the Reich and Yates (1988) studies found evidence for specific risk, other studies have found more complicated pathways, finding evidence that a variety of parental mental illnesses, including panic disorder and especially major depression, can predict SAD in offspring (Horwath and Weissman 1995; Biederman et al. 2001; Lieb et al. 2000). Inheritance of SAD demonstrates concordance or nonsignificant differences in heritability between monozygotic and dizygotic twins (Kendler et al. 1992; Skre et al. 1993). Stein and Stein 2008 has suggested that genetic inheritance of internalizing disorders may be best characterized as the passing on of broad, nonspecific traits that are predictive of anxiety disorders in general rather than of SAD in particular.

A key inherited nonspecific set of traits appears to be behavioral inhibition to the familiar (BI), first identified by Kagan and colleagues (1988; Kagan 1989). BI was used to describe observation of generalized emotional and behavioral tendencies among 10–15 % of Caucasian infants to withdraw or become upset when presented with new or otherwise unfamiliar stimuli. In the youngest children, BI might look like withdrawal, looking to parents or becoming upset when presented with a new toy. In preschool-aged and elementary school-aged children, this temperamental tendency might manifest as constricted emotional expression, hesitancy when speaking or approaching a new situation, and/or reluctance to engage in conversation with peers or adults. In a meta-analytic review of the link between BI and SAD, researchers indicated that BI predicted a three- to sevenfold increase in risk, translating to 40 % of children with BI developing SAD (Clauss and Blackford 2012). However, it is worth noting that the same study concluded that BI was best construed as a generalized risk factor for SAD, not an early precursor; in support of this contention, Clauss and Blackford (2012) cite that the majority of children with BI do not develop SAD, and children with BI do not automatically suffer from the same deficits in emotional regulation and pervasive fear of negative evaluation seen in children with SAD. On the other hand, as noted by Perez-Edgar and Guyer (2014), the precise relationship between BI and SAD has not been definitively established by any direct research.

Multiple studies have supported the stability of BI from infancy through toddlerhood and into middle and late childhood (Caspi and Silva 1995; Asendorph 1994; Fordham and Stevenson-Hinde 1999; Goldsmith and Lemery 2000). Kagan and colleagues (1988) posited that the observed emotional and behavioral correlates of BI were a function of a lower response threshold of the basolateral and central nuclei of the amygdala and projections to the striatum, hypothalamus, and the sympathetic chain and cardiovascular system. This hypothesis has been supported in some studies, although not consistently (Hirshfeld et al. 1992; also, for a review, see Ollendick and Hirshfeld-Becker 2002). Similarly, BI and SAD have been frequently linked in the literature. Among the children from the original Kagan et al. studies, the rates of generalized SAD were found to be substantially higher among those who demonstrated highest BI as toddlers, as compared with the adolescents who were most extroverted as toddlers (34 % vs. 9 %, respectively) (Schwartz et al. 1999). The differences were even starker among girls (44 % vs. 6 %). A separate study found that adolescents with childhood BI were four to five times more likely to develop social anxiety disorder than adolescents without childhood BI (Biederman et al. 2001). At least one study suggested that BI was uniquely predictive of lifetime SAD (as opposed to being more generally predictive of the presence of any anxiety disorder) (Chronis-Tuscano et al. 2009).

Consistent with the BI hypothesis, researchers have also noted significant links between hyperreactivity of the amygdala in response to emotional expression in others and SAD (Battaglia et al. 2012; Blair et al. 2011; Guyer et al. 2008). The first critical fMRI study of adolescents found evidence for significantly higher amygdala and fusiform gyrus activation in response to fearful faces; in addition to the amygdala's role coordinating fear activities, the fusiform gyrus is implicated in facial recognition (Guyer et al 2008). Battaglia and colleagues (2012) were able to successfully predict onset of SAD in a group of 14- to 15-year-olds by measuring brain reactivity (particularly in the amygdala) to angry and fearful faces at the age of 8–9 years old. Blair and colleagues (2011) reported significantly increased reactivity in the amygdala and rostral anterior cingulate cortex in both adolescents and adults with SAD in response to others' emotional expression. The authors went on to note that the failure to find any significant interactions except in the context of SAD and reactivity to target emotion suggested a developmentally stable disruption (as opposed to a developmental deterioration) (Blair et al. 2011). That is, the disruption associated with SAD appears to be an independent interference on the normal development of facial recognition and recognition of emotion in others' faces. Although these studies offer important support for long-held conventional wisdom around the role of the amygdala in anxiety disorders, it is worth noting that each of these studies suffers from relatively small samples and accompanying power difficulties.

Addressing Biological Risk Factors in Clinical Treatment

In effective evidence-based treatment, consideration of biological vulnerabilities can influence both assessment and psychoeducation about the nature of the disorder. Clinicians may want to attend in particular to adolescents endorsing early onset of SAD or families endorsing high prevalence of anxiety among first-degree relatives. These adolescents may be at particularly high risk for high levels of social anxiety and avoidance, and referral for psychiatric consultation or more intensive treatment options may be appropriate to consider at an earlier point in treatment. In our clinic, for example, adolescents with earlier onset and higher family loading for anxiety and youth with greater functional impairment may be offered individual and group therapy to occur concurrently as a means of giving a higher "dose" of intervention.

Of equal, or perhaps even more importance, appropriately educating families about genetic and temperamental risk for anxiety disorders is crucial. As noted previously, SAD can manifest as more of a trait personality factor rather than an illness with a more chronic or intermittent course (Wittchen and Fehm 2003). Accordingly, many individuals can interpret the notion that SAD is partially heritable as more or less a "life sentence" or that their symptoms are not amenable to psychosocial change. Given the importance placed on developing a strong sense of identity during this stage, defining oneself as an "anxious person," as our patients all too frequently do, can be an especially sticky and pernicious form of self-fulfilling prophecy. It can be important to engage and challenge these ideas. It can be worth noting that it was only among the extreme 10–15 % of individuals with BI that Kagan and his team saw stability of symptoms into adulthood, and even among that 10–15 %, quite a few demonstrated apparently spontaneous shifts toward increased comfort with the unfamiliar or even extroversion. As noted above, even the largest estimate of individuals identified with BI who later develop SAD peaks at 48 % (Clauss and Blackford 2012). During the psychoeducation process, therefore, it is crucial for clinicians to discuss the overall plasticity of the brain, especially in these early years, and that early trends toward distress and dysfunction are amenable to amelioration or even radical change. It is also crucial to help those adolescents who have a nascent, or even well-developed notion of themselves as "anxious people" to use cognitive restructuring to challenge this inaccurate (and often self-fulfilling) label and help them become more aware of other constructive aspects of identity.

There is a diametric peril for the psychoeducating clinician, of course. While communicating optimism or the potential for change, the clinician should be careful not to share an overly rosy perspective; increasing numbers of clinicians are considering the possibility that while anxiety can be regulated effectively, it may also require a lifelong commitment to challenging one's anxiety and using skills gained in treatment to sustain gains from therapy.

SAD and Family Organization

In early childhood, parents assume a crucial role, from facilitating to disrupting the arc of development. For example, parents can influence positive growth during early life by directly and indirectly promoting social skills, encouraging peer interactions through supervision and direct facilitation (such as scheduling play dates), and offering feedback on appropriate and inappropriate types of play (Masia and Morris 1998). In contrast to nonaffected individuals, adults and teens with social anxiety disorder are more likely to report memoires of less affectionate parents who were more socially isolated and hyperconcerned about the opinions of others, who behaved in both overprotective and in rejecting or neglectful ways, who were ashamed of their own shyness and poor social performance, who tended to discipline by shaming, and who tended to isolate their children as well (Arrindell et al. 1989; Bogels et al. 2001; Bruch and Heimberg 1994; Burgess et al. 2001; Caster et al. 1999; Lieb et al. 2000; Parker 1979). In complement to these retrospective reports, other studies have found that parents of anxious children have demonstrated both impaired ability to help their children engage with peers and are more likely to encourage avoidance of potentially threatening situations (Barrett et al. 1996b; Finnie and Russell 1988). Notably, these problematic parental behaviors appear to be uniquely predictive of difficulties in their offspring. One study found that while parental lack of emotional warmth and family dysfunction were both uniquely predictive of adolescent SAD, parental psychopathology only predicted SAD in the context of other vulnerability factors (although the authors added that psychopathology may be crucial to disorder onset, they qualified that this variable likely plays a more secondary role in contributing to the maintenance of symptoms over time) (Knappe et al. 2009).

Given that so many of these studies have a limited frame of reference or rely on self-report or memories of past interactions, the possibility cannot be ruled out that the nascent vulnerability to anxiety may have influenced (or even coerced) parental responses. Still, these conclusions are bolstered by the results of some work focusing on parental and sibling impressions of their own behaviors and observational studies, which find that parents of anxious youth also view themselves as overprotective and relatively more rejecting than the average parent (Garcia-Lopez et al. 2009, 2014; Gulley et al. 2014; Hudson and Rapee 2001, 2005; Lieb et al. 2000; Rubin and Mills 1990; Siqueland et al. 1996; also, see Wong and Rapee, Chap. 2; Knappe et al., Chap. 4, this volume, for a comprehensive review). It is also worth noting that in this literature, "parenting" is often code for the relationship with the mother; fathers remain underrepresented in these research studies. Among the few studies that have focused in particular on father nurturing behaviors, there is little consistency. One study supported a connection between overcontrolling parenting behaviors and social anxiety (Greco and Morris 2002), while another study failed to find any clear link between a father's parenting style and social anxiety (Hudson and Rapee 2002).

More recently, researchers have begun to address this deficit—Bogels and colleagues (2011) suggested that the behavior of fathers might be more impactful on the anxiety of their children than maternal behaviors. In contrast, Knappe et al. (2012) reported distinct and contrasting patterns of parental dysfunction, such that maternal overprotection and paternal rejection and lower emotional warmth predicted SAD in their children. Interestingly, the crossover relationships were not found to be true—paternal overprotection and maternal rejection or lack of warmth failed to significantly predict SAD in their children (Knappe et al. 2012).

Intervening at the Familial Level

Research indicates that the nature of parenting of children with SAD can be ambivalent and inconsistent, reflecting patterns of overprotectiveness, overcontrolling behaviors and neglect, and tendency to encourage avoidance or social isolation. Clinically, we often see other complicated parental emotions underlying these patterns. A representative sample can include emotions such as concern and anxiety over their child's future; anger or upset around the teen's failure to take responsibility or initiative; confusion over the "can't vs. won't" issue (i.e., whether their child is avoiding or truly incapable of engaging with a particular task or challenge), and therefore when to push and when to be understanding; and sadness in recognizing similar patterns or struggles from their own past or present lives. We have seen these emotional responses, and many others, in the course of treating adolescents (and, in turn, their parents) in our clinic.

These clinical observations have been borne out in research. Garcia-Lopez and colleagues (2009) reported that in a clinical sample of 16 adolescents with SAD, adolescents with parents who were high in parental overinvolvement, criticism, and hostility (a construct known as expressed emotion) failed to benefit from a school-based CBT intervention. Garcia-Lopez and colleagues (2009) also emphasized that this pattern differentiated socially anxious adolescents from their adult counterparts, for whom outside criticism was less of a variable.

These parental emotions can lead to a variety of other mutually detrimental patterns. Frequently, parents can become overly intrusive, offering instrumental support or even solutions as opposed to encouraging independence or efficacy on the part of the child and offering support only when needed. All too often we have seen parents complete therapy and school homework assignments or otherwise advocate for their anxious adolescent because they were afraid to let the adolescent negotiate the situation on his or her own. Another common pattern is inconsistency in parenting behaviors, as parents often attempt to compensate for their ambivalence and confusion by vacillating between disciplinary and supportive approaches in unpredictable ways. The inconsistency can come at the between-parent level, where father and mother have different points of view and apply those perspectives simultaneously, resulting in confusion for the child and bringing the parents into conflict. Inconsistency can also come at the within-parent level, where a mother or father can apply supportive approaches until suddenly losing temper at the lack of progress, or meet the child's avoidance with strong discipline only to immediately retreat into support or apologies. Parents frequently struggle with the paradox of knowing they need to encourage independence but being afraid to let the child struggle, and on occasion fail, or being unsure how to encourage or discipline because they cannot discern willful violations of expectations or rules from impairing symptoms of anxiety.

Given that, developmentally, the hope is that parents are becoming somewhat less involved during adolescence, bringing them into treatment can seem somewhat counterintuitive. The truth is, parents can still play crucial roles as allies; the important part is helping them to become more involved in constructive ways as a support system (as opposed to a strict authority) and help the entire family unite around a shared goal and purpose, with clearer understanding of the best skills to help the child move forward.

Albano and colleagues (1991) understood the importance of involving parents in CBGT-A in transitional sessions. By directly involving parents in treatment at key times, parents could get crucial instruction in the skills their children were using in order to help support their adolescent's practice and use of those skills. Involving parents in goal setting helps them better direct their efforts. For example, as opposed to "shotgunning" feedback—that is, giving reactive and inconsistent feedback in a variety of areas, often in the form of criticism—feedback could be more focused around specific goal areas. In other words, feedback could be strategically directed at supporting improvement within two or three specific domains where the child could consistently challenge him or herself, and the parent could give both praise and constructive feedback in a consistent manner, building better reinforcement of gains. In concert, by observing exposures, parents could gain valuable insight into their child's independent capabilities and challenges as well as see how facilitating exposure with effective application of cognitive restructuring and processing of the situation critically differs from simply compelling a child to engage in an anxiety-provoking situation. Each of these is a key technique to help parents become more constructively involved, while also allowing the teen significant independence and authority over their own treatment and life choices.

Other treatment models involve parents in different ways. In a small, randomized, controlled trial examining the efficacy of social skills training (SST; Spence 1995) in treating children and adolescents, a clinical sample of socially anxious children and adolescents (ages 7–14) were assigned either to SST plus parental involvement (PI; $n=17$), SST with no parent involvement (NPI; $n=19$) or a wait list control group (WLC; $n=14$) (Spence et al. 2000). In the PI condition, parents viewed all child-focused SST sessions through a one-way mirror and simultaneously received 12 weekly group parent training sessions. Children and adolescents who received SST with either PI or NPI both improved compared to WLC. Although no significant differences were found in outcomes between PI or NPI SST groups at either posttreatment or 12-month follow-up time points, investigators noted a trend toward superior results when parents were involved in treatment.

A third use of parents can be simply involving them at the outset of treatment, during the orientation and psychoeducation phases. Beidel and colleagues employed such a model in their social effectiveness training for children (SET-C; Beidel et al. 1998). In this case, although the treatment was found to be effective overall in both immediate and long-term follow-ups, the contributions of the parental component were not directly assessed. This treatment also targeted children slightly before the teen years (age 8–12), further complicating the direct comparison with other models.

Another school-based intervention also incorporated targeting parents high in expressed emotion in the form of high overinvolvement, criticism, and hostility. This treatment program, called Intervencion en Familias & Adolescentes con Fobia Social (IFAFS; Garcia-Lopez et al. 2014), was an adaptation of a program targeting social anxiety in adolescents without directly targeting families. The original program consisted of 12 weekly group sessions of 90 min each and incorporated psychoeducation, social skills training, cognitive restructuring, and exposure through use of peer assistants and video feedback, all during school hours and with additional, optional individual sessions. IFAFS built on this previous clinical program by incorporating five additional 120-min group sessions specifically for parents, offering psychoeducation about social anxiety and expressed emotion, and giving parents feedback on communication skills and use of contingency management to help them better manage their child's anxiety. In direct comparison of the derivative and parent component-enhanced IFAFS programs, adolescents in the IFAFS program reported somewhat higher diagnosis remission rates (although not statistically significant).

Still, one may reasonably conclude as a result of the research that parents play a crucial role in the development of SAD and may also be a crucial component of treatment. However, as we can see here, there are several models for how one might approach this issue (not to mention the numerous trials that fail to include parents at all), and more research is critical to determine whether one model offers greater benefits and change relative to the others.

Conditioning Events

During adolescence, the research focus has narrowed on the role of conditioning events, proximal events that lead directly to the manifestation of social anxiety, or cause a nascent vulnerability to flower (Higa-McMillan and Ebesutani 2011). Consistent with behavioral learning models of anxiety, anxiety arises in response to direct classical or operant conditioning (e.g., a child is ridiculed or bullied by peers, leading to social withdrawal or avoidance) or through modeling or observational learning (e.g., a child observes parental social withdrawal and apes that avoidance among peers). Previously unthreatening events, such as raising a hand in class, speaking to unfamiliar people, or talking to peers can become a fraught and complicated situation as the awareness of others increases in tandem with the ability to abstractly reason. Indeed, a single instance of physiological hyperarousal and real or perceived social humiliation can be enough to poison performance in a narrow or wide array of social performance situations (Higa-McMillan and Ebesutani 2011). Estimates of adults with social anxiety disorder who can recall their anxiety rising in response to a single social performance failure range between 23 and 58 %, although evidence is generally in favor of the majority of adults recalling a conditioning incident (Kendler et al. 2002; Öst and Hugdahl 1981; Öst 1985; Stemberger et al. 1995).

Active peer rejection appears to be a significant proximal risk factor or conditioning event for SAD (Inderbitzen et al. 1997; La Greca and Lopez 1998). Adolescents with social anxiety tend to have fewer close friends and often view the quality of the friendships they do have to be low (La Greca and Lopez 1998). Prospective studies have linked peer victimization to increasing rates of both the experience of social anxiety and the onset of SAD in adolescence (Siegel et al. 2009; Storch et al. 2005). Although peer victimization has been linked with onset of a number of disorders, including depression, its relationship with SAD appears to be unique and pernicious. Ranta and colleagues (2009) reported that adolescents meeting criteria for SAD were more likely to report past episodes of peer victimization than adolescents who did not have SAD; although higher levels of peer victimization were more prevalent among adolescents with both depression and SAD, peer victimization and depression were not directly related. Follow-up work in this area drew patterns in longitudinal development (Ranta et al. 2013). Direct peer victimization at the age of 15 predicted SAD in boys at the age of 17, and SAD also predicted later peer victimization. Ranta and colleagues (2013) proposed a reciprocal and mutually reinforcing relationship between these variables, such that social avoidance led to risk in victimization, which in turn predicted avoidance and again victimization. In girls, only relational victimization was predictive of SAD. Persistence of victimization was also reported to be four to five times more frequent in boys than it was in girls in the sample.

Addressing Conditioning Events in Treatment

Whereas learning theory predicts the development of a disorder, it can also play a crucial role in helping overcome those learning events through effective use of exposure. Given the key role of conditioning events in kindling SAD and social avoidance during adolescence, it is no surprise that every empirically effective treatment for SAD in adolescence employs some form of exposure (Albano et al 1995; Beidel et al. 2000; Gallagher et al. 2004; Garcia-Lopez 2000, 2007; Hayward et al. 2000; Spence et al. 2000).

Additionally, the focus on group treatments and social skill development reinforces the importance that treatment research has placed on engaging potential deficits in functioning and the need to overcome social neglect and improve overall social functioning. As previously mentioned, CBGT-A places social skill development as a core priority of treatment (Albano et al. 1991). Spence's SST places even greater emphasis on social skills training through modeling, role-playing, prompts, and reinforcement, first taught didactically as "micro-skills" and later in the context of in-session practice. The 12-week program consists of weekly, hour-long group sessions followed by 30 min of social practice "games." Beidel and colleagues' (1998) SET-C goes even further still; during the 24 twice-weekly treatment sessions spanning 12 weeks, participants attend both a 60-min individual exposure session and a 60-min social skills training group. In addition, immediately following each social skills training group, children participate in a 90-min peer generalization session with a group of outgoing, unfamiliar peers. These sessions are designed to provide participants with opportunities to practice social skills with nonanxious peers through collaborative group activities (e.g., bowling, pizza parties, etc.).

Masia and colleagues (1999) developed Skills for Academic and Social Success (SASS) program, which was primarily derived from SET-C with adaptations for practical delivery in a high school environment (e.g., briefer sessions, incorporation of teachers) and developmental modifications for an adolescent population (e.g., age-appropriate social skills training, addition of training in "realistic thinking"). The SASS program consists of 14 group sessions: one session of psychoeducation and orientation, one session of instruction in realistic thinking, five sessions each of social skills training and exposure, and the remaining sessions focusing on relapse prevention and the opportunity to practice skills in the context of two unstructured social activities (e.g., pizza parties). Another unique aspect of the protocol pertains to direct involvement of teachers who were asked to conduct practice exposure exercises with group members (e.g., spontaneously calling them in class).

Although bullying and peer victimization have received significant study as their own phenomena, they have never been directly studied in the context of treatment for SAD. However, there is recent work by La Greca et al. (2014) on the development of the PEERS/UTalk program for the prevention of depression and SAD among adolescents with elevated social anxiety and depressive symptoms. This interpersonal treatment program also includes components that are aimed at enhancing adolescents' strategies for dealing with interpersonal peer victimization (see Chap. 11). Even among the social skills groups mentioned here, it is unclear how much focus has been given to negotiating peer victimization. Again, we see that there is a sound empirical basis for attention to intervention in challenging the impact of conditioning events through the use of exposure, social skills training, and other forms of adaptive skills. What remains unclear are what components might be most vital or what approaches might be most effective in accomplishing this goal.

Future Directions: Developmental Functioning as a Target of Treatment Intervention

Although one can reasonably find evidence for a building consensus around the development, phenomenology, and effective treatment of SAD in adolescence, a close examination of these issues will reveal substantial issues. Definitions of basic constructs and populations of interest have shown considerable variability. SAD first appeared in the third edition of the *Diagnostic and Statistical Manual for Mental Disorders* (*DSM*; APA 1980). Since then, the diagnostic construct has undergone substantial revisions in every edition, and *DSM-5* (APA 2013) is no exception. Children and adolescents did not receive diagnoses of social phobia (the former SAD) in *DSM-III* and *DSM-III-R*, instead receiving a diagnosis of avoidant disorder of childhood or adolescence. *DSM-5* officially changed the name from social phobia to social anxiety disorder in an attempt to better communicate the scope and consequence of the disorder. *The DSM-5* also expanded the definition of SAD to include fear of any form of negative evaluation (as opposed to fear of only humiliation or embarrassment), as well as the role of clinician judgment in evaluating how disproportionate the individual's fears might be in sociocultural context (Heimberg et al. 2014). In a similar vein, definitions of periods of childhood and adolescence have also varied in research samples, contributing to complexity in making direct comparisons of results across research studies.

What this means is that the definitions of SAD and adolescence have been somewhat moving targets, and although many of these results have been presented here as equivalent, they can include somewhat different groups and fail to include others who perhaps had flawed understanding of their condition. For example, rather than the generalized/nongeneralized subtype frequently alluded to in this paper, *DSM-5* has opted for a new specifier, "performance only," emphasizing a narrower range of the condition in a subgroup of individuals. The implications of these definitions and redefinitions have unclear and understudied implications for the operationalization of SAD both in the past and in the future.

One may also note that despite *DSM-III*'s early suggestion that SAD in childhood might be somewhat different from adult SAD, most techniques represent downward extensions of adult models. Adult models have hypothesized that social anxiety is maintained through mental imagery or schema defining what is expected as a performance standard in a given social situation and then evaluating all the ways in which the mental image of self deviates from that ideal standard (Rapee and Heimberg 1997). What is less clear is how well these adult models describe SAD in adolescence; given that SAD primarily onsets in adolescence, the reader may be forgiven for thinking this process has a bit of a backwards quality.

A number of studies have found evidence that, relative to their nonsocially anxious counterparts, socially anxious teens generate more negative interpretations of ambiguous and neutral social performance situations, worry about negative outcomes, and have flawed representations of both social threat and their own ability to perform effectively in social situations (Cartwright-Hatton et al. 2005; Miers et al. 2008; Muris et al. 2000; Rheingold et al. 2003; Spence et al. 1999). Higa and Daleiden (2008) reported that heightened SAD was associated with heightened self-focus in teens, but experimental manipulation of self-imagery to heighten negative self-awareness did not influence ratings of social anxiety in nonanxious teens, whether self- or observer reported (Alfano et al. 2008). Such events can be further complicated by cognitive factors; socially anxious children and teens have been found to be hypervigilant for threatening social-evaluative cues relative to their less anxious peers (Foa et al. 1996; Lucock and Salkovskis 1988; Muris et al. 2000). Socially anxious teens also demonstrate deficits in executive control, such as finding it more difficult to eliminate no longer relevant material from memory in a directed forgetting task (Gomez-Ariza et al. 2013). And, although interest in selective attention for threatening stimuli has become an area of hot research interest over the last decade, thus far no studies have examined adolescents for these biases (Higa-McMillan and Ebesutani 2011).

Besides concerns over the gaps in research that might help us further understand SAD, we must also consider that even the extensive extant research on SAD in adolescence, particularly of the biological and especially neurological underpinnings of SAD, is plagued by small and overwhelmingly white samples. In addition to the concerns over sufficient power, especially as the ambitions and analyses of these samples grow ever more complex, we must be concerned over the homogeneity of the samples as well. In their seminal review regarding the study of anxiety disorders in African-American populations, Neal and Turner (1991) noted that the mode of nonwhite participants in research studies on anxiety was zero. Lamentably, a cursory review of the literature will indicate that in the ensuing two decades, this situation has not improved much.

With these major caveats in mind, we can note that the last two decades have also generated exciting progress in understanding SAD in adolescence, and we can best regard these as challenges and directions for growth. The chronic and often deteriorating lifetime course of SAD makes a strong case for early recognition and early intervention in this disorder. As we have come to use more developmentally informed approaches in the conceptualization and targeting of the illness, our own understanding has grown exponentially. Treatment models have shown great foresight in emphasizing a multidimensional approach to this multifaceted problem. Further armed with research about the early risk factors and stressors that cause social anxiety to take hold over the individual, we are now able to think of the period in a way that is even more embedded in the specific developmental tasks and challenges of adolescence. To that end, treatment of the adolescent (ages 13–17) and the emerging adult (ages 18–28) in our clinic now involves a multifaceted, exposure and family-based approach that is patient-centered with intervention components prescribed according to functional and developmental impairments.

The launching emerging adults program (LEAP; Albano A.M. (unpublished)) incorporates our earlier model of CBGT-A and expands upon the role and tasks of development in the healthy transition from adolescence to independent adult functioning. It is well established that an interaction of adolescent avoidance of social-anxiety provoking situations and parental overprotection (e.g., inadvertent or deliberate reinforcement of avoidance, assisting with task completion) serves to maintain anxiety. This parental involvement also prevents or delays the adolescent's development of the ability to take on situations and tasks that are normative for their emerging independent functioning (see Table 9.1). These tasks involve everyday activities from shopping for one's self to arranging for healthcare visits, to seeking out opportunities for education or employment, to effectively managing social and romantic relationships and their ups and downs, without parental intervention. If parents continue to be centrally engaged in the completion of behaviors, on adolescent's behalf, that promote the adolescent's development, then the teen is compromised not just with greater anxiety but also with having less skill and ability to function independently over time. Indeed, through a pattern of parental leveling and even removal of essential opportunities for developmentally appropriate challenge and growth, it is proposed that this cycle takes the adolescent off of the track of normal or typical development, fostering a greater and longer dependency on the

Table 9.1 The tasks of adolescent development and associated behavioral indicators of accomplishment

Task	Behavioral indicators
Establish emotional independence from parents	Soothes self when confronted with disappointment or challenge; seeks advice appropriately and weighs options; able to own feeling states and reactions
Develop self-identity	Affirmatively describes self in terms of aspirations, interests, abilities, and skills; recognizes own limits
Establish behavioral independence from parents	Completes tasks on own; takes initiative; asserts self to meet needs
Manage money responsibly	Spends money in relation to budget and awareness of meeting responsibilities; makes own purchases for food, clothing, and other needs; manages finances so that relaxation/hobbies/interests are pursued with little financial tension
Make and keep long-term friendships	Engages with others and pursues relationships on own
Controls personal self-care	Regulates own sleep patterns; aware of and engages in healthy diet and exercise routine; self-soothes appropriately
Controls personal medical/health care	Makes regular appointments in timely way (annual physical, mental health visits); seeks healthcare consultations as needed and in timely way; manages medications on own
Engage and accept sexual identity	Is engaged in pursuing sexual knowledge and understands own sexual identity; accepts sexual identity
Form romantic relationships	Has interest in and pursues romantic partner(s) in a healthy and meaningful way
Formulate and engage in long-term vocational goals	Able to articulate interests and pursue education or training in areas related to the interest; develops set of skills/abilities to pursue goals
Complete educational requirements	Completes compulsory educational requirements of high school or equivalent; seeks further education to pursue goals for career/vocation
Establish financial independence	Earns and saves own money
Lives independently	Moves away from home (potentially in stages, such as for college or with housemates until independent); establishes own residence and maintains all aspects (financial, upkeep) on own

parents and inhibiting their transition to adult functioning. Therefore, effective treatment needs to address not only the adolescent's anxiety but also the context of parent-adolescent interactions that maintain anxiety and stalls development. Figure 9.1 presents a schematic representation of the LEAP treatment model, whereby adolescents engage in individual and/or group CBT, with specific "transition sessions" designed to address parent-adolescent interactions.

LEAP is in development in response to the absence of a focus in CBT programs on developmental tasks of transition from one stage to the next and, specifically, to increase independent functioning as the adolescent prepares for adulthood. Few CBT programs explicitly address autonomy issues and the implications for the transfer of

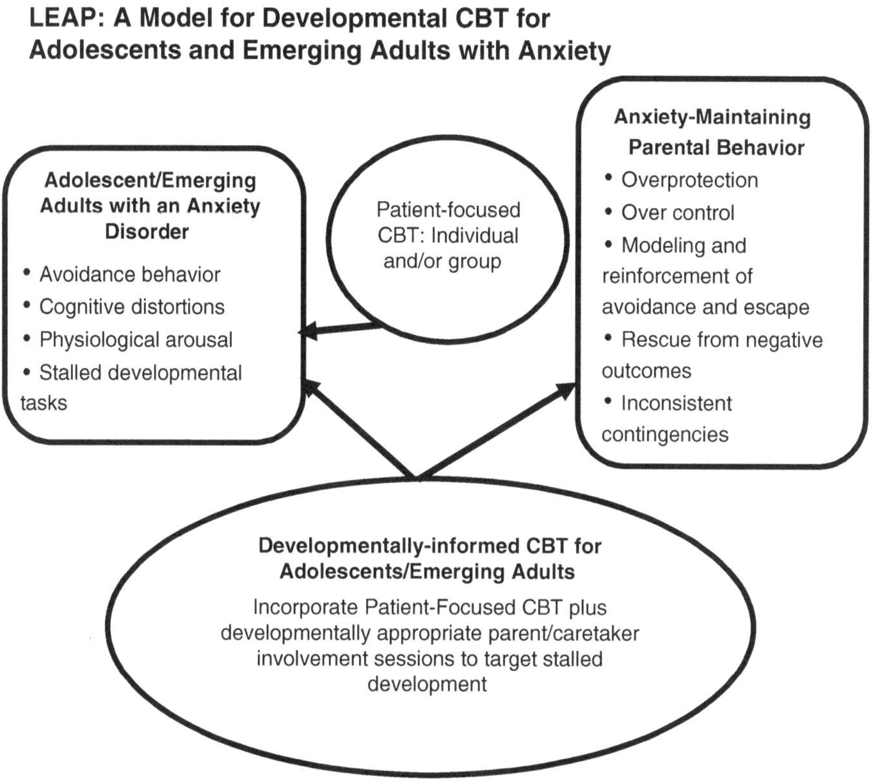

Fig. 9.1 A model for developmentally informed CBT for adolescents and emerging adults with social anxiety disorder: The launching emerging adults program (From Detweiler et al. (2014), with permission of Elsevier)

responsibility for everyday tasks but also for managing the youth's social anxiety (and related disorders) from parent to the adolescent. Adolescents (or young adults) are offered individual CBT, with the traditional anxiety exposures being largely conducted in group format, as in CBGT-A (Albano et al. 1991). This allows for individualized attention to the adolescent's needs and for establishing a therapeutic alliance along with goal setting and cognitive work, while simultaneously capitalizing on the rich ecological validity of the group format with similar-aged peers for conducting exposures. These exposure groups are initially conducted within the clinic, using mainly the role-play format found in CBGT-A and in the Heimberg model. However, exposures then move to an in vivo format, to situations and activities found in the local environment, such as in stores, on subways, restaurants, and other public settings. The idea is to capitalize on the contextual elements of real situations to enhance the validity of the exposure and the unpredictability of the real world.

In addition, LEAP involves a series of parent-adolescent "transition sessions." In these sessions conducted by an individual therapist, a developmental hierarchy is created in collaboration with the adolescent and parent, and then subsequent contextual exposures make explicit the parents' stepping back to allow for focus on remediating the adolescent's functional impairment while addressing anxiety and arrested development. Further, in these supportive contexts, adolescents and parents discuss their beliefs, frustration, wishes, and other aspects of emotion that they experience with each other, and through communication training and family problem-solving, they co-negotiate action plans for allowing more autonomy and acceptance of responsibility on the part of the adolescent for managing age-appropriate tasks. We often address the parents' fear of their child "failing" in a given situation and work through the value of allowing "mess ups" to occur for the learning experience. In this way, parents are taught how to reduce the tendency to respond impulsively and emotionally and instead assume the role of effective, planful coaches and how to assist the adolescent without taking over the situation.

Related work by Garcia-Lopez and colleagues (2014) found promising results for adding a parent training component to a school-based treatment for social anxiety in adolescents (ages 13–18). For parents who evidenced high expressed emotion (EE), training to reduce EE via communication skills and appropriate contingency management led to greater decreases in social distress, avoidance, and social anxiety in their adolescents, as compared to the group treatment without parent training. Similarly, LEAP is designed to address family communication in the context of development. The ultimate goals of LEAP are to improve the adolescent's management of anxiety, decrease avoidance, change family interaction patterns to be supportive rather than enabling, and to improve developmental outcomes that support independent functioning over the long term. Evaluation of the LEAP approach is underway.

In conclusion, viewing SAD and its treatment through a developmentally informed lens can help us tighten our operationalization of what SAD is and provide for the most rigorous scientific examination of the phenomenology and etiology associated with this disorder. Armed with this greater understanding and as we increase the size and diversity of our samples to reflect the true complexity of this condition, we can insure that our findings remain both flexibly cognizant of the intense variability inherent in this condition and robust to the challenges of measuring shifts in our understanding of what is happening for these at-risk teens and what is the best thing to do about it. The context of the family, within which the adolescent lives and is dependent upon for meeting his or her needs, needs to be a focus of evaluation and treatment for youth with social anxiety, despite the prevailing and commonplace ideas that a wide boundary between therapist and parents is necessary for engaging adolescents during treatment. And finally, exposure remains the cornerstone of effective treatment for SAD. We advocate for using enhanced, ecologically valid, and contextually rich exposures to maximize the potential for improvement in symptoms but also in overall adaptive functioning.

References

Albano AM, Barlow DH (1996) Breaking the vicious cycle: cognitive-behavioral group treatment for socially anxious youth. In: Hibbs ED, Jensen PS (eds) Psychosocial treatments for child and adolescent disorders: empirically-based strategies for clinical practice. APA, Washington, DC, pp 43–62

Albano AM, Marten PA, Holt CS (1991) Cognitive-behavioral group treatment of adolescent social phobia: therapist manual. Unpublished manuscript, State University of New York at Albany
Albano AM, Marten PA, Holt CS, Heimberg RG, Barlow DH (1995) Cognitive-behavioral treatment for social phobia in adolescents: a preliminary study. J Nerv Ment Dis 183:649–656
Alfano CA, Beidel DC, Turner SM (2008) Negative self-imagery among adolescents with social phobia: a test of the adult model of the disorder. J Clin Child Adolesc Psychol 37:327–336
American Psychiatric Association (1980) Diagnostic and statistical manual of mental disorders, 3rd edn. American Psychiatric Association, Washington, DC
American Psychiatric Association (2013) Diagnostic and statistical manual of mental disorders, 5th edn. American Psychiatric Association, Washington, DC
Arrindell WA, Kwee MG, Methorst GJ, Van der Ende J, Pol E, Moritz BJ (1989) Perceived parental rearing styles of agoraphobic and socially phobic in-patients. Br J Psychiatry 155:526–535
Asendorph JB (1994) The malleability of behavioral inhibition: a study of individual developmental function. Dev Psychol 30:912–919
Barrett PM, Rapee RM, Dadds MM, Ryan SM (1996b) Family enhancement of cognitive style in anxious and aggressive children. J Abnorm Child Psychol 24:187–203
Battaglia M, Zanoni A, Taddei M, Giorda R, Bertoletti E, Lampis V, Scanini S, Cappa S, Tettamanti M (2012) Cerebral responses to emotional expressions and the development of social anxiety disorder: a preliminary longitudinal study. Depress Anxiety 29:54–61
Beatty MJ, Heisel AD, Hall AE, Levine TR, La France BH (2002) What can we learn from the study of twins about genetic and environmental influences on interpersonal affiliation, aggressiveness, and social anxiety? A meta-analytic study. Commun Monogr 69:1–18
Beidel DC, Turner SM, Morris TL (1998) Social effectiveness therapy for children: a treatment manual. Medical University of South Carolina, Charleston
Beidel DC, Turner SM, Morris TL (2000) Behavioral treatment of childhood social phobia. J Consult Clin Psychol 68:1072–1080
Biederman J, Hirshfeld-Becker DR, Rosenbaum JF, Herot C, Friedman D, Snidman N, Kagan J, Faraone SV (2001) Further evidence of association between behavioral inhibition and social anxiety in children. Am J Psychiatry 158:1673–1679
Blair KS, Geraci M, Korelitz K, Otero M, Towbin K, Ernst M, Leibenluft E, Blair RJR, Pine DS (2011) The pathology of social phobia is independent of developmental changes in face processing. Am J Psychiatry 168:1202–1209
Bogels SM, van Oosten A, Muris P, Smulders D (2001) Familial correlates of social anxiety in children and adolescents. Behav Res Ther 39:273–287
Bogels S, Stevens J, Madiandzic M (2011) Parenting and social anxiety: fathers' versus mothers' influence on their children's anxiety in ambiguous situations. J Child Psychol Psychiatry 52:599–606
Brown TA, Campbell LA, Lehman CL, Grisham JR, Mancill RB (2001) Current and lifetime comorbidity of the DSM-IV anxiety and mood disorders. J Abnorm Psychol 110:49–58
Bruch MA, Heimberg RG (1994) Differences in perceptions of parental and personal characteristics between generalized and nongeneralized social phobics. J Anxiety Disord 8:155–168
Buote VM, Pancer SM, Pratt MW, Adams G, Birnie-Lefcovitch S, Polivy J, Wintre MG (2007) The importance of friends: friendship and adjustment among 1st-year university students. J Adolesc Res 22:665–689
Burgess K, Rubin KH, Cheah C, Nelson L (2001) Socially withdrawn children: parenting and parent-child relationships. In: The self, shyness and social anxiety: a handbook of concepts, research, and interventions. Wiley, New York
Burstein M, He J-P, Kattan G, Albano AM, Avenevoli S, Merikangas KR (2011) Social phobia and subtypes in the national comorbidity survey-adolescent supplement: prevalence, correlates, and comorbidity. J Am Acad Child Adolesc Psychiatry 50:870–880
Cartwright-Hatton S, Tschernitz N, Gomersall H (2005) Social anxiety in children: social skills deficit, or cognitive distortion? Behav Res Ther 43:131–141
Caspi A, Silva PA (1995) Temperamental qualities at age three predict personality traits in young adulthood: longitudinal evidence from a birth cohort. Child Dev 66:486–498

Caster JB, Inderbitzen HM, Hope D (1999) Relationship between youth and parent perceptions of family environment and social anxiety. J Anxiety Disord 13:237–251
Chronis-Tuscano A, Degnan KA, Pine DS, Perez-Edgar K, Henderson HA, Diaz Y, Raggi VL, Fox NA (2009) Stable early maternal report of behavioral inhibition predicts lifetime social anxiety disorder in adolescence. J Am Acad Child Adolesc Psychiatry 48:928–935
Clauss JA, Blackford JU (2012) Behavioral inhibition and risk for developing social anxiety disorder: a meta-analytic study. J Am Acad Child Adolesc Psychiatry 51:1066–1075
Compas BE (2004) Processes of risk and resilience during adolescence: Linking contexts and individuals. In Lerner RM, Steinberg L (Eds.) Handbook of Adolescent Psychology, 2nd ed. John Wiley & Sons
Compton SN, Nelson AH, March JS (2000) Social phobia and separation anxiety symptoms in community and clinical samples of children and adolescents. J Am Acad Child Adolesc Psychiatry 39:1040–1046
Detweiler MF, Comer JS, Crum KI, Albano AM (2014) Social anxiety in children and adolescents: biological, developmental and social considerations. In: Hofmann SG, DiBartolo PM (eds) Social anxiety: clinical, developmental and social perspectives, 3rd edn. Academic Press, Amsterdam, pp 254–309
Elkind D (1967) Egocentrism in adolescence. Child Dev 38:1025–1034
Erikson EH (1959) Identity and the life cycle (Vol. 1). *Psychological Issues. Monograph*, 1. International Universities Press, New York
Finnie V, Russell A (1988) Preschool children's social status and their mothers' behavior and knowledge in the supervisory role. Dev Psychol 24:789
Foa EB, Franklin ME, Perry KJ, Herbert JD (1996) Cognitive biases in generalized social phobia. J Abnorm Psychol 105:433
Fordham K, Stevenson-Hinde J (1999) Shyness, friendship quality, and adjustment during middle childhood. J Child Psychol Psychiatry 40:757–768
Fyer AJ, Mannuzza S, Chapman TF, Liebowitz MR, Klein DF (1993) A direct interview family study of social phobia. Arch Gen Psychiatry 50:286–293
Fyer AJ, Manuzza S, Chapman TF, Martin LY, Klein DF (1995) Specificity in familial aggregation of phobic disorders. Arch Gen Psychiatry 52:564–573
Gallagher HM, Rabian BA, McCloskey MS (2004) A brief group cognitive behavioral intervention for social phobia in childhood. J Anxiety Disord 18:459–479
Garcia-Lopez LJ (2000, 2007) Examining the efficacy of three cognitive-behavioural treatments aimed at overcoming social anxiety in adolescents. University of Murcia: Publication Service
Garcia-Lopez LJ, Olivares J, Turner SM, Albano AM, Beidel DC, Sanchez-Meca J (2002) Results at long-term among three psychological treatments for adolescents with generalized social phobia (II): clinical significance and effect size. Psicol Conductual Behav Psychol 10:371–385
Garcia-Lopez LJ, Olivares J, Beidel DC, Albano AM, Turner SM, Rosa AI (2006) Efficacy of three treatment protocols for adolescents with social anxiety disorder: a five-year follow up assessment. J Anxiety Disord 20:175–191
Garcia-Lopez LJ, Muela JM, Espinosa-Fernandez L, Diaz-Castela M (2009) Exploring the relevance of expressed emotion to the treatment of social anxiety disorder in adolescence. Journal of Adolescence 32:1371–1376
Garcia-Lopez LJ, Diaz-Castela MM, Muela-Martinez JA, Espinosa-Fernandez L (2014) Can parent training for parents with high levels of expressed emotion have a positive effect on their child's social anxiety improvement? J Anxiety Disord 28:812–822
Goldsmith HH, Lemery KS (2000) Linking temperamental fearfulness and anxiety symptoms: a behavior–genetic perspective. Biol Psychiatry 48:1199–1209
Gomez-Ariza CJ, Iglesias-Parro S, Garcia-Lopez LJ, Diaz-Castela M, Espinosa-Fernandez L, Muela JA (2013) Selective intentional forgetting in adolescents to social anxiety disorder. Psychiatry Res 208:151–155
Greco L, Morris T (2002) Paternal child-rearing style and child social anxiety: investigation of child perceptions and actual father behavior. J Psychopathol Behav Assess 24:259–267
Gulley LD, Oppenheimer CW, Hankin BL (2014) Associations among negative parenting, attention bias to anger, and social anxiety among youth. Developmental Psychology 50:577–585

Guyer AE, Lau JY, McClure-Tone EB, Parrish J, Shiffrin ND, Reynolds RC, Chen G, Blair RJR, Leibenluft E, Fox NA, Ernst M, Pine DS, Nelson EE (2008) Amygdala and ventrolateral prefrontal cortex function during anticipated peer evaluation in pediatric social anxiety. Arch Gen Psychiatry 65:1303–1312

Hall GS (1904) Adolescence, vol 2. Appleton, New York

Hayward C, Varady S, Albano AM, Thienemann M, Henderson L, Schatzberg AF (2000) Cognitive-behavioral group therapy for social phobia in female adolescents: results of a pilot study. J Am Acad Child Adolcsc Psychiatry 39:721–726

Heimberg RG, Becker RE, Goldfinger K, Vermilyea JA (1985) Treatment of social phobia by exposure, cognitive restructuring, and homework assignments. J Nerv Ment Dis 173: 236–245

Heimberg RG, Dodge CS, Hope DA, Kennedy CR, Zollo L, Becker RE (1990) Cognitive behavioral group treatment for social phobia: comparison to a credible placebo control. Cognit Ther Res 14:1–23

Heimberg RG, Hofmann SG, Liebowitz MR, Schneier FR, Smits JAJ, Stein MB, Hinton DE, Craske MG (2014) Social anxiety disorder in DSM-5. Depress Anxiety 31:472–479

Higa CK, Daleiden EL (2008) Social anxiety and cognitive biases in non-referred children: the interaction of self-focused attention and threat interpretation biases. J Anxiety Disord 22:441–452

Higa-McMillan CK, Ebesutani C (2011) The etiology of social anxiety disorder in adolescents and young adults. In: Alfano CA, Beidel DC (eds) Social anxiety in adolescents and young adults: translating developmental science into practice. American Psychological Association, Washington, DC, pp 29–51

Hirshfeld DR, Rosenbaum JF, Beiderman J, Bolduc EA, Faraone SV, Snidman N, Reznick JS, Kagan J (1992) Stable behavioral inhibition and its association with social anxiety disorder. J Am Acad Child Adolesc Psychiatry 31:103–111

Hope DA, Heimberg RG (1993) Social phobia and social anxiety. In: Barlow DH (ed) Clinical handbook of psychological disorders: a step-by-step treatment manual. Guilford Press, New York, pp 99–136

Horwath E, Weissman MM (1995) Epidemiology of depression and anxiety disorders. In: Textbook in psychiatric epidemiology. Wiley-Liss, New York, pp 317–344

Hudson JL, Rapee RM (2001) Parent–child interactions and anxiety disorders: an observational study. Behav Res Ther 39:1411–1427

Hudson JL, Rapee RM (2002) Parent-child interactions in clinically anxious children and their siblings. J Clin Child Adolesc Psychol 31:548–555

Hudson JL, Rapee RM (2005) Parental perceptions of overprotection: specific to anxious children or shared between siblings? Behav Change 22:185–194

Hughes AA, Furr JM, Sood ED, Barmish AJ, Kendall PC (2009) Anxiety, mood, and substance use disorders in parents of children with anxiety disorders. Child Psychiatry Hum Dev 40: 405–419

Inderbitzen HM, Walters KS, Bukowski AL (1997) The role of social anxiety in adolescent peer relations: differences among sociometric status groups and rejected subgroups. J Clin Child Psychol 26:338–348

Juster HR, Heimberg RG (1995) Social phobia: longitudinal course and long-term outcome of cognitive-behavioral treatment. Psychiatr Clin North Am 18:821–842

Kagan J (1989) Temperamental contributions to social behavior. Am Psychol 44:668–674

Kagan J, Reznick JS, Snidman N (1988) Biological bases of childhood shyness. Science 240:167–171

Kendler KS, Neale MC, Kessler RC, Heath AC, Eaves LJ (1992) The genetic epidemiology of phobias in women: the interrelationship of agoraphobia, social phobia, situational phobia, and simple phobia. Arch Gen Psychiatry 49:273–281

Kendler KS, Myers J, Prescott CA (2002) The etiology of phobias: an evaluation of the stress-diathesis model. Arch Gen Psychiatry 59:242–248

Knappe S, Beesdo K, Fehm L, Hofler M, Lieb R (2009) Do parental psychopathology and unfavorable family environments predict the persistence of social phobia? J Anxiety Disord 23:986–994

Knappe S, Beesdo-Baum K, Fehm L, Lieb R, Wittchen H-U (2012) Characterizing the association between parenting and adolescent social phobia. J Anxiety Disord 26:608–616
La Greca AM, Lopez N (1998) Social anxiety among adolescents: linkages with peer relations and friendships. J Abnorm Child Psychol 26:83–94
La Greca AM, Prinstein MJ (1999) Peer group. In: Silverman WK, Ollendick TH (eds) Developmental issues in the clinical treatment of children. Allyn & Bacon, Needham Heights, pp 171–198
La Greca AM, Mufson L, Ehrenreich-May J, Girio-Herrera E, Chan S (2014) Developing an evidence-based preventive intervention for peer victimized adolescents at risk for social anxiety disorder and/or depression. Presented at the biennial meeting of the International Society for Affective Disorders, Berlin, Apr 2014
Lieb R, Wittchen HU, Höfler M, Fuetsch M, Stein MB, Merikangas KR (2000) Parental psychopathology, parenting styles, and the risk of social phobia in offspring: a prospective-longitudinal community study. Arch Gen Psychiatry 57:859–866
Lucock MP, Salkovskis PM (1988) Cognitive factors in social anxiety and its treatment. Behav Res Ther 26:297–302
Manuzza S, Schneier FR, Chapman TF, Liebowitz MR, Klein DF, Fyer AJ (1995) Generalized social phobia: reliability and validity. Arch Gen Psychiatry 52:230–237
Masia CL, Beidel DC, Albano AM, Rapee RM, Turner SM, Morris TL, et al. (1999) Skills for academic and social success. Available from Carrie Masia-Warner, New York
Masia CL, Morris TL (1998) Parental factors associated with social anxiety: methodological limitations and suggestions for integrated behavioral research. Clin Psychol Sci Pract 5:211–228
Miers AC, Blöte AW, Bögels SM, Westenberg PM (2008) Interpretation bias and social anxiety in adolescents. J Anxiety Disord 22:1462–1471
Muris P, Merckelbach H, Damsma E (2000) Threat perception bias in nonreferred, socially anxious children. J Clin Child Psychol 29:348–359
Neal AM, Turner SM (1991) Anxiety disorders research with African Americans: current status. Psychol Bull 109(3):400
Olivares J, Garcia-Lopez LJ, Beidel DC, Turner SM, Albano AM, Hidalgo M (2002) Results at long-term among three psychological treatments for adolescents with generalized social phobia (I): statistical significance. Psicol Conductual 10:147–164
Ollendick TH, Hirshfeld-Becker DR (2002) The developmental psychopathology of social anxiety disorder. Biol Psychiatry 51:44–58
Öst LG (1985) Ways of acquiring phobias and outcome of behavioral treatments. Behav Res Ther 23:683–689
Öst LG, Hugdahl K (1981) Acquisition of phobias and anxiety response patterns in clinical patients. Behav Res Ther 19:439–447
Parker G (1979) Reported parental characteristics in relation to trait depression and anxiety levels in a non-clinical group. Australas Psychiatry 13:260–264
Perez-Edgar KE, Guyer AE (2014) Behavioral inhibition: temperament or prodrome? Curr Behav Neurosci Rep 1:182–190
Prenoveau JM, Craske MG, Zinbarg RE, Mineka S, Rose RD, Griffith JW (2011) Are anxiety and depression just as stable as personality during late adolescence? Results from a three-year longitudinal latent variable study. J Abnorm Psychol 120:832–843
Puklek Levpušček M (2006) Adolescent individuation in relation to parents and friends: age and gender differences. Eur J Dev Psychol 3:238–264
Ranta K, Kaltiala-Heino R, Pelkonen M, Marttunen M (2009) Associations between peer victimization, self-reported depression and social phobia among adolescents: the role of comorbidity. J Adolesc 32:77–93
Ranta K, Kaltiala-Heino R, Frojd S, Marttunen M (2013) Peer victimization and social phobia: a follow-up study among adolescents. Soc Psychiatry Psychiatr Epidemiol 48:533–544
Rapee RM, Heimberg RG (1997) A cognitive-behavioral model of anxiety in social phobia. Behav Res Ther 35:741–756

Reich J, Yates W (1988) Family history of psychiatric disorders in social phobia. Compr Psychiatry 29:72–75

Reich J, Goldenberg I, Vasile R, Goisman R (1994) A prospective follow-along study of the course of social phobia. Psychiatry Res 54:249–258

Rheingold AA, Herbert JD, Franklin ME (2003) Cognitive bias in adolescents with social anxiety disorder. Cognit Ther Res 27:639–655

Rosellini AJ, Rutter LA, Bourgeois ML, Emmert-Aronson BO, Brown TA (2013) The relevance of age of onset to the psychopathology of social phobia. J Psychopathol Behav Assess 35:356–365

Rubin KH, Mills RS (1990) Maternal beliefs about adaptive and maladaptive social behaviors in normal, aggressive, and withdrawn preschoolers. J Abnorm Child Psychol 18:419–435

Schwartz CE, Snidman N, Kagan J (1999) Adolescent social anxiety as an outcome of inhibited temperament in childhood. J Am Acad Child Adolesc Psychiatry 38:1008–1015

Siegel RS, La Greca AM, Harrison HM (2009) Peer victimization and social anxiety in adolescents: prospective and reciprocal relationships. J Youth Adolesc 38:1096–1109

Siqueland L, Kendall PC, Steinberg L (1996) Anxiety in children: perceived family environments and observed family interaction. J Clin Child Psychol 25:225–237

Skre I, Onstad S, Torgersen S, Lygren S, Kringlen E (1993) A twin study of DSM-III-R anxiety disorders. Acta Psychiatr Scand 88:85–92

Smetana JG (1997) Parenting and the development of social knowledge reconceptualized: a social domain analysis. In: Grusec JE, Kuczynski L (eds) Parenting and the internalization of values. New York, Wiley, pp 162–192

Spence SH (1995) Social skills training: enhancing social competence with children and adolescents. NFER-Nelson, Windsor

Spence SH, Donovan C, Brechman-Toussaint M (1999) Social skills, social outcomes, and cognitive features of childhood social phobia. J Abnorm Psychol 108:211

Spence SH, Donovan C, Brechman-Toussaint M (2000) The treatment of childhood social phobia: the effectiveness of a social skills training-based, cognitive-behavioral intervention, with and without parental involvement. J Child Psychol Psychiatry 41:713–726

Stein MB, Stein DJ (2008) Social anxiety disorder. Lancet 371:1115–1125

Stein M, Chartier M, Hazen A, Kozak M, Tancer M, Lander S (1998) A direct-interview family study of generalized social phobia. Am J Psychiatry 155:90–97

Steinberg L (2001) We know some things: parent–adolescent relationships in retrospect and prospect. J Res Adolesc 11(1):1–19

Steinberg L (2004) Risk taking in adolescence: what changes, and why? Ann N Y Acad Sci 1021(1):51–58

Stemberger RT, Turner SM, Beidel DC, Calhoun KS (1995) Social phobia: an analysis of possible developmental factors. J Abnorm Psychol 104(3):526–531

Storch EA, Masia-Warner C, Crisp H, Klein RG (2005) Peer victimization and social anxiety in adolescence: a prospective study. Aggress Behav 31:437–452

Vasey MW, Dadds MR (2001) The developmental psychopathology of anxiety. Oxford University Press, New York

Wittchen H-U, Fehm L (2003) Epidemiology and natural course of social fears and social phobia. Acta Psychiatr Scand Suppl 108:4–18

Cognition-Focused Interventions for Social Anxiety Disorder Among Adolescents

10

Lauren F. McLellan, Candice A. Alfano, and Jennifer L. Hudson

Introduction

Social anxiety disorder (SAD) typically onsets during mid-adolescence (Cohen et al. 1993). This is no surprise given the increased relevance of the social environment during this developmental period. Dependence on parents reduces; peer relationships and romantic relationships become more important (Furman and Buhrmester 1992). Even so, adolescents with SAD have fewer and poorer friendships (Greco and Morris 2005; La Greca and Moore 2005), have fewer romantic relationships (see also Chaps. 5 and 8), are more likely to marry their first partner, and are less likely to have a regular partner (Caspi et al. 1988). Furthermore, the impact of social anxiety is significant, and ongoing (Wittchen and Fehm 2003), and socially fearful adolescents need not meet full diagnostic criteria for SAD to experience distress and impairment (Essau et al. 1999; Inderbitzen et al. 1997). Adolescents with social anxiety are also likely to experience anxiety into adulthood and may develop related mood or substance use problems (Beesdo et al. 2007; Pine et al. 1998; Zimmermann et al. 2003). With such widespread impact, effective treatment is vital.

The focus of this chapter is on cognitive interventions for SAD among adolescents. We will briefly review the models of SAD as they relate to cognitive interventions, identify the important aspects of clinical assessments that inform a comprehensive cognitive intervention approach, and provide a detailed description of interventions that target cognitions and/or cognitive processes. This description includes both cognitive and cognitive behavioural interventions. To facilitate this,

L.F. McLellan, PhD (✉) • J.L. Hudson, MClinPsych, PhD
Department of Psychology, Centre for Emotional Health,
Macquarie University, Sydney, NSW, Australia
e-mail: lauren.mclellan@mq.edu.au; jennie.hudson@mq.edu.au

C.A. Alfano, PhD
Department of Psychology, University of Houston, Houston, TX, USA

K. Ranta et al. (eds.), *Social Anxiety and Phobia in Adolescents: Development, Manifestation and Intervention Strategies*, DOI 10.1007/978-3-319-16703-9_10

we will present a typical case and review how these interventions can be used to treat SAD among adolescents.

Cognitive Aspects of Social Anxiety Models

As outlined in Chap. 2, models of SAD indicate that the disorder is associated with biases in social information processing, attention, and cognitions that trigger and maintain anxious affect and behaviour (Rapee and Heimberg 1997; Clark and Wells 1995; Rapee and Spence 2004). When this occurs, there is reduced opportunity for positive social interactions, and the biases and anxiety are reinforced. Cognitive models also acknowledge the important role of biases about *other* people in ongoing symptoms. For example, SAD is associated with the belief that other people are critical and evaluate others negatively (Rapee and Heimberg 1997). Research suggests that the cognitive processes underlying social anxiety are similar in children, adolescents, and adults (Rapee and Spence 2004). Youth with SAD report more negative social cognitions than nonclinical youth, particularly self-focused negative cognitions (Ranta et al. 2014). In particular, studies show that socially anxious youth anticipate more negative consequences, expect to perform worse in social situations, and rate their social performance more negatively than non-anxious peers (Alfano et al. 2006; Spence et al. 1999).

Although factors like genetics, life experiences/events, and parent/peer interactions are considered to be important in the aetiology of SAD (Rapee and Spence 2004, Chap. 2 by Wong and Rapee), cognitive biases play a crucial role in the maintenance of social anxiety. Assessment and treatments that focus on cognitions and other cognitive phenomena have good efficacy (James et al. 2013). Best practice for the assessment and treatment of social anxiety targeting cognitions will be presented below.

Assessment

As outlined in Chap. 6 by Garcia-Lopez et al., a comprehensive assessment of social anxiety is important. The assessment process will allow differential diagnosis, provide information about severity of symptoms, and determine the impact of symptoms on an adolescent's functioning. Importantly, assessment informs treatment planning and so requires a focus on factors that may maintain symptoms. Commonly used diagnostic interviews (e.g. Anxiety Disorders Interview Schedule for DSM-IV for Children and Parents (ADIS-C/P); Silverman and Albano 1996) provide information about social anxiety and other anxiety disorders and allow an accurate diagnosis to be made. Questionnaire measures of adolescent anxiety enable peer comparison of symptoms using normative data (e.g. March et al. 1997), reflect degree of impairment, and are sensitive to treatment effects. Questionnaires measuring broad anxiety concerns, as well as instruments focusing on social anxiety more specifically provide useful information as part of a thorough assessment.

Comprehensive assessment involves gathering multi-method and multi-informant data. Research shows that adolescents may under-report anxiety because of social desirability factors (Comer and Kendall 2004; DiBartolo et al. 1998), a phenomenon that may be more prominent for adolescents with social concerns. Furthermore, research also indicates that adolescents and their parents differ in their understanding of anxiety (Achenbach et al. 1987; De Los Reyes and Kazdin 2005). At a minimum, separate interviews with the adolescent and their primary caregiver, along with self-report and parent-report questionnaires, provide desired information. In addition, teacher and/or peer reports may be used to collect information about symptoms and impairment in functioning. Given the focus of this chapter is on cognitive interventions, this section will briefly review methods for assessing cognitions in socially anxious adolescents.

Assessing Cognitions

Clinical Interview

A thorough clinical interview is an important starting point for any clinical intervention for SAD and especially cognitive intervention (see Garcia-Lopez et al. this volume, Chap. 6). Several reliable and validated structured and semi-structured diagnostic interviews are available for use with anxious children and adolescents (Schniering et al. 2000). The ADIS-C/P is commonly used because it provides detailed assessment of individual anxiety disorders according to the DSM categories as well as differential diagnoses for other common difficulties in youth. Although typically used in research clinic settings, reliable and valid diagnoses of SAD can be made using the ADIS-C/P in non-research settings (Rapee et al. 1994; Wood et al. 2002).

In addition to structured interviews, a comprehensive clinical interview will include collecting information about an adolescent's cognitions, that is, their expectations in social situations, their perceptions of threat during or in anticipation of social situations, beliefs about other people's evaluations of them, and/or their own judgements about their social performances. In order to understand whether their interpretations and expectations are biased, it is also important that a clinical interview collect information about social skills, performance ability, and negative experiences in social situations, for example, experiences of bullying, negative feedback in social situations, etc. There is a complex interplay between social skills/experiences, interpretations of social situations, and social anxiety in youth. Some research has found that youth with high levels of social anxiety have poorer social skills when rated by independent observers and that socially anxious youth are at risk of peer victimisation (Miers et al. 2011). Information about social skills and experiences with peers may be collected via direct questioning during a clinical interview and also by observation of the adolescent's social skills and ability during the interview. Such information provides clinicians an understanding of how maladaptive cognitions or biased interpretations have developed and should be targeted in therapy.

Questionnaires

While many questionnaires assess anxiety symptoms in children, fewer have been developed for use in adolescents. However, the Multidimensional Anxiety Scale for Children (March et al. 1997; March and Parker 1999) and the Screen for Child Anxiety Related Emotional Disorders (Birmaher et al. 1997, 1999) measure broad anxiety symptoms, including social anxiety symptoms, and can be used reliably for adolescents. Instruments specifically measuring social anxiety symptoms in adolescents include the Social Anxiety Scale for Adolescents (SAS-A; La Greca and Lopez 1998) and the Social Phobia and Anxiety Inventory (SPAI). The SAS-A provides a measure of an adolescent's fear of negative evaluation and their social avoidance and distress. The SPAI measures social fears in multiple settings, focusing on cognitions, behaviour, and physiological responses and has good psychometric properties in adolescents and young adults (Clark et al. 1994; Garcia-Lopez et al. 2001, 2009, 2014, 2015; Olivares et al. 1999; Piqueras et al. 2012; Vieira et al. 2013). Further, a brief version of SPAI (SPAI-B; Garcia-Lopez et al. 2008) has been developed for adolescents with social anxiety (see Garcia-Lopez et al. this volume, Chap. 6). A measure of particular clinical utility for cognitive interventions is the Children's Automatic Thoughts Scale (CATS; Schniering and Rapee 2002). This measure has been used in anxious adolescents with strong psychometric properties (Schniering and Rapee 2004; Schniering and Lyneham 2006, 2007) and provides a general measure of an adolescent's negative self-statements as they relate to both internalising and externalising problems. In particular, the social threat subscale of the CATS measures cognitions related to social anxiety that inform cognitive interventions targeting the disorder. For example, social threat items include 'Kids will think I'm stupid', 'Kids are going to laugh at me', and 'I'm going to look silly'.

Cognitive Bias

As previously outlined, cognitive theories of social anxiety suggest that biased attention and processing of threat lead to anxiety-related affect and behaviour. In SAD, attention bias might involve selectively attending to threat (e.g. negative facial expressions of others) or self-focused attention (e.g. negative aspects of one's own appearance). Furthermore, interpretation biases might involve viewing social cues (e.g. responses from someone in the audience) as a sign of social threat (e.g. someone yawning is because the talk is boring not because the person had a poor night sleep). Biased attention to threat (Bar-Haim et al. 2007) and biased social interpretations (Miers et al. 2008) have been found in socially anxious children and adolescents.

In general, a number of experimental cognitive psychology paradigms have been designed to detect attention and interpretation bias and empirically investigate causal relationships between cognitive bias and anxiety symptoms (Muris and Field 2008). Attention biases have been identified in tasks where faster processing of stimuli takes place following a probe that replaces threat stimuli vs neutral or positive stimuli. In attention bias tasks, stimuli are typically pictures or words (threat/neutral/positive), and participants respond by making a quick response. In the visual dot-probe task, the stimuli are presented followed by a dot located behind either the negative or neutral image. Bias towards threat is detected when the child is faster at locating the dot when it appears behind the threatening image. Interpretation bias tasks typically involve generating a response to a stimulus where the stimulus is a word, sentence, or paragraph that is ambiguous, and the response involves recall or comprehension question that requires removing the ambiguity. For example, to assess interpretation bias with a focus on social situations, a child may be provided with a hypothetical situation ambiguous to threat (e.g. a group of children are playing a game and as you approach you notice they are laughing). The child is asked to provide an interpretation of the situation, 'Why are the children laughing?' A child who believes the children were laughing at them (e.g. as opposed to the game itself) would demonstrate an interpretational threat bias. Research has found that clinically anxious children show attention and interpretation biases towards negative or threat information, and in adults, inducing negative cognitive biases increases anxiety symptoms (MacLeod and Mathews 2012). Recently, Gomez-Ariza et al. (2013) have found adolescents suffer from deficits in their ability to intentionally inhibit irrelevant memories.

Psychosocial Interventions

Cognitive Behavioural Therapy

Background and Overview

Cognitive behavioural therapy (CBT) for SAD aims to provide techniques that directly target excessive and interfering fears regarding social performance, social evaluations, and negative social outcomes. The goal of the intervention is not to remove anxiety completely, but instead, to reduce an adolescent's anxiety to a manageable level so that anxiety does not impact on daily functioning. This distinction is particularly important for SAD in adolescents since self-awareness and related anxiety in social situations increase normatively during the teenage years (Westenberg et al. 2004). There are at present several evidence-based CBT treatments developed for adolescent anxiety disorders including Cool Kids (Rapee et al. 2006) and Coping C.A.T. (Kendall and Hedtke 2006) which have been among the rigorous studied. Programmes developed for SAD specifically, including Social Effectiveness Training for Children (SET-C; Beidel et al. 2000) and Cognitive-Behavioral Group Treatment for Adolescents (CBGT-A; Albano et al. 1995; Hayward et al. 2000; Herbert et al. 2009), the original IAFS (Intervención en Adolescentes con Fobia Social-Treatment for Adolescents with Social Phobia; Garcia-Lopez 2000, 2007); SASS (Skills for Academic and Social Success; Masia et al., 2001); the protocol entitled "To be myself among the others" (Salvador & Pinto-Gouveia, 2009); and Cognitive-Behavioral Group Therapy for Social Anxiety (Aydin et al. 2010), also continue to emerge (see Chaps. 9 and 13). Some treatment components differ across these manualised CBT interventions, but most share the same common elements. Programmes which have been specifically designed for targeting cognitive symptoms of SAD typically include additional strategies like attention training techniques and video feedback exercises (Garcia-Lopez 2000, 2007; Melfsen et al. 2011). Below we describe common components across CBT treatment programmes for SAD and later turn to how specific SAD treatment strategies might provide benefit.

Individual Treatment Components

Treatment Rationale/Psychoeducation

The initial step in a cognitive-behavioural intervention is to provide adolescents and their families with information about social anxiety. Educational information about anxiety includes explanation that anxiety is a normal response accompanied by (i) bodily feelings (physiological symptoms), (ii) thoughts (cognitions), and (iii) actions (behaviours) (Rapee and Heimberg 1997). While a normal response to actual danger or threat, excessive anxiety can interfere with someone's ability to function and cope. For example, being concerned about what your school principal thinks of you might be a problem if it creates such a high level of anxiety that an adolescent experiences intense physical symptoms and avoids going to school all together. Psychoeducation also shows adolescents that the core components of treatment are skills that can be used to manage all three aspects of anxiety. That is, treatment helps adolescents manage their bodily feelings/physical symptoms through awareness and relaxation, think in more helpful and realistic ways through cognitive restructuring, and change behaviour to reduce avoidance through gradual exposure. Cognitive restructuring is supported by gradual exposure and other related techniques like problem-solving and social skills training.

Relaxation Training

Relaxation training is sometimes used as a strategy to assist the adolescent to manage and cope with their arousal in social situations and provide the adolescent with skills to cope with challenging social situations. Encouraging the adolescent to identify the bodily symptoms they experience in social situations (e.g. blushing, stomach distress) can also be useful as these symptoms can then be used as a cue or warning sign for using relaxation techniques. Progressive muscular relaxation (PMR), originally described by Jacobsen (1929), is a common form of relaxation training in which individuals are instructed to alternate between tensing and relaxing different muscle groups. Several scripts for PMR are available and can help guide adolescents through these techniques both in session and at home. PMR is also sometimes paired with a second relaxation technique called controlled or deep breathing. For more information on these skills, see Rapee et al. (2000).

Cognitive Restructuring

Cognitive restructuring is an important treatment component. Cognitive restructuring involves questioning the accuracy of anxious thoughts and evaluating and challenging negative or unhelpful thoughts. The objective of cognitive restructuring is to move from often unrealistic and unhelpful thinking to more realistic and helpful thinking that enables an adolescent to more effectively manage their anxiety. Importantly, the objective of cognitive restructuring is not to arrive at positive thinking but rather realistic thinking. The 'realistic thinking' process involves the following steps: (1) identifying the event/situation causing anxiety; (2) identifying the thought behind the anxiety; (3) evaluating how realistic the thought is, for example, by looking for evidence; (4) considering how realistic the expected consequence is; and (5) identifying a realistic thought to replace the unrealistic/unhelpful anxious thought (Beck 1970; Heimberg et al. 1990).

To effectively use cognitive restructuring, an adolescent must first understand the connection between thoughts and feelings/behaviour. That is, the way you think affects how you feel and what you do (or don't do). In the case of SAD, an adolescent may identify thoughts like 'others will think badly of me', 'I'll do something embarrassing', 'everyone will laugh at me', or 'they'll think I'm stupid/boring/silly/dumb/a joke'. It can also be useful for adolescents to become aware of any patterns in their thinking. Examples of common 'thinking traps' particularly relevant for individuals with SAD include mind-reading, looking for the negative, or personalising. The mind-reading trap refers to the adolescent's misperception that they know what another person is thinking. For example, 'my friend didn't say anything about the dress I am wearing because she doesn't like it and doesn't like me anymore'. In this case, the adolescent believes she knows what her friend is thinking. This is also an example of personalising because the teen has made the assumption that the reason her friend did not say anything about her outfit was because of negative feelings about her or her outfit. Through the process of understanding and identifying common thinking traps, an adolescent can more easily make a connection between expecting negative evaluation in social situations and their own anxiety (Albano 1995).

For adolescents with social phobia, there is an underlying belief system that drives anxious thoughts. For example, the adolescent may believe that 'all individuals must like me' or perhaps another belief that 'I am unlikeable' or 'people are mean'. Working with core beliefs is an advanced cognitive technique that involves challenging the underlying core belief. Using the same process described above, the therapist can assist the adolescent to find evidence for and against the core belief. Successfully challenging the core belief can lead to a shift in a range of anxious thoughts linked to the same core belief.

Gradual Exposure

Gradual exposure is considered a cornerstone of CBT for SAD. During exposure tasks, individuals face anxiety-provoking situations/stimuli that elicit symptoms of anxiety/arousal with the primary goal of reducing anxiety. The goal is to facilitate cognitive change by showing that feared consequences are less negative than imagined. Exposure tasks also serve secondary goals of increasing confidence that the feared situation can be faced with success and that anxiety symptoms, although uncomfortable, will eventually diminish.

Most exposure-based interventions for adolescents with SAD utilise a gradual approach. Adolescents first identify specific social fears and worries according to the degree of fear/worry they provoke. For example, a socially anxious adolescent may find starting conversations mildly anxiety provoking, giving speeches or presentations at school moderately difficult, and being assertive extremely anxiety provoking. Exposure tasks for this adolescent would begin by having the teen engage in conversations with others. Once these situations no longer produce significant anxiety, other (i.e. more anxiety provoking) social fears are targeted. Adolescents are assisted in developing a hierarchy of 'steps' for each fear/worry. In many cases, more intense fears are broken down into smaller steps allowing the adolescent to gradually face their fear.

It is important to identify the cognitions and predictions that occur in these situations as well (e.g. 'What do you think will happen if you start a conversation?') and to find out what makes the situation more difficult (e.g. starting a conversation with a stranger might be easier than starting a conversation with a peer). Any number of factors may make conversing more or less difficult, and creating steps that address these factors will help to produce a hierarchy that begins with easier steps and gets progressively more difficult. For example, the first step in 'starting conversations' might be to say hello to a stranger. More difficult steps might be to say hello (or goodbye) to peers and to ask questions to a stranger. The most difficult step might be to approach a peer who looks like they are in a rush and begin a conversation.

Importantly, an adolescent should be able to successfully complete a step (i.e. feel significantly less or minimal anxiety) before progressing to the next step on their hierarchy. A good hierarchy will include tasks that are practical so they can be repeated regularly and allow the adolescent to stay in the situation long enough for them to experience a reduction in their anxiety levels before leaving the situation or completing the step. By repeatedly facing their fears, adolescents break the cycle of avoidance, learn that they can cope with anxiety, and, importantly, have first-hand evidence about the accuracy of their anxious vs realistic thoughts. Generally, adolescents learn that (1) what they thought was going to happen (e.g. everyone will laugh at them) is unlikely and (2) that even if the feared consequence occurs, they can handle it. A further strategy that integrates the cognitive restructuring and gradual exposure techniques is behavioural experiments (see Bennett-Levy et al. 2004). Behavioural experiments involve making a prediction (e.g. everyone will laugh at me when I give the speech), testing out the veracity of the prediction by conducting an experiment (e.g. speak in front of the class, and note down the number of people who laugh), reviewing the results of the experiment (e.g. actually no one laughed while I was speaking), and using the results to inform the initial prediction and come to a more realistic and helpful expectation (e.g. it is unlikely that people will laugh at me when I am speaking). In this way, gradual exposure supports the cognitive restructuring process and assists the adolescent to hold more helpful coping beliefs.

Problem-Solving

The aim of problem-solving is to assist adolescents to arrive at alternate, less avoidant, and more adaptive solutions to a given situation. Problem-solving can help youth to cope more adaptively in anxiety-provoking situations and refrain from their usual maladaptive avoidant response. Problem-solving has been used in efficacious cognitive and cognitive behavioural interventions for youth anxiety (Albano et al. 1995; Hayward et al. 2000; Rapee et al. 2006). An adolescent is taught to identify a specific problem/situation (e.g. not understanding the tasks required for an assignment due in 2 weeks) and brainstorm possible responses to the problem (e.g. figure it out on my own, find out more about the assignment, ask for extra time). In the brainstorming phase, the adolescent is encouraged to list all possible responses without evaluating them. Evaluation is encouraged once the brainstorming process is complete, that is, the therapist encourages the adolescent to consider the advantages and disadvantages associated with each response and select the most ideal response. It is important to consider the short-term and long-term consequences of each solution. For example, an avoidant solution like 'say no to the party invitation' may reduce the child's anxiety in the short term but in the long term it maintains it. Problem-solving skills are most effectively taught by working through a real-life example.

Social Skills (Assertiveness)

While nonclinical levels of social anxiety are not necessarily associated with social skill deficits, substantial evidence documents the presence of social skill deficits among adolescents with SAD (Alfano et al. 2006; Beidel et al. 2007, 2014; Spence et al. 1999). Specific deficits vary but commonly pertain to voice volume, eye contact, speech length, social assertiveness, initiating and maintaining conversations, and listening skills. Fortunately, adolescents with SAD have been shown to benefit from being taught specific skills for increasing social competence (Beidel et al. 2000; Masia et al. 2001; Garcia-Lopez et al. 2002, 2006, 2009, 2014; Olivares et al. 2002). A description of treatments with social skills training modules can be found in Chaps. 12 and 13. Social skills training is generally conducted in a group format, though individual training may also be used. Typically, areas of difficulty are discussed, followed by instruction and clinician modelling of skills. Adolescents are then provided opportunities to practise these new skills and receive feedback on their performance. In-session role-plays and feedback are particularly important in shaping new skill development in that they allow for repeated practise in a structured, supportive environment prior to use in real-world settings. Specific skills might include using a confident posture (e.g. not slouching), appropriate tone and volume of voice (e.g. not quiet and monotone), appropriate eye contact (e.g. not always looking away or on the ground), and appropriate conversation content (e.g. polite and pleasant rather than submissive or aggressive and demanding) (Beidel et al. 2000).

Given the important influence of peers during adolescence and the impact of social anxiety on the development of adaptive peer relationships, strategies to deal with teasing and bullying might also be an important aspect in the treatment of SAD. Adolescents are taught strategies to respond in a way that shows they are confident and are not bothered by the teasing. Achieving this requires mastery of the above-mentioned social and assertiveness skills. Ignoring, getting an audience, and making confident responses or behaviours are encouraged. Youth are encouraged to practise their responses in a safe situation (e.g. using role plays) before using them in real-life situations. Of course, when bullying becomes violent in anyway, the adolescent should be taught to involve appropriate authority figures (parents, school personnel, etc.).

Cognitive Bias Modification

Given the causal links identified between cognitive bias and anxiety symptoms, research has increasingly turned to using cognitive bias modification (CBM) tasks as an intervention to alter these maladaptive cognitive biases. CBM interventions involve modifying existing negative biases away from threat with repeated practise. The interventions either focus on attentional bias or interpretation bias. In attention bias modification, during repeated practise, the individual is rewarded for moving their attention away from threatening images/faces and towards happy/positive/neutral images.

The evidence in support of the use of attention bias modification is promising. For example, Bar-Haim et al. (2011) showed that children with high levels of anxiety reported lower anxiety levels in response to a stressful puzzle task following a single attention bias modification task. The effects of extended attention bias modification has been assessed in a group of high school students, where those trained not to attend to negative stimuli responded with less anxiety to a stressor than those in the control group (See et al. 2009). Similarly, in a sample of socially anxious and test anxious high school students, CBM led to a greater reduction in negative automatic associations compared to CBT and a control (Sportel et al. 2013). Yet, CBT led to the significantly greater reductions in social anxiety symptoms.

CBM has been used in clinical samples. Rozenman et al. (2011) showed that youth (10–17 years of age) diagnosed with an anxiety disorder (social anxiety, separation anxiety, or generalised anxiety) responded to 4 weeks of attention bias modification training: only 25 % of youth met diagnostic criteria for an anxiety disorder following CBM. In a sample of 37 7–13-year-olds, Waters and colleagues (2013) were successfully able to train children to develop a bias towards happy faces in a visual search paradigm and were able to show greater reductions in anxiety diagnoses and severity (50 % free of their principal diagnosis), compared to children in a control condition (8 % diagnosis free). These findings are consistent with studies utilising CBM training in socially anxious adults (Schmidt et al. 2009).

Even more positive results have been found for interpretation bias modification tasks and especially for individuals with SAD. Socially anxious adults who received eight sessions of CBM over 4 weeks were less likely to interpret ambiguity negatively and reported reductions in social anxiety symptoms (Beard and Amir 2008). Similar results were found for socially anxious children who received three sessions of CBM (Vassilopoulos et al. 2009). At Macquarie University's Centre for Emotional Health, we have also trained benign interpretations in clinically anxious children between 7 and 12 years of age. Over a 2-week period, children were asked to finish scenarios that were related to either social threat, general threat, or separation threat. Unlike children in the neutral condition, children in the positive training showed a significant reduction in interpretation bias on the social threat scenarios after training. All children showed lower self-reported social anxiety and generalised anxiety independent of training condition. However, parents reported a significant reduction of social anxiety in their children in the positive training group but not in the neutral group. This study provides support for remediation of negative interpretation biases among clinically anxious youth (Hudson et al. 2012).

Studies using CBM interventions, particularly for social anxiety, are promising, yet most report change in symptoms using self-report measures, and few use observational or diagnostic measures of anxiety (MacLeod and Mathews 2012). The latter is an important issue based on the results of a recent randomised, controlled study utilising CBM training among adults with SAD (Bunnell et al. 2013). Specifically, based on a multimodal assessment of anxiety and functioning, adults assigned to eight sessions of CBM did not differ from those assigned to a placebo control condition based on self, clinician, or behavioural measures at posttreatment (Bunnell et al. 2013). Another important question is whether, in addition to statistically significant change, interpretation and attentional changes are in fact clinically meaningful. That is, while social anxiety symptoms may decrease, distress, avoidance, and skill deficits may be less affected. Finally, there remain questions as to whether results are maintained over time. Future research needs to address these limitations before this form of cognitive intervention can be considered 'evidence based'. This style of intervention may be a useful addition to therapy or option for those that do not respond to standard cognitive interventions described above.

Efficacy of Cognitive Behavioural Therapy

Review of the Efficacy of CBT for Adolescent Anxiety

Cognitive behavioural treatment (CBT) is an evidence-based treatment and typically the first line of treatment for youth anxiety. Comprehensive reviews of randomised controlled trials consistently show that CBT is effective in reducing anxiety symptoms in children and adolescents (Silverman et al. 2008). On average, 59 % of anxious children and adolescents who receive CBT will experience remission in anxiety symptoms following brief CBT (James et al. 2013). The effects of CBT are also generally considered to persist over time (Barrett et al. 2001) although additional controlled follow-up studies are necessary to confirm this finding (James et al. 2013).

In general, research has not yet identified consistent factors that predict which children respond favourably to a standard course of CBT and which children may require additional treatment. For example, treatment format (individual, group, family/parental), treatment length, gender, age, comorbidity, parental psychopathology, and initial anxiety severity have not consistently predicted response to CBT for anxious youth (James et al. 2013; Knight et al. 2014). However, although inconsistent, comorbid depression and externalising disorder have been associated with poorer CBT outcome (Knight et al. 2014). Greater pretreatment anxiety symptoms tend to predict greater symptom change but poorer endpoint for anxious youth following CBT (Knight et al. 2014). An important area of enquiry and relevant to the focus of the current chapter is whether the child's initial anxiety diagnosis predicts differential outcome. That is, do children with SAD respond as well to treatment protocols as children with other anxiety disorders like generalised anxiety disorder or separation anxiety disorder? There has become increasing evidence that children with a diagnosis of social anxiety disorder have a slower response to CBT as well as poorer endpoints compared to children with other anxiety disorders (Crawley et al. 2008; Compton et al. 2014; Hudson et al. 2015). This is not to say that the treatments are not effective for children with social anxiety disorder, rather it says that it is less effective than for children with other types of anxiety. The question remains as to how we can make cognitive and cognitive behavioural interventions more effective for children with social anxiety.

Given the continually increasing number of CBT protocols for anxious youth (including adolescents with SAD), researchers (e.g. Kashdan and Herbert 2001) have pointed out the need for (1) controlled treatment research that utilises active, alternative interventions (e.g. rather than waitlist conditions) in establishing efficacy and (2) study designs that provide a better understanding of critical (i.e. essential) treatment components. For example, all CBT programmes for adolescents with SAD begin with psychoeducation about anxiety and its symptoms (cognitions, behaviours, and bodily sensations). Similarly, virtually all interventions include some form of exposure to feared situations, thoughts, or outcomes. Other aspects of treatment, however, differ in line with distinct theoretical models. For example, based on cognitive models of SAD (Rapee and Heimberg 1997; Clark and Wells 1995), cognitions are considered fundamental to the experience and maintenance of SAD and are therefore directly targeted during treatment. Other intervention programmes have focused more on social skill deficits. For example, Social Effectiveness Training for Children (SET-C; Beidel et al. 2000) the original *Intervención en Adolescentes con Fobia Social—Therapy for Adolescents with Social Phobia* (IAFS; Garcia-Lopez 2000, 2007, 2013) and Skills for Academic and Social Success (SASS; Masia et al. 2001) specifically include social skills training and peer experiences for practising new skills. Unfortunately, direct comparisons of these treatments are generally absent from the literature at present. There is, however, some evidence from child self-report data that effect sizes for disorder-specific treatments are greater than generic treatments for anxiety (Reynolds et al. 2012).

With regard to cognitive-focused interventions for youth with SAD, attention retraining skills and video feedback have been used. With video-assisted feedback (e.g. Garcia-Lopez 2007; Rapee and Hayman 1996), patients view recordings of their social performances as a means of challenging self-focused negative thoughts (i.e. the video provides objective information about performance). This treatment component targets a common cognitive bias in SAD whereby individuals believe their performance is worse than it actually is. In using video feedback, clients firstly identify what they expect to see in their social performance, complete the task while being video recorded, and then observe their performance as objectively as possible. Although there is mixed evidence (Ramos et al. 2008; Smits et al. 2006), video feedback has been found to add benefit to treatment for social anxiety in adults (Rodebaugh et al. 2010) and reduce anticipatory anxiety in adolescents (Parr and Cartwright-Hatton 2009). Studies comparing CBT enhanced with both attention retraining and video feedback to standard CBT programmes have found significantly better outcomes for adults with SAD using the enhanced CBT (Rapee et al. 2009). With the exception of a pilot study by Melfsen et al. (2011), few studies have examined the use of video-assisted feedback among socially anxious teens. Using attention training and video feedback components, Melfsen et al. showed significant differences compared to waitlist on both symptom measures and diagnoses.

One additional limitation of existing treatment research among youth with SAD is that many studies have focused on treatments for children *and* adolescents, with little differentiation between these two developmentally distinct periods. Although the specific symptoms and impairments observed among adolescents with SAD overlap to a large extent with those observed in children (e.g. social isolation and school avoidance), unique impairments also may exist (e.g. related to romantic interests, dating, part-time jobs, and college preparation) (Alfano et al. 2006). Thus, the appropriateness of treatments developed for socially anxious children should not automatically assumed for teens. Nevertheless, there have been several controlled studies using specifically adolescent populations that allow conclusions about the value of these treatments in this developmental period (Baer and Garland 2005; Garcia-Lopez et al. 2006, 2014; Olivares et al. 2002; Hayward et al. 2000; Herbert et al. 2009; Masia-Warner et al. 2005, 2007; Tillfors et al. 2011).

Possible Barriers to Treatment for Adolescents with Social Anxiety Disorder

While it is important to consider methods of enhancing treatment by targeting the important cognitive aspects of etiological models of social anxiety, it is also important to consider other factors that may be influencing poorer response to CBT for youth with SAD compared to other anxiety disorders and so attempt to minimise the impact of these on treatment.

Treatment length may need to be extended to allow for the gradual development of social competence and confidence. Standard treatment length may mean that exposure exercises are attempted too quickly (i.e. before social confidence can build), and so rather than being experienced as positive learning opportunities confirm social threat and negative evaluation from others. Thus, rather than learning the feared expectation is unfounded, the exposure may lead to a strengthening of the fear belief (e.g. people don't like me, or people will think I am stupid). Evidence from treatment studies suggests that loneliness and poor social skills in fact mediate treatment outcome for children with social anxiety (Alfano et al. 2009).

Additionally, treatment may require more in-session time to facilitate practice, including role plays, before youth can effectively implement the skills outside of the treatment context. Not only may it be beneficial to extend the length of treatment (total number of sessions), but it may be beneficial to spread out the treatment sessions so that skills can be implemented (see Chap. 12) in real-life social situations before moving on to new, additive skills in treatment.

Importantly, treatment itself is a social situation. That is, the socially anxious adolescent is engaging in exposure and facing their fears by virtue of just meeting with the clinician each week. Higher levels of anxiety about the therapist and treatment may impair their ability to engage with the therapist and engage with the treatment programme. In the adult literature, there is evidence to suggest that social anxiety can impact on interpersonal closeness and disclosure (Kashdan and Wenzel 2005; Meleshko and Alden 1993). Thus, clinicians should be mindful of a teen's social anxiety levels in session, reduce expectations for disclosure, prioritise efforts to establish and build rapport, and endeavour to minimise social anxiety levels in session.

These are a few of the important factors that should be considered when treating a socially anxious adolescent. Careful consideration of the impact of social anxiety on the treatment relationship and setting is an important aspect of treating this population.

Case Example: Model of Assessment and Treatment

Case Presentation

Mark and his parents presented to the clinic for treatment. Mark (16), the youngest of three children, has always been extremely shy according to his parents. In primary school, Mark was often teased and excluded by other children. Although this hasn't happened in high school, Mark is very reluctant to stand up for himself, so he has missed out on activities he enjoys for fear of what the other students will think of him. Mark's school reports indicate that he does not participate in class. While he is coping well academically, Mark and his parents report that he experiences a lot of distress leading up to tests and performances. Mark also agreed that he rarely volunteers to answer questions in class, prefers not to ask for help from the teacher, and feels like he clams up when taking tests because he is worried about coming last in the class. Mark stated that he worries that everyone will notice his anxiety, that he'll go bright red in the face and stutter, or that his mind will go blank.

Mark's parents indicated that he only has a small group of friends and doesn't often attend social gatherings or outings with them. Mark also indicated that he would like to be more comfortable around his peers, girls in particular. He likes a girl at his school and would like to ask her out, but he is sure that she thinks he is a loser and will say no. Mark also worries a great deal about his appearance, spending significant amounts of time ensuring that he will not stand out or look different to others. Although interactive and confident at home, when with people Mark does not know well, with peers, or in crowded situations, he is very quiet and does not voluntarily participate. Mark and his parents indicated that they would most like to work on his inability to speak in the classroom or give presentations, distress during activities involving performance or sport, and desire for deeper friendships including romantic relationships.

Cognitive Intervention: Step-By-Step Guidelines

The following pages outline the session-by-session treatment for Mark based on the Cool Kids (Chilled) programme for adolescent anxiety (Rapee et al. 2006). In the programme delivered in an individual format, each session involves Mark, and at times the therapist reviews skills and home practice with his parents.

Session 1

The aim of session 1 is to develop rapport, provide the rationale for treatment, normalise anxiety, introduce the link between thoughts and feelings, and identify the bodily symptoms associated with anxiety.

Because Mark is very shy talking to new people, the therapist chooses to include Mark's parents in the beginning of the session and doesn't start by talking about anxiety. Instead, they talk about the family, their interests, and hobbies. The therapist tries to find some common interests with him. Mark is initially a little reserved, giving brief answers but begins to speak more openly after some time.

After getting to know Mark and his parents, the therapist begins to talk about treatment giving the family information about what to expect and providing the rationale for treatment. Then, the therapist spends time with the parents and Mark separately. During the time with Mark's parents, the therapist emphasises the treatment rationale and their role in the programme. Mark's mother is particularly concerned to know 'where anxiety comes from' and worries that she has passed on her own anxieties to Mark. The therapist provides some information about the causes of social anxiety and emphasises that the causes of anxiety are not as important as what Mark can do to help manage his anxiety. Importantly, the family are provided information about how the programme will help Mark to face gradually the social situations he has been avoiding.

During her time with Mark, the therapist asks Mark to generate specific goals for the treatment programme. Mark reports that he would like to (1) be able to get involved in classroom discussions; (2) give a confident speech as part of his English assessment; and (3) develop closer friendships, even with girls. The therapist then talks about 'feelings' and discusses with Mark a range of different feelings, including anxiety and fear. The 'feelings scale' is introduced: a 0–10-point scale that Mark will use to indicate how severe his anxiety/worry is: 0, no worry at all; to 10, the most worry he has ever felt. The therapist asks Mark to think about different situations that would evoke different levels of anxiety to show how the feelings scale is used. For example, Mark says that he feels a '3' when the teacher asks questions he is certain he knows the answer to and an '8' when he has to read from a novel or play in front of the class.

Using a worksheet with thought bubbles from the workbook, the therapist then introduces a discussion about 'thoughts'. The worksheet helps Mark to see that different people have different thoughts in the same situation and that certain thoughts are associated with certain feelings. For example, if Mark thinks, 'The guys are going to laugh at me' when I ask the teacher for help, then he feels anxious. But if he thinks, 'I'll get a good grade if I know what to do with this assignment', then Mark might feel excited. Mark quickly understands the link between thoughts and feelings, so they move on to talk about what happens in his body when he feels anxious. To help Mark feel less anxious, the therapist also talks about her own physical feelings when she gets nervous. The therapist normalises Mark's bodily feelings (sickly feeling in his stomach, heart beating quickly, a little blushing, tension in his neck, and shaky legs) and provides information about how these bodily symptoms play an important role in keeping him alive.

At the end of the session, the therapist gives Mark a practice task for the week, which is to record daily his thoughts and feelings (using the feelings scale) during situations that occur each day.

Session 2

The aim of session 2 is to introduce cognitive restructuring/'realistic' thinking. The therapist will spend most of the session with Mark and only briefly introduce the idea of realistic thinking to Mark's parents towards the end of the session. To start the session, the therapist reviews Mark's week and practice task.

During the week, Mark was supposed to go to a party with his friends but spent so long getting ready that his parents couldn't drop him off before going out to a function they had. In his practice task, Mark reports that he was anxious about having conversations at the party and that he was feeling worried ('6' on the feelings scale) that no one would speak to him. He also reports feeling anxious ('5' on the feelings scale) that he would look silly and stand out and that the other people at the party would talk about him behind his back. Mark had kept a good record of his thoughts and feelings. The therapist informs Mark she will come back to this situation at the end of the session, after they learn 'realistic' thinking. The therapist acknowledges Mark's hard work on the practice.

The therapist talks about thinking styles and identifies the different thinking traps. Mark comes up with some examples of each type of thinking trap. The therapist then introduces cognitive restructuring to Mark, as a skill to look for evidence for his thoughts. Using a realistic thinking sheet with four columns (situation/thought, evidence, realistic consequences, realistic thought based on the evidence), the therapist leads Mark through his first realistic thinking exercise.

For the first realistic thinking exercise, the therapist uses a less threatening situation to get Mark started with the realistic thinking: answering a question in class. In this situation, the anxious thought is 'I will get the question wrong and everyone will laugh'. The therapist works through this example with Mark. First, they work on the evidence for the thought, 'I will get it wrong', then separately, 'If I get it wrong, everyone will laugh'. The therapist gives Mark lots of prompting questions, such as 'What happens when other people in the class get the answer wrong?' 'How many times have you got the answer wrong before?' and 'What else could happen?' The therapist reminds Mark about how easy it is to fall into the trap of mind-reading, that is, thinking you know what other people are thinking. The therapist challenges Mark's belief that he knows what other people are thinking. Rather than providing Mark with the evidence, the therapist encourages Mark to find the answers and the evidence for himself. They then work on a more difficult example: giving a presentation at school. In this situation, the anxious thought is 'People will notice how embarrassed I am, and they'll talk about me behind my back'. Again, the therapist and Mark work on the evidence for the thought, 'People will notice how embarrassed I am' and then separately, 'People will talk about me behind my back'. The therapist gives Mark lots of prompting questions, such as 'What have people told you when you have given presentations before?', 'Have they actually commented that you look embarrassed?', 'What do you notice when other people give presentations?', 'How many people do you think feel anxious giving talks?', 'When you have noticed signs of anxiety in others, have you spoken about them behind their back?', 'Have you heard other people speak about your peers that seem anxious giving presentations?', and 'What else could happen?' After this process, Mark records down a realistic thought based on the evidence 'People might notice that I'm a little embarrassed, but most people in my class don't like giving presentations so it probably won't be a big deal'.

The therapist briefly explains cognitive restructuring to Mark's parents and uses examples in their own life to review the process. Mark's parents indicate that the strategy will be useful in their day-to-day lives, because they both tend to think the worst in difficult situations. Mark's mother identifies that she worries a lot about what other people think of her and can get quite stressed about managing the children. Mark's father notes that he worries about running late for work and important meetings. The therapist encourages the parents to use these thinking strategies on their own worry and stress and to help coach Mark to come up with evidence against his worries when he might get stuck or needs extra assistance.

Bringing Mark and his parents together, the therapist leads Mark through his thoughts from the previous week and examines the evidence for his thought that he will stand out in what he is wearing at the party. At the end of the exercise, there is some evidence that, yes, maybe someone might have commented on his outfit, but it was more likely to be a positive than a negative comment and that there was no way to know whether people were talking about him behind his back. By doing realistic thinking, Mark brought his worry down from a '5' to a '2' on the feelings scale. The therapist then briefly explores the 'So what?' of the situation and asks Mark to think about the following reaction: 'Well, so what if someone doesn't like what I was wearing? What would be so bad about that?'

The practice task for the week is to use the realistic thinking sheet daily to get as much practice as possible. Mark's parents are also encouraged to complete a realistic thinking sheet on their worries during the week.

Session 3

The purpose of this session is to (1) review realistic thinking skills, (2) introduce rewards, and (3) provide the rationale and start planning for facing fears using gradual exposure. Mark's practice tasks are reviewed. Mark has used realistic thinking during the week and has come up with a couple of pieces of evidence for each situation. The therapist helps Mark to think of a few more pieces of evidence to write down for each situation. Again, Mark reports that anxiety impacted his week. Mark had a test during the week and panicked the night before, because he had been sick and missed some of the content for one of the test topics. He had an argument with his parents, because his parents had tried to use realistic thinking with him but he felt they were being dismissive. The therapist notes that she will review with Mark's parents how they have been assisting him with realistic thinking at home. The therapist encourages Mark for his good efforts using realistic thinking during the week.

The therapist then talks to Mark explicitly about rewards and how important it is to praise himself for the times when he tries hard in a test or is brave in answering even the easiest of questions. They talk about what makes a good reward, and Mark writes down some rewards that he could award himself for working on better ways to manage his anxiety.

Table 10.1 Mark's fears and worries list

	Get involved in class discussions – give opinion
I find these things really hard to do	Talking to girls
	Doing a solo at the school talent quest
	Give a presentation in English
I find these things hard to do	Ask my friends if they want to do something with me on the weekend
	Taking a test
	Not being bothered by what I wear when I go out
I find these things make me a little worried	Answering questions that I know the answer to
	Talking to my friends if they are already talking
	Starting conversations

Having had some success with realistic thinking and some examples of remaining fears, the therapist introduces gradual exposure (stepladders). They talk about the best way to learn to swim or ride a bike. These tasks involve overcoming fears or concerns about safety, yet are often mastered by gradual attempts in the situation. The therapist proposes that they work together on a plan to help 'Paul' face his fear of heights. Paul is scared of heights and has been invited to a friend's birthday party on the top floor of 'Millennium Tower', a skyscraper in the city. While Paul wants to go to the party, he is reluctant because of his fear. The therapist asks Mark how he first learned to swim, and whether he could use any lessons from this experience to help Paul learn to tolerate heights. Mark suggests that Paul first practise standing on a balcony of a two-story building or going up and down in the elevators of smaller buildings before the party as practice for the skyscraper. Using this example, the therapist talks about the principles of gradual exposure and begins to develop a list of the things that Mark worries about and would like to be able to do (see Table 10.1).

The therapist finds out how Mark's parents have been helping him with realistic thinking. They tell the therapist that they told Mark that he always did well, and it was only a test. The parents report that the realistic thinking 'didn't help'. The therapist works through this example with Mark's parents, reminding them that to begin with it is much easier to practise the realistic thinking skill leading up to or after rather than 'during' the anxiety-provoking situation. The therapist encourages them not to provide the evidence for Mark but to prompt him with the questions and, if he will allow them, to sit down together to work on a realistic thinking sheet in a more systematic way. The therapist talks with Mark's parents about their role in rewarding his attempts to manage his anxiety. The therapist also encourages both parents to continue using their realistic thinking sheets, so that they can model courageous behaviour. Mark's mother talks about the stress she experiences in social situations and that she would prefer to stay at home. The therapist encourages Mark's mother to use the strategies Mark has been learning to face her own social fears in the coming weeks.

The practice task for this week is for Mark to record times when he rewards himself and to continue to use realistic thinking for worries that come up during the week. Mark is also encouraged to practise realistic thinking on some of his bigger worries, even if they don't come up this week.

Session 4

The purpose of this session is to (1) review practice tasks, (2) review gradual exposure, and (3) begin to develop some stepladders for Mark's fears and worries.

The therapist asks Mark what he remembers about gradual exposure/stepladders, and they review the concepts through a review of the stepladder that they put together for Paul's fear of heights the previous session. They also review Mark's list of fears and worries.

From this list, Mark and the therapist choose something relatively easy on his list to begin developing the first stepladder: 'Starting conversations'. The therapist asks Mark a number of questions to help determine what makes 'starting conversations' easier rather than harder, so that Mark can manipulate the steps easily. Mark reports that the having more people around makes it harder than just approaching someone one-on-one. Knowing in advance what he will talk about helps, as does talking to a male rather than a female. After brainstorming these steps and ordering them in order from steps likely to cause the least anxiety to most anxiety, Mark's first exposure stepladder is complete. At the end of the session, Mark agrees with his family to complete steps daily between now and the next session. The therapist encourages Mark to use realistic thinking before he completes the steps and to record what he learns after completing the steps for future realistic thinking exercises.

Session 5–9

The purpose of these sessions is to continue working on gradual exposure and extending or simplifying realistic thinking. Additionally, in session 7, the therapist works with Mark on problem-solving and in sessions 8–9 on assertiveness strategies and dealing with teasing and bullying. Each week, the therapist reviews the stepladder tasks set the previous week and realistic thinking completed as part of this process. When Mark forgets to do his practice during the week, the therapist and Mark complete the practice in session. When Mark completes practice tasks between sessions, the therapist praises his efforts.

Mark is making good progress with his 'starting conversations' stepladder and adds another step at the end of the ladder, in which he is required to start a conversation and intentionally allowing silence in the conversation. In this exposure task, Mark is able to face his fear that he will not have anything to say to the person, and they will not continue with the discussion. Before completing this task, the therapist and Mark come up with a plan to help Mark feel less anxious during the silence. Worry surfing is introduced as a useful strategy to tolerate anxiety rather than avoid it, as is, 'acting-as-if' you are not worried/anxious. Worry surfing involves firstly acknowledging the anxiety Mark experiences and rather than avoiding the anxiety, encouraging Mark to ride the wave of anxiety without fighting it, but instead focusing on the task at hand and persisting in the situation.

In session 5, Mark starts work on a second stepladder: 'Answering questions in class'. With this stepladder, Mark starts with 'Answering questions that I know' and works up to being able to 'Deliberately answer the question incorrectly'. The

Table 10.2 Mark's stepladder about seeing friends more

	Goal: to go out with friends more at weekends
1	Ring Max and ask about some homework details
2	Ask friends what they did at the weekend, and extend the conversation by finding out more about what they did
3	Invite Max over for dinner with the family
4	Walk around to Max's house to see if he is home
5	Look interested when friends are talking about the weekend, ask to be included
6	Arrange to meet a friend at 'Intencity' to play video games
7	Ring Sam and ask him to go to the movies
8	Go to a party when invited

purpose of these steps is to help Mark realise that it is okay to get the answer wrong and observe that his peers and teacher will generally react more positively than he expects. By the end of session 9, Mark is working through a number of stepladders, including 'Going out with friends more at weekends', 'Not being bothered by how I look when I go out', and Giving a presentation'. An example is provided in Table 10.2.

Throughout treatment, the therapist and Mark continue to work on realistic thinking. In particular, they work on challenging Mark's core beliefs that people will be unkind to him and that he is unlikeable or different. Using the realistic thinking sheets, Mark is able to generate evidence that he is a likeable person, and even if someone does not like him, it is not the end of the world.

In session 6, the therapist talks to Mark about simplifying realistic thinking so that it can be more effectively used 'in the moment'. To use 'in-your-mind realistic thinking', Mark creates cue cards with the questions he has found most useful to gather realistic evidence.

In session 7, the therapist introduces the problem-solving technique. The therapist discusses with Mark how to brainstorm as many potential solutions to a problem, then to review the pros and cons of each before selecting a solution to try, and, finally, to evaluate the solution (and if necessary select another).

In sessions 8–9, the therapist introduces assertiveness training. Mark is able to use appropriate social skills when he is not anxious, but he becomes less confident and less able to use skills like eye contact and voice volume in anxiety-provoking situations. The therapist discusses with Mark the difference between assertive, passive, and aggressive behaviour. Mark and the therapist role play different scenarios as if they are responding assertively, passively, and aggressively. Mark identifies that he almost always acts in a passive way (except with his parents), because he does not want people to pick on him if he puts himself forward. The therapist suggests that by being assertive, Mark could challenge these thoughts and in the process be more likely to have people like and respect him and to have his own needs met rather than always making sure others' needs are met. The therapist and Mark develop a stepladder for being assertive. Because of Mark's previous history with teasing, the therapist works with him to develop strategies to deal with teasing if it were to occur in the future. Using role plays where the therapist initially models an appropriate response, Mark is able to give assertive responses to the teasing, with the intent of letting the bully know he does not care about what they are saying.

During the second half of the programme, it becomes increasingly important for Mark's mum to also use exposure to reduce her own social fears. The therapist assists Mark's mother in working on a series of stepladders to increase her social confidence. Some of the steps include starting conversations with work colleagues, talking to family members she has lost touch with (initially over the phone and then at family gatherings), accepting social invitations, inviting people over for dinner, and being assertive at work when requesting annual leave. Mark and his mother work together on assertiveness role-plays, and Mark's father helps to encourage both Mark and his wife to practise facing their fears.

Session 10

The purpose of session 10 is to review the strategies covered in the programme, review goals, set future objective, and discuss relapse prevention.

Upon review of the goals Mark set out in session 1, Mark and his parents report that most have been achieved. Mark reports that he still feels some anxiety doing these things, but that the anxiety is manageable and no longer stops him from doing what he would like to do. The family plans future stepladders that Mark might work on, including talking to girls. Mark agrees that he still needs to continue working on the last few steps of some of the stepladders and is keen to continue with his assertiveness stepladder.

The therapist asks Mark and his parents to look to the future and think about how he (and they) will respond if stressful or anxiety-provoking situations arise. For example, the therapist asks Mark to imagine that he wants to ask a girl out. What would he do? Or what if Mark starts feeling anxious in an aeroplane? What would he do? The purpose of these scenarios is to review the skills Mark and his parents have learned and to encourage them to apply these skills to future, unknown scenarios. The therapist reminds the family that situations, even anxiety-provoking ones, in the future can be managed by remembering and applying the skills from the programme.

Conclusion

Cognitive behavioural interventions are efficacious in treating social anxiety disorder in adolescents. This chapter has provided an overview of a range of treatment strategies that are currently used to modify socially anxious cognitions and behaviour to reduce anxious affect. Research suggests that additional enhancements may be required to improve the efficacy of these interventions. The field is at a critical point as it is imperative that we develop and evaluate enhanced treatment programmes that will lead to improved outcomes for socially anxious youth (Hudson et al. 2015). There is some emerging evidence that cognitive bias modification paradigms may be effective in reducing social anxiety and that treatments specifically target discrete disorders may lead to larger effect sizes. There is also evidence from the treatment of social anxiety in adults that suggests additional treatment components such as video feedback and attention training may be useful (Amir et al. 2009; Melfsen et al. 2011; Ramos et al. 2008). It is also possible that all that is required to improve outcomes is a longer dose of the same treatment. Given the long-term implications of untreated social anxiety symptoms, these questions are of great clinical importance and need to be evaluated in future randomised clinical trials.

References

Achenbach TM, McConaughy SH, Howell CT (1987) Child/adolescent behavioural and emotional problems: implications of cross-informant correlations for situational specificity. Psychol Bull 101:213–232

Albano AM (1995) Treatment of social anxiety in adolescents. Cogn Behav Pract 2:271–298

Albano AM, Marten PA, Holt CS, Heimberg RG, Barlow DH (1995) Cognitive behavioral group treatment for social phobia in adolescents: a preliminary study. J Nerv Ment Dis 183:685–692

Alfano CA, Beidel DC, Turner SM (2006) Cognitive correlates of social phobia among children and adolescents. J Abnorm Child Psychol 34:182–194

Alfano CA, Pina AA, Villalta IK, Beidel DC, Ammerman RT, Crosby LE (2009) Mediators and moderators of outcome in behavioural treatment of childhood social phobia. J Am Acad Child Adolesc Psychiatry 48:945–953

Amir N, Beard C, Taylor CT, Klumpp H, Elias J, Burns M, Chen X (2009) Attention training in individuals with generalized social phobia: a randomized controlled trial. J Consult Clin Psychol 77(5):961

Aydin A, Tekinsav S, Sorias O (2010) Evaluation of the effectiveness of a cognitive-behavioral therapy program for alleviating the symptoms of social anxiety in adolescents. Turkish Journal of Psychiatry, 21:25–36

Baer S, Garland EJ (2005) Pilot study of community-based cognitive behavioral group therapy for adolescents with social phobia. J Am Acad Child Adolesc Psychiatry 44:258–264. doi:10.1097/00004583-200503000-00010

Bar-Haim Y, Lamy D, Pergamin L, Bakermans-Kranenburg MJ, van IJzendoorn MH (2007) Threat-related attentional bias in anxious and nonanxious individuals: a meta-analytic study. Psychol Bull 133:1–24

Bar-Haim Y, Morag I, Glickman S (2011) Training anxious children to disengage attention from threat: a randomized controlled trial. J Child Psychol Psychiatry 52:861–869

Barrett PM, Duffy AL, Dadds MR, Rapee RM (2001) Cognitive-behavioral treatment of anxiety disorders in children: long-term (6-year) follow-up. J Consult Clin Psychol 69:135–141

Beard C, Amir N (2008) A multi-session interpretation modification program: changes in interpretation and social anxiety symptoms. Behav Res Ther 46:1135–1141

Beck AT (1970) Cognitive therapy: nature and relation to behaviour therapy. Behav Ther 1:184–200

Beesdo K, Bittner A, Pine DS, Stein MB, Hofler M, Lieb R, Wittchen HU (2007) Incidence of social anxiety disorder and the consistent risk for secondary depression in the first three decades of life. Arch Gen Psychiatry 64:903–912

Beidel DC, Turner SM, Morris TL (2000) Behavioral treatment of childhood social phobia. J Consult Clin Psychol 68:1072–1080

Beidel DC, Turner SM, Young BJ, Ammerman RT, Sallee RF, Crosby L (2007) Psychopathology of adolescent social phobia. J Psychopathol Behav Assess 29:47–54

Beidel DC, Alfano CA, Kofler MJ, Rao PA, Scharfstein L, Wong N (2014) The impact of social skills training for social anxiety disorder: a randomized controlled trial. J Anxiety Disord 28: 908–918. doi: 10.1016/j.janxdis.2014.09.016

Bennett-Levy J, Butler G, Fennell M, Hackmann A, Mueller M, Westbrook D (eds) (2004) Oxford guide to behavioural experiments in cognitive therapy. Oxford University Press, Oxford

Birmaher B, Khetarpal S, Brent D, Cully M, Balach L, Kaufman J, Neer SM (1997) The Screen for Child Anxiety Related Emotional Disorders (SCARED): scale construction and psychometric characteristics. J Am Acad Child Adolesc Psychiatry 36:545–553

Birmaher B, Brent DA, Chiappetta L, Bridge J, Monga S, Baugher M (1999) Psychometric properties of the Screen for Child Anxiety Related Emotional Disorders (SCARED): a replication study. J Am Acad Child Adolesc Psychiatry 38:1230–1236

Bunnell B, Beidel DC, Mesa F (2013) A randomized trial of attention training for generalized social phobia: does attention training change social behavior? Behav Ther 44:662–673

Caspi A, Elder GH Jr, Bem DJ (1988) Moving away from the world: life-course patterns of shy children. Dev Psychology 24:824–831

Clark DM, Wells A (1995) A cognitive model of social phobia. In: Liebowitz MR (ed) Social phobia: diagnosis, assessment, and treatment. Guilford Press, New York, pp 69–93

Clark DB, Turner S, Beidel D, Donovan J, Kirisci L, Jacob RG (1994) Reliability and validity of the social phobia and anxiety inventory for adolescents. Psychol Assess 6:135–140

Cohen P, Cohen J, Kasen S, Velez CN, Hartmark C, Johnson J, Rojas M, Brook J, Streuning EL (1993) An epidemiological study of disorders in late childhood and adolescents: 1. Age- and gender-specific prevalence. J Child Psychol Psychiatry 34:851–867

Comer JS, Kendall PC (2004) A symptom-level examination of parent–child agreement in the diagnosis of anxious youths. J Am Acad of Child Adolesc Psychiatry 43:878–886

Compton SN, Peris TS, Almirall D, Birmaher B, Sherrill J, Kendall PC, March JS, Gosch EA, Ginsburg GS, Rynn MA (2014) Predictors and moderators of treatment response in childhood anxiety disorders: results from the CAMS trial. J Consult Clin Psychol 82(2):212

Crawley SA, Beidas RS, Benjamin CL, Martin ED, Kendall PC (2008) Treating socially phobic youth with CBT: differential outcomes and treatment considerations. Behav Cogn Psychother 36:379–389

De Los Reyes A, Kazdin AE (2005) Informant discrepancies in the assessment of childhood psychopathology: a critical review, theoretical framework, and recommendations for further study. Psychol Bull 131:483–509

DiBartolo PM, Albano AM, Barlow DH, Heimberg RG (1998) Cross-informant agreement in the assessment of social phobia in youth. J Abnorm Child Psychol 26:213–220

Essau CA, Conradt J, Petermann F (1999) Frequency and comorbidity of social phobia and social fears in adolescents. Behav Res Ther 37:831–843

Furman W, Buhrmester D (1992) Age and sex differences in perceptions of networks of personal relationships. Child Dev 63:103–115

Garcia-Lopez LJ (2000, 2007) Examining the efficacy of three cognitive-behavioural treatments aimed at overcoming social anxiety in adolescents. University of Murcia: Publication Service

Garcia-Lopez LJ, Olivares J, Hidalgo MD, Beidel DC, Turner SM (2001) Psychometric properties of the social phobia and anxiety inventory, the social anxiety scale for adolescents, the fear of negative evaluation scale, and the social avoidance and distress scale in an adolescent Spanish-speaking sample. J Psychopathol Behav Assess 23:51–59

Garcia-Lopez LJ, Olivares J, Turner SM, Beidel DC, Albano AM, Sánchez-Meca J (2002) Results at long-term among three psychological treatments for adolescents with generalized social phobia (II): clinical significance and effect size. Psicologia Conductual [Behav Psychol] 10:165–179

Garcia-Lopez L-J, Olivares J, Beidel D, Albano A, Turner S, Rosa AI (2006) Efficacy of three treatment protocols for adolescents with social anxiety disorder: a 5-year follow-up assessment. J Anxiety Disord 20:175–191. doi:10.1016/j.janxdis.2005.01.003

Garcia-Lopez LJ, Beidel DC, Hidalgo MD, Olivares J, Turner SM (2008) Brief form of the social phobia and anxiety inventory for adolescents. Eur J Psychol Assess 24:150–156. doi:10.1027/1015-5759.24.3.150

Garcia-Lopez LJ, Muela JA, Espinosa-Fernández L, Diaz-Castela MM (2009) Exploring the relevance of expressed emotion to the treatment of social anxiety disorder in adolescence. J Adolesc 32:1371–1376. doi:10.1016/j.adolescence.2009.08.001

Garcia-Lopez LJ (2013) Tratando…trastorno de ansiedad social [Treating…social anxiety disorder]. Piramide, Madrid

Garcia-Lopez LJ, Diaz-Castela MM, Muela-Martinez JA, Espinosa-Fernandez L (2014) Can parent training for parents with high levels of expressed emotion have a positive effect on their child's social anxiety improvement? J Anxiety Disord 28:812–822. doi:10.1016/j.janxdis.2014.09.001

Garcia-Lopez LJ, Beidel DC, Muela-Martinez JM (2015) Optimal cut-off score for detecting social anxiety disorder and DSM-5 specifier with the Social Phobia and Anxiety Inventory-Brief form. Eur J Psychol Assess (in press)

Garcia-Lopez LJ, Saez-Castillo A, Beidel DC, La Greca AM (in press). Brief measures to screen for social anxiety in Spanish adolescents. J Dev Behav Pediatr

Gómez-Ariza CJ, Iglesias-Parro S, Garcia-López LJ, Díaz-Castela MM, Espinosa-Fernández L, Muela JA (2013) Selective intentional forgetting in adolescents with social anxiety disorder. Psychiatry Res 208:151–155

Greco LA, Morris TL (2005) Factors influencing the link between social anxiety and peer acceptance: contributions of social skills and close friendships during middle childhood. Behav Ther 36:197–205

Hayward C, Varady S, Albano AM, Thienemann M, Henderson L, Schatzberg AF (2000) Cognitive-behavioral group therapy for social phobia in female adolescents: results of a pilot study. J Am Acad Child Adolesc Psychiatry 39:721–726

Heimberg RG, Dodge CS, Hope DA, Kennedy CR, Zollo LJ, Becker RE (1990) Cognitive behavioural group treatment for social phobia: comparison with a credible placebo control. Cogn Ther and Res 14:1–23

Herbert JD, Gaudiano BA, Rheingold AA, Moitra E, Myers VH, Dalrymple KL, Brandsma LL (2009) Cognitive behaviour therapy for generalized social anxiety disorder in adolescents: a randomized controlled trial. J Anxiety Disord 23:167–177

Hudson JL, Klein AM, Rapee RM, Schniering CA, Wuthrich V, Kangas L, Rinck M (2012) Interpretation modification training reduces interpretation bias and anxiety in clinically anxious children. Paper presented at the European Association of Cognitive Behaviour Therapy, Geneva

Hudson JL, Rapee RM, Lyneham H, McLellan L, Wuthrich V, Schniering C (2015) Cognitive behavioural therapy outcomes for children with specific anxiety disorders. Manuscript submitted for publication

Inderbitzen HM, Walters KS, Bukowski AL (1997) The role of social anxiety in adolescent peer relations: differences among sociometric status groups and rejected subgroups. J Clin Child Psychol 26:338–348

Jacobsen E (1929) Progressive relaxation. Univ. of Chicago Press, Oxford

James AACJ, James G, Cowdrey FA, Soler A, Choke A (2013) Cognitive behavioural therapy for anxiety disorders in children and adolescents. Cochrane Database Syst Rev (4). doi:10.1002/14651858

Kashdan TB, Herbert JD (2001) Social anxiety disorder in childhood and adolescence: current status and future directions. Clin Child Fam Psychol Rev 4:37–61

Kashdan TB, Wenzel A (2005) A transactional approach to social anxiety and the genesis of interpersonal closeness: self, partner, and social context. Behav Ther 36(4):335–346

Kendall PC, Hedtke K (2006) Coping cat workbook, 2nd edn. Workbook Publishing, Ardmore

Knight A, McLellan L, Jones M, Hudson J (2014) Pre-treatment predictors of outcome in childhood anxiety disorders: a systematic review. Psychopathol Rev 1:77–129

La Greca AM, Lopez N (1998) Social anxiety among adolescents: linkages with peer relations and friendships. J Abnorm Child Psychol 26:83–94

La Greca AM, Moore HH (2005) Adolescent peer relations, friendships, and romantic relationships: do they predict social anxiety and depression? J Clin Child Adolesc Psychol 34:49–61

MacLeod C, Mathews A (2012) Cognitive bias modification approaches to anxiety. Annu Rev Clin Psychol 8:189–217

March JS, Parker J (1999) Chapter 2: the multidimensional anxiety scale for children (MASC). In: Maruish ME (ed) The use of psychological testing for treatment planning and outcome assessment, vol 2. Lawrence Erlbaum Associates, Mahwah, pp 39–62

March J, Parker J, Sullivan K, Stallings P, Conners C (1997) The Multidimensional Anxiety Scale for Children (MASC): factor structure, reliability and validity. J Am Acad Child Adolesc Psychiatry 36:554–565

Masia CL, Klein RG, Storch E, Corda B (2001) School-based behavioral treatment for social anxiety disorder in adolescents: results of a pilot study. J Am Acad Child Adolesc Psychiatry 40:780–786

Masia-Warner C, Klein RG, Dent HC, Fisher PH, Alvir J, Albano AM, Guardino M (2005) School-based Intervention for adolescents with social anxiety disorder: results of a controlled study. J Abnorm Child Psychol 33:707–722

Masia-Warner C, Fisher PH, Shrout PE, Rathor S, Klein RG (2007) Treating adolescents with social anxiety disorder in school: an attention control trial. J Child Psychol Psychiatry 48:676–686. doi:10.1111/j.1469-7610.2007.01737.x

Meleshko KG, Alden LE (1993) Anxiety and self-disclosure: toward a motivational model. J Pers Soc Psychol 64(6):1000

Melfsen S, Kuhnemund M, Schwieger J, Warnke A, Stadler C, Poustka F, Stangier U (2011) Cognitive behavioural therapy of socially phobia children focusing on cognition: a randomised wait-list control study. Child Adolesc Psychiatry Ment Health 5:5

Miers AC, Blote AW, Bögels SM, Westenberg PM (2008) Interpretation bias and social anxiety in adolescents. J Anxiety Disord 22:1462–1471

Miers AC, Blote AW, Westenberg PM (2011) Negative social cognitions in socially anxious youth: distorted reality or a kernel of truth? J Child Fam Stud 20:214–223. doi:10.1007/s10826-010-9423-2

Muris P, Field AP (2008) Distorted cognition and pathological anxiety in children and adolescents. Cogn Emotion 22:395–421. doi:10.1080/02699930701843450

Olivares J, Garcia-Lopez LJ, Hidalgo MD, Turner SM, Beidel DC (1999) The social phobia and anxiety inventory: reliability and validity in an adolescent Spanish population. J Psychopathol Behav Assess 21:67–78

Olivares J, Garcia-Lopez LJ, Beidel DC, Turner SM, Albano AM, Hidalgo MD (2002) Results at long-term among three psychological treatments for adolescents with generalized social phobia (I): statistical significance. Psicología Conductual [Behav Psychol] 10:147–164

Parr CJ, Cartwright-Hatton S (2009) Social anxiety in adolescents: the effect of video feedback on anxiety and the self-evaluation of performance. Clin Psychol Psychother 16:46–54

Pine DS, Cohen P, Gurley D, Brook J, Ma Y (1998) The risk of early-adulthood anxiety and depressive disorders in adolescents with anxiety and depressive disorders. Arch Gen Psychiatry 55:56–64

Piqueras JA, Espinosa-Fernandez L, Garcia-Lopez LJ, Beidel DC (2012) Validaci.n del Inventario de Ansiedad, & Fobia Social-Forma Breve en j.venes adultos espa.oles [Validation of the SPAI-B in young adults]. Behav Psychol 20:505–528

Ramos V, Piqueras JA, Garcia-Lopez LJ (2008) Análisis de la eficacia y eficiencia del empleo del videofeedback en el tratamiento de adolescentes con un trastorno de ansiedad social Efficacy and efficiency of the use of video-feedback in the cognitive-behavioral treatment of young people with social anxiety disorder. Clínica y Salud19:249–264

Ranta K, Tuomisto MT, Kaltiala-Heino R, Rantanen P, Mattunen M (2014) Cognition, imagery and coping among adolescents with social anxiety and phobia: testing the Clark and Wells model in the population. Clin Psychol Psychother 21:252–263. doi:10.1002/cpp.1833

Rapee RM, Hayman K (1996) The effects of video feedback on the self-evaluation of performance in socially anxious subjects. Behav Res Ther 34:315–322. doi:10.1016/0005-7967(96)00003-4

Rapee RM, Heimberg RG (1997) A cognitive-behavioral model of anxiety in social phobia. Behav Res Ther 35:741–756

Rapee RM, Spence SH (2004) The etiology of social phobia: empirical evidence and an initial model. Clin Psychol Rev 24:737–767

Rapee RM, Barrett PM, Dadds MR, Evans L (1994) Reliability of the DSM-III-R childhood anxiety disorders using structured interview: interrater and parent–child agreement. J Am Acad Child Adolesc Psychiatry 33:984–992

Rapee RM, Spence SH, Cobham VE, Wignall A (2000) Helping your anxious child: a step-by-step guide for parents. New Harbinger, Oakland

Rapee RM, Lyneham HJ, Schniering C, Wuthrich V, Abbott M, Hudson JL, Wignall A (2006) Centre for emotional health. Macquarie University, Sydney

Rapee RM, Gaston JE, Abbott MJ (2009) Testing the efficacy of theoretically derived improvements in the treatment of social phobia. J Consult Clin Psychol 77:317–327

Reynolds S, Wilson C, Austin J, Hooper L (2012) Effects of psychotherapy for anxiety in children and adolescents: a meta-analytic review. Clin Psychol Rev 32(4):251–262

Rodebaugh TL, Heimberg RG, Schultz LT, Blackmore M (2010) The moderated effects of video feedback for social anxiety disorder. J Anxiety Disord 24:663–671

Rozenman M, Weersing V, Amir N (2011) A case series of attention modification in clinically anxious youths. Behav Res Ther 49:324–330

Schmidt NB, Richey J, Buckner JD, Timpano KR (2009) Attention training for generalized social anxiety disorder. J Abnorm Psychol 118:5–14

Salvador MC, Pinto-Gouveia J (2009) Helping adolescents with social phobia: A new treatment protocol to empower them is social situations. Europ Psychiatry, 24 (Suppl 1):S335. doi: 10.1016/S0924-9338(09)70568-1
Schniering CA, Lyneham H (2006) The children's automatic thoughts scale in a clinical sample: reliability, validity and sensitivity to treatment changes. Behav Res Ther 45:1931–1940
Schniering CA, Lyneham HJ (2007) The children's automatic thoughts scale in a clinical sample: psychometric properties and clinical utility. Behav Res Ther 45(8):1931–1940
Schniering CA, Rapee RM (2002) Development and validation of a measure of children's automatic thoughts: the children's automatic thoughts scale. Behav Res Ther 40:1091–1109
Schniering CA, Rapee RM (2004) The structure of negative self-statements in children and adolescents: a confirmatory factor analytic approach. J Abnorm Child Psychol 32:95–109
Schniering CA, Hudson JL, Rapee RM (2000) Issues in the diagnosis and assessment of anxiety disorders in children and adolescents. Clin Psychol Rev 20:453–478
See J, MacLeod C, Bridle R (2009) The reduction of anxiety vulnerability through the modification of attentional bias: a real-world study using a home-based cognitive bias modification procedure. J Abnorm Psychol 118:65–75
Silverman WK, Albano AM (1996) The anxiety disorders interview schedule for children for DSM-IV: child and parent versions. Psychological Corporation, San Antonia
Silverman WK, Pina AA, Viswesvaran C (2008) Evidence-based psychosocial treatments for phobic and anxiety disorders in children and adolescents. J Clin Child Adolesc Psychol 37:105–130
Smits JA, Powers MB, Buxkamper R, Telch MJ (2006) The efficacy of videotape feedback for enhancing the effects of exposure-based treatment for social anxiety disorder: a controlled investigation. Behav Res Ther 44:1773–1785
Spence SH, Donovan C, Brechman-Toussaint M (1999) Social skills, social outcomes, and cognitive features of childhood social phobia. J Abnorm Psychol 108:211–221
Sportel BE, de Hullu E, de Jong P, Nauta MH (2013) Cognitive bias modification versus CBT in reducing adolescent social anxiety: a randomized controlled trial. PLoS One 8:e64355. doi:10.1371/journal.pone.0064355
Tillfors M, Andersson G, Ekselius L, Furmark T, Lewenhaupt S, Karlsson A, Carlbring P (2011) A randomized trial of internet-delivered treatment for social anxiety disorder in high school students. Cogn Behav Ther 40:147–157. doi:10.1080/16506073.2011.555486
Vassilopoulos SP, Banerjee R, Prantzalou C (2009) Experimental modification of interpretation bias in socially anxious children: changes in interpretation, anticipated interpersonal anxiety, and social anxiety symptoms. Behav Res Ther 47:1085–1089
Vieira S, Salvador MC, Matos AP, Garcia-Lopez LJ, Beidel D (2013) Inventario de Fobia, & Ansiedad Social- Versi.n Breve: Propiedades psicom.tricas en una muestra de adolescentes portugueses [SPAI-B: Psychometric properties in a sample of Portuguese adolescents]. Behav Psychol 21:25–38
Waters AM, Pittaway M, Mogg K, Bradley BP, Pine D (2013) Attention training to positive stimuli in childhood anxiety disorders. Dev Cogn Neurosci 4:77–84
Westenberg PM, Drewes MJ, Goedhart A, Siebelink BM, Treffers PD (2004) A developmental analysis of self-reported fears in late childhood through mid-adolescence: social-evaluative fears on the rise? J Child Psychol Psychiatry 45:481–495
Wittchen H-U, Fehm L (2003) Epidemiology and natural course of social fears and social phobia. Acta Psychiatr Scand 108(Suppl 417):4–18. doi:10.1034/j.1600-0447.108.s417.1.x
Wood J, Piacentini JC, Bergman RL, McCraken J, Barrios V (2002) Concurrent validity of the anxiety disorders section of the anxiety disorders interview schedule for DSM-IV: child and parent version. J Clin Child Adolesc Psychol 31:335–342
Zimmermann P, Wittchen HU, Hofler M, Pfister H, Kessler RC, Lieb R (2003) Primary anxiety disorders and the development of subsequent alcohol use disorders: a 4-year community study of adolescents and young adults. Psychol Med 33:1211–1222. doi:10.1017/S0033291703008158

Interpersonal Approaches to Intervention: Implications for Preventing and Treating Social Anxiety in Adolescents

11

Laura Mufson, Annette M. La Greca, Jami F. Young, and Jill Ehrenreich-May

Both social anxiety disorder (SAD) and depression are prevalent among adolescents and are often comorbid (Beesdo et al. 2007; Costello et al. 2011; Dalrymple and Zimmerman 2011; Lewinsohn et al. 1999; Rapee et al. 2009; Stein et al. 2001). Rates of SAD and depression increase across the adolescent years and are associated with significant impairment (Birmaher et al. 1996; Costello et al. 2003; Garcia-Lopez et al. 2008; Grant et al. 2005). When comorbid, the onset of SAD often precedes that of major depressive disorder, and adolescent onset SAD is associated with a more severe and chronic course of depressive illness than is adult-onset SAD (Dalrymple and Zimmerman 2011).

These findings suggest that an integrative approach to the treatment and/or prevention of SAD and depression in adolescents may be useful. At present, however, evidence-based interventions for adolescent SAD are scarce, and existing studies predominantly focus on improving youths' social skills and reducing social inhibition (Beidel et al. 2007; Garcia-Lopez et al. 2002, 2006, 2009, 2014; Masia-Warner et al. 2001, 2005; Silverman et al. 2008), but not on coping with feelings of depression (Masia-Warner 2009; Masia-Warner et al. 2007). Similarly, evidence-based interventions for treating and preventing adolescent depression do not explicitly

L. Mufson, PhD (✉)
Department of Psychiatry, College of Physicians and Surgeons, and New York State Psychiatric Institute, CUMC, Columbia University, New York, NY, USA
e-mail: mufsonl@nyspi.columbia.edu

A.M. La Greca, PhD
Department of Psychology, University of Miami, Coral Gables, FL, USA

J.F. Young, PhD
Graduate School of Applied and Professional Psychology, Rutgers University, Piscataway, New Brunswick, NJ, USA

J. Ehrenreich-May, PhD
Department of Psychology, University of Miami, Coral Gables, FL, USA

K. Ranta et al. (eds.), *Social Anxiety and Phobia in Adolescents: Development, Manifestation and Intervention Strategies*, DOI 10.1007/978-3-319-16703-9_11

address issues of adolescent social anxiety (Garber et al. 2009; Stice et al. 2008), although recent work suggests that interpersonal approaches to preventing and treating adolescent depression may have a positive impact on adolescents who have co-occurring social anxiety (Young et al. 2006b, 2012a, b).

In our view, interpersonal approaches to treating and preventing adolescent depression have much to offer for helping youth with clinical or subclinical levels of social anxiety, whether or not the social anxiety co-occurs with depression. Thus, the purpose of this chapter is to describe interpersonal approaches to treating and preventing adolescent depression and to consider how these approaches might be adapted or modified for treating or preventing adolescent SAD. Because interpersonal approaches have focused primarily on the treatment or prevention of depression, evidence of their efficacy and effectiveness for treating adolescent social anxiety is scant at this point, but emerging. We hope that the material in this chapter will encourage others to develop and evaluate interpersonal approaches for treating and preventing social anxiety in youth.

The chapter content is organized as follows. The initial sections review the importance of interpersonal relations for understanding adolescent depression and SAD. Next, we cover theory and empirical support for Interpersonal Psychotherapy for Adolescents (IPT-A), an evidence-based treatment for adolescent depression; we also describe work that supports the use of IPT for treating social anxiety in adults. In the last sections of the chapter, we describe how the IPT-A model has been adapted for preventing adolescent depression and how we are extending the prevention model to address issues of adolescent social anxiety.

Importance of Interpersonal Relations for Depression and Social Anxiety

Interpersonal Factors Related To Depression

The onset and maintenance of depression have been strongly linked to interpersonal factors in both adults and adolescents (Hammen 1999; Lewinsohn et al. 1994; Puig-Antich et al. 1993; Rudolph et al. 2000; Sheeber et al. 2001; Stader and Hokanson 1998). In adults, stressors such as marital distress, reduced social support, social isolation, or excessive need for emotional support from others have been identified as antecedents to depression (Barnett and Gotlib 1988; Hammen 1999). Once depressed, adults engage people differently, which can result in relationship difficulties or loss that further exacerbates the depression (Coyne 1976; Weissman and Paykel 1974).

Similarly, interpersonal problems with peers and family are associated with depression in adolescents. Interpersonal stressors are linked to depression (Blechman et al. 1986; Rudolph et al. 2000), especially for girls (Hankin et al. 2007). This relationship is reciprocal in that depression also has been found to precipitate interpersonal stress (Hammen 1991; Rudolph et al. 2000). For adolescents, problems with family members and peers place them at risk for depression (Hammen and Brennan

2001; Kobak et al. 1991; Sheeber et al. 2007). In general, consistent with Bowlby's attachment theory, a loss or paucity of relationships seems to be a significant risk factor for adolescent depression (Allen et al. 2006).

With respect to family issues, the relationship problems commonly associated with adolescent depression are characterized by conflictual and unsupportive relationships with parents or other primary caregivers. Given that adolescents are negotiating their individuation from their parents, it makes sense that conflicts and problems in this significant attachment are associated with depression (Sheeber et al. 2007). In addition, depressed adolescents display more negative affect during interactions with their parents than do healthy adolescents (Sanders et al. 1992; Sheeber et al. 2000). This expressed negative affect may hinder adolescents' ability to communicate or problem-solve effectively, which may result in a vicious cycle of interpersonal conflict leading to depressive symptoms and more negative affect, which in turn results in more interpersonal difficulties (Bosquet and Egeland 2006; Gotlib and Hammen 1992).

The negative effects of depressive symptoms are also evident in adolescents' peer relationships (Brunstein-Klomek et al. 2007). Peer relationship problems such as rejection, unpopularity, teasing/bullying, peer victimization, and poor communication patterns are all associated with depression in adolescents (Allen et al. 2006; Galambos et al. 2004; Brunstein-Klomek et al. 2007; La Greca et al. 2009; La Greca and Harrison 2005; Nolan et al. 2003; Ranta et al. 2009). Adolescent social withdrawal can be both an antecedent and consequence of depression. When adolescents withdraw socially, they often fall behind in their social development and the interpersonal skills needed for effective peer interactions, which makes it difficult for them to establish new relationships; in turn, this can lead to feelings of inadequacy and further social withdrawal (Allen et al. 2006).

Many of the interpersonal risk factors for depression, such as negative interpersonal concerns and stressful life events that are interpersonal and uncontrollable, are heightened for females and may contribute to the higher rates of depression for adolescent girls (Galambos et al. 2004). The experience or perception of peer rejection may contribute to low self-esteem, which increases an adolescent's vulnerability to depression; in particular, early adolescents are especially self-conscious and concerned about the opinion of others (Nolan et al. 2003). Given the interpersonal difficulties associated with adolescent depression, an interpersonal approach to intervention seems like a natural fit. As discussed below, Interpersonal Psychotherapy for Adolescents (IPT-A) targets adolescents' communication and problem-solving impairments in both family and peer relationships and appears to be an effective treatment for depressed adolescents. IPT-A provides adolescents with skills that will be helpful in both current and future interpersonal contexts.

Interpersonal Factors Related to Social Anxiety

Anxiety disorders also are characterized by significant interpersonal difficulties (Heerey and Kring 2007; La Greca and Landoll 2011), as discussed here and elsewhere in this volume. Adults with anxiety disorders, especially SAD, typically have fewer relationships, greater marital distress, less satisfaction in their relationships, and difficulties asserting their own needs (Alden and Taylor 2004). SAD in adults has been associated with significant impairment in social functioning, characterized by excessive dependence, lack of assertiveness, and avoidance of conflict (Alden and Taylor 2004; Grant et al. 2007; Plasencia et al. 2011).

Adolescents with social anxiety similarly are characterized as having fewer friendships, fewer supportive relationships, more negative peer interactions, poor social skills, lower levels of assertiveness, greater conflict avoidance, greater social distress, and more avoidance of emotional expression within relationships in comparison to non-anxious youth (Davila and Beck 2002; Ginsburg et al. 1998; La Greca and Landoll 2011; La Greca and Lopez 1998; Storch and Masia-Warner 2004; Vernberg et al. 1992). Socially anxious adolescents are also less likely to date and be engaged in romantic relationships than their non-anxious peers (Glickman and La Greca 2004; Hebert et al. 2013; La Greca and Mackey 2007, see also Chap. 8). For socially anxious youth, difficulties with self-assertion also may result in greater vulnerability to negative peer interactions and bullying and consequently lead to even more social anxiety (Davila and Beck 2002; Garcia-Lopez et al. 2011; Ranta et al. 2009, 2013; Storch and Masia-Warner 2004; Storch et al. 2005).

In fact, some studies have found similar vulnerability factors for both social anxiety and depression. For example, problematic family relationships, especially when the child feels rejected or negatively judged, can generalize to peer relationships; such youth may expect peers to react similarly and consequently may avoid social situations in anticipation of encountering negative experiences. However, an avoidant coping strategy can maintain and exacerbate anxiety symptoms (Festa and Ginsburg 2011). As another example, community studies find that peer-rejected youth have substantial interpersonal and emotional difficulties (Coie et al. 1990) and report greater social anxiety than their peers (Kingery et al. 2010; La Greca and Lopez 1998), as well as more depressive symptoms (Prinstein and Aikins 2004). Similarly, peer victimization experiences have an impact on adolescents' anxious and depressive symptoms (see La Greca and Lai 2013 for a review). In particular, relational forms of peer victimization (i.e., being left out or socially excluded by peers) are strongly associated with both social anxiety and depression (e.g., La Greca and Harrison 2005; Siegel et al. 2009; Storch and Masia-Warner 2004; Vernberg 1990). The association between low peer acceptance, poor social skills, and social anxiety has been found in both normative and clinical samples of youth (Kingery et al. 2010; La Greca and Landoll 2011; Puklek and Berce 2012). Similar to findings for depressed adolescents, socially anxious youth demonstrate poorer social skills and tend to interpret social cues in a personally threatening manner, which may result in social avoidance and increased social anxiety (Kingery et al. 2010).

In summary, there is substantial evidence that interpersonal problems, especially those involving peer relationships, play an important role in social anxiety disorder (e.g., Festa and Ginsburg 2011; Gazelle and Ladd 2003; Kingery et al. 2010; La Greca and Landoll 2011; La Greca and Lai 2013, see also Chaps. 5 and 8). This body of evidence supports the use of interpersonal approaches to treatment. IPT-A, with its focus on interpersonal problem areas and improving communication and affect management within relationships, may be well suited to address the interpersonal deficits that contribute to and maintain social anxiety.

Theory and Empirical Support for Interpersonal Psychotherapy with Adolescents (IPT-A)

In this section, we describe the theory and background for the development of IPT-A. We also review evidence supporting its efficacy and effectiveness.

Theory and Background

IPT-A is adapted from Interpersonal Psychotherapy (IPT), which is an empirically validated, brief, time-limited, psychosocial treatment that originally was developed for depressed, nonpsychotic, unipolar adult outpatients (Weissman et al. 2000a, b). IPT focuses on relationship difficulties and bases the treatment on the premise that a person's mood and relationships are intertwined and that when there are difficulties in significant relationships, symptoms of depression can arise or be exacerbated. IPT adheres to the idea that, regardless of the underlying cause of the depression, the disorder occurs within an interpersonal context. There is a large body of research demonstrating the efficacy of IPT for depressed adults (Cuijpers et al. 2011; van Hees et al. 2013; (Weissman et al. 2000a, b). In fact, a recent meta-analysis (Cuijpers et al. 2011) concluded that IPT efficaciously treats depression and "deserves its place in treatment guidelines as one of the most empirically validated treatments for depression" (p. 581).

The premise of IPT is based on Sullivan's interpersonal theory of psychiatry (1953), which espoused the belief that a significant component of psychiatric illness develops out of and is perpetuated by problems in interpersonal interactions. Meyer (1957) expanded on that theory to include his belief that psychopathology arises from the manner in which a person attempts to adapt to his or her environment, including relationships and other stressors. Therefore, IPT examines the role of contextual factors and stressful life events surrounding the individual's interpersonal interactions and how they relate to the onset and maintenance of depression. In addition, IPT has its roots in Bowlby's attachment theory (1969) which stated that people have an innate need to develop strong bonds with significant others. When these bonds are disrupted in some way, the individual experiences emotional distress that often manifests itself in symptoms of depression. Depression is a result, in part, of a loss of social support, and IPT aims to improve and expand the individual's social support network as one of its treatment goals.

The specific goal of IPT is to decrease depressive symptoms by focusing on current interpersonal difficulties and helping the individual improve his or her relationships and interpersonal interactions. Four specific problem areas may be targeted depending on the individual's interpersonal circumstances: grief, role transitions, role disputes, and interpersonal deficits. *Grief* is defined as an abnormal reaction to the loss of a significant other (e.g., delayed or chronic reaction) due to an actual death. *Role transition* refers to difficulties adjusting to changes in life status (e.g., divorce, changing schools or jobs). *Role disputes* refer to significant conflicts with another person due to differing expectations. Finally, *interpersonal deficits* are identified when the individual is socially isolated, lonely, and lacking in social skills necessary to cultivate new relationships and a support system (Weissman 2006). These four problem areas are a focus of both the adult and adolescent adaptation of IPT, described below.

Adaptation of IPT for Depressed Adolescents

Mufson and colleagues (2004a) adapted IPT for use with adolescents with mild to moderate depression. IPT-A maintains the same four problem areas as IPT, but takes into consideration developmental issues unique to this age group. Adolescence is a time of increased autonomy and significant change in all facets of life, particularly relationships with family and peers (Erikson 1968). Adolescents must learn to negotiate changes in their relationships with friends, family members, romantic partners, and teachers, among others. The family is often a focus of treatment because it is a time when adolescents struggle to negotiate their individuation while also desiring to maintain some element of closeness with their parents (Steinberg 1990). IPT-A skills and strategies can facilitate successful achievement of these adolescent developmental tasks.

For IPT-A, several specific adaptations were made to IPT (Mufson et al. 2004a), including involvement of parents, contact with the school when necessary, the use of a 1–10 mood scale to help adolescents monitor their mood, and the use of a closeness circle to help adolescents identify significant relationships and the nature of their attachment and interactions. IPT-A is an active treatment with a large psychoeducational component and a skill-building component aimed at facilitating adolescents' communication and problem-solving skills. Since being in therapy is not a normative role for adolescents, IPT-A is an especially good fit given its short duration (once a week for 12–16 weeks) and its focus on what is presently happening in the adolescents' current significant relationships.

Empirical Support for IPT-A

IPT-A for depressed adolescents has been studied in four clinical trials (Mufson et al. 1999, 2004b; Rosselló and Bernal 1999; Rosselló et al. 2008). The initial efficacy study (Mufson et al. 1999) was conducted with 48 adolescents (12–18 years of age) with clinical depression who were randomly assigned to either IPT-A or clinical monitoring. Results indicated an average effect size of 0.54; 75 % of those receiving IPT-A compared to 46 % in the control group were recovered, with a score of ≤ 6 on the Hamilton Rating Scale for Depression at week 12.

Rosselló and Bernal (1999) and Rosselló et al. (2008) have examined a different adaptation of IPT designed specifically for depressed adolescents in Puerto Rico. Rosselló and Bernal (1999) compared IPT, cognitive-behavioral therapy (CBT), and a wait-list control condition for 71 depressed adolescents in Puerto Rico. Findings revealed that both IPT and CBT reduced depressive symptoms compared with the control condition and that IPT also improved adolescents' self-esteem and social adaptation. Overall, 82 % of adolescents in IPT and 59 % of those in CBT were functional after treatment. In both of the above studies, adolescents receiving IPT experienced reductions in depression symptoms, increases in self-esteem, and improvements in social functioning.

In addition to these efficacy studies, Mufson and colleagues (2004b) conducted an effectiveness study of IPT-A in school-based health clinics with 63 adolescents (mean age = 15.1 years) who were predominantly female (84 %), Hispanic (71 %), of low socioeconomic status, and clinically depressed. Youth were randomly assigned to IPT-A versus usual care. Results indicated an average effect size of 0.50 for IPT-A compared to usual care, which was individual supportive psychotherapy. Thus, across studies, the IPT-A results showed a moderate to large effect size for decreasing depression symptoms and improving global and social functioning in comparison to control groups that include clinical monitoring, treatment as usual (TAU), and wait-list (Mufson et al. 1999, 2004b; Rosselló and Bernal 1999).

In further analyses of the Mufson et al. (2004b) IPT-A effectiveness study described above, Young et al. (2006b) examined outcomes of adolescents with comorbid depression and anxiety who received IPT-A or treatment as usual. Three anxiety disorders (SAD, generalized anxiety disorder, and panic disorder) were grouped together because of their high level of comorbidity; supplemental analyses also looked at each of these disorders separately. Regarding depression outcomes, Young et al. (2006b) found that among adolescents with comorbid depression and anxiety, those who received IPT-A had significantly lower posttreatment depression scores (on the HRSD) than those who received TAU, suggesting that IPT-A may be particularly effective for youth with comorbid depression and anxiety. However, in the supplemental analyses looking specifically at youth with comorbid depression and SAD, this finding did not hold up. Rather, there was only evidence of a main effect. Specifically, adolescents with SAD had higher depression scores post-intervention than adolescents without SAD regardless of intervention condition.

Regarding anxiety outcomes, for adolescents with an anxiety disorder at baseline, approximately half no longer had an anxiety diagnosis at the end of treatment regardless of treatment condition, despite the fact that treatment specifically targeted depression. This held across the various anxiety disorders. Among the 20 youth with comorbid SAD, 11 of the 20 no longer met criteria for SAD at post-intervention. Further, those youth who showed improvements in their social anxiety demonstrated significantly greater improvements in depression and overall functioning than youth whose social anxiety did not improve. Taken together these findings suggest that anxiety and depression symptoms improve together. This supports the use of IPT and other interventions to address comorbid depression and SAD but suggests that some modifications may need to be made to these interventions to maximize the effects of these programs on depression and anxiety symptoms in comorbid youth.

In summary, the IPT-A-manualized treatment used in the Mufson studies (1999, 2004b) meets criteria for a "probably efficacious intervention" as defined by the American Psychological Association Task Force on the Promotion and Dissemination of Psychological Procedures guidelines (David-Ferdon and Kaslow 2008) because all the IPT-A studies were conducted by one research group, that of the treatment developer. The two studies in Puerto Rico were considered to have used a different manual. However, as a theoretical orientation, IPT-A meets the criteria of a "well-established treatment" for adolescent depression according to the same task force report (David-Ferdon and Kaslow 2008). Most importantly, IPT-A is one of a few evidence-based psychotherapies that has been transported and implemented in community settings with demonstrated effectiveness when delivered by community therapists. IPT-A is now included in SAMHSA's National Registry of Evidence-Based Programs and Practices (http://www.nrepp.samhsa.gov/ViewIntervention.aspx?id=198) and is considered to be an effective, evidence-based treatment for adolescent depression by the Society of Clinical Child and Adolescent Psychology (http://effectivechildtherapy.com/content/depression).

Based on the findings described above, further study of the impact of IPT-A on adolescent social anxiety would be important and desirable. At this point, it appears that depressed adolescents with comorbid social anxiety show improvements in their levels of depression following IPT-A treatment (Young et al. 2006b), but the impact of treatment on social anxiety as an outcome is not as clear. In addition, the question of whether IPT-A is effective with socially anxious adolescents without comorbid depression remains to be evaluated.

Use of IPT Model for Social Anxiety in Adults

Although IPT-A has not been evaluated directly with socially anxious adolescents, the adult-oriented IPT for depression has been adapted to treat adult social phobia (Borge et al. 2008; Lipsitz et al. 1999, 2008; Stangier et al. 2011). Like the model for depression, the SAD adaptation espouses the premise that the anxiety disorder develops within an interpersonal context and is impacted by a person's level of interpersonal functioning and interpersonal stressors and that the resulting interpersonal problems further perpetuate social anxiety (see (Weissman et al. 2000a, b).

Lipsitz and colleagues (1999) specifically adapted IPT for the treatment of social phobia (IPT-SP), with the same goal as in IPT: to decrease symptoms of social anxiety by improving social functioning. Social dysfunction can be situation specific, or it can manifest itself in a global social withdrawal, lack of assertiveness, or avoidance of conflict and expression of feelings (Lipsitz and Markowitz 2006). The modifications of IPT for SAD included a refocus of psychoeducation on symptoms of social anxiety as treatable and the interplay of social anxiety and relationship problems. IPT-SP also redefined the problem area of interpersonal deficits as a problem area called "role insecurity," because the problem area of interpersonal deficits, which overlaps with the core symptoms of SAD, may cause individuals with SAD to feel demoralized rather than hopeful that treatment can lead to improvements (Lipsitz 2012). Thus, for individuals with SAD, the problem area of role insecurity emphasizes that their social skills are impeded by anxiety and will likely emerge as their interpersonal approach is refined in treatment and their anxiety dissipates (Lipsitz and Markowitz 2006).

Lipsitz and colleagues (1999, 2008) conducted both an open trial and a randomized controlled trial (RCT) of IPT-SP. In the pilot open trial of 9 adults with SAD, 78 % were much or very much improved on the Liebowitz Social Anxiety Scale (Heimberg et al. 1999) by the end of the 14-week treatment. A larger RCT with 70 adults with SAD compared 14 weeks of IPT to psychodynamic supportive therapy (Lipsitz et al. 2008); the investigators found that both treatments led to decreases in social anxiety symptoms and impairment. IPT was superior to supportive psychotherapy only for addressing concerns about negative evaluation (Lipsitz et al. 2008). However, it should be noted that the comparison treatment of psychodynamic psychotherapy has been efficacious for SAD, which may explain the finding of improvements in both conditions (Markowitz et al. 2014). Also, a possible study limitation is that the same therapists administered both the supportive and the IPT treatments; as such, there may have been contamination between the treatment conditions.

More recent studies of IPT for SAD conducted by other investigators have not found superiority for IPT in comparison to cognitive therapy (CT). In fact, some studies found that CT resulted in significantly greater improvements in outcomes than did IPT (Borge et al. 2010; Stangier et al. 2011). Although IPT was not found to be superior to its comparison treatments, treatment with IPT did consistently result in a reduction of social anxiety symptoms, suggesting that the interpersonal focus may have some benefit in the treatment of social anxiety (Markowitz et al. 2014) but may require more adaptation.

In summary, the efficacy of IPT for social anxiety has only been studied in adults and remains undetermined given the current mixed findings. Although existing findings are promising, further research is needed to better evaluate the efficacy of IPT for adults with SAD and to determine whether it can be used for adolescents with SAD (who are not also depressed).

A Prevention Framework for the IPT Model

Use of IPT as a Preventive Intervention for Adolescent Depression

Despite efficacious treatments, the treatment response rate for adolescent depression ranges from 50 to 70 % (e.g., Clarke et al. 1999; Brent et al. 1997; Curry et al. 2011; Goodyer et al. 2007; Mufson et al. 1999, 2004b), which leaves room for improvement. Add to that the problem of access to efficacious treatments for many adolescents (Meredith et al. 2009) and it seems important to turn attention to the possibility of preventing depressive episodes and disorder whenever possible.

One challenge for depression prevention is identifying vulnerable adolescents. In this regard, it appears that one of the biggest risk factors for developing a depressive disorder is elevated levels of depressive symptoms (e.g., Fergusson et al. 2005). Elevated depressive symptoms can be chronic and are associated with considerable psychosocial impairment (Lewinsohn et al. 2000). Thus, targeting adolescents with elevated, but subclinical, levels of depressive symptoms for preventive interventions may be a useful and viable strategy. Another challenge for prevention studies is providing interventions in an easily accessible setting with minimal stigma. An IPT-based prevention program for adolescent depression, called Interpersonal Psychotherapy-Adolescent Skills Training, was designed to be delivered in school settings, where adolescents are most likely to receive services (e.g., Hoagwood and Olin 2002; Hogan 2003).

Interpersonal Psychotherapy-Adolescent Skills Training (IPT-AST) (Young and Mufson 2006) is a group-oriented preventive intervention for adolescents identified with subthreshold symptoms of depression. IPT-AST has 2 individual sessions and 8 weekly 90-min group sessions. The group focuses on teaching adolescents interpersonal and communication skills that can be applied to their current relationships, with the idea that these skills will enable adolescents to weather future stressful interpersonal events without developing a depressive disorder.

Empirical Evidence for IPT-AST

There have been two randomized controlled trials of IPT-AST for youth with elevated symptoms of depression (see Young et al. 2006a, 2010 for further details on depression and functioning outcomes). In the first study, 41 adolescents, aged 11–16 years, with elevated depressive symptoms were randomized to IPT-AST or usual school counseling (SC). Adolescents in IPT-AST had significantly fewer depressive symptoms and greater overall functioning than adolescents in SC at post-intervention and through a 6-month follow-up. They also reported significantly fewer depression diagnoses than youth in SC over the follow-up period (Young et al. 2006a). The second study included 57 adolescents, aged 13–17 years, with elevated symptoms. Youth in IPT-AST reported significantly greater reductions in depressive symptoms and greater improvements in overall functioning than youth in SC (Young et al. 2010) and significantly greater improvements in total social functioning and functioning with friends (Young, Kranzler et al. 2012).

In addition to evaluating the impact of IPT-AST on adolescent depressive symptoms and functioning, Young and colleagues (2012a, b) also examined anxiety outcomes in the two randomized controlled trials of IPT-AST versus school counseling, which involved 98 adolescents. Although the youth were selected on the basis of elevated depressive symptoms, 40 % of the youth in the two studies had elevated anxiety symptoms as defined by a score of 25 or higher on the Screen for Child Anxiety Related Emotional Disorders (SCARED; Birmaher et al. 1999). There was a significant association between adolescents' anxiety scores at baseline and change in depressive symptoms (i.e., as assessed by the Center for Epidemiologic Studies Depression Scale) over the course of intervention, with youth who were low in anxiety showing more rapid and greater reductions in depression symptoms than youth high in anxiety; however, the youth with high anxiety caught up over time. When looking at three specific subscales on the SCARED (panic/somatic symptoms, generalized anxiety, and social anxiety), panic/somatic symptoms and generalized anxiety symptoms predicted change in depressive symptoms over time, but baseline social anxiety symptoms did not. Thus, within a prevention context, unlike the treatment literature, comorbid depression and anxiety symptoms did not mean worse depression outcomes over time, but rather delayed intervention effects. Perhaps anxious adolescents are initially hesitant to use the skills learned from the prevention programs, but gradually implement the skills in their day-to-day lives, resulting in a reduction in depressive symptoms over time.

Regarding anxiety outcomes, adolescents who received IPT-AST reported significantly greater reductions in total anxiety symptoms, generalized anxiety symptoms, and panic/somatic symptoms during the course of the intervention than adolescents who received standard care (SC; Young et al. 2012a, b). There were no significant differences between IPT-AST and individual SC in rates of change in social anxiety symptoms; adolescents in both conditions showed a small, but significant, reduction in social anxiety during the course of the intervention with continued reductions through the 12-month follow-up period. These findings suggest that both IPT-AST and individual counseling are effective at reducing social anxiety symptoms in youth with elevated depressive symptoms.

Although IPT-AST focuses on improving interpersonal relationships, which is an area of concern for socially anxious adolescents (La Greca and Landoll 2011), IPT-AST requires adolescents to work on their relationships outside of the session. Enhancing the effectiveness of IPT-AST for socially anxious youth may involve helping adolescents confront their feelings of social anxiety and reduce their social avoidance, so they can engage in interpersonal work both inside and outside of group that will lead to improvements in their social functioning and reduce symptoms of social anxiety. Further modifications of IPT-AST for socially anxious youth may be desirable, and we discuss current efforts in this regard in the next chapter section.

Nevertheless, the post-intervention effect sizes for total anxiety symptoms, generalized anxiety symptoms, and panic/somatic symptoms were medium to large and larger than those found for anxiety outcomes in past depression treatment studies (Chu and Harrison 2007; Weisz et al. 2006). Furthermore, the effects of IPT-AST on depressive symptoms are strong even in the face of comorbid depression and anxiety. Given the frequent comorbidity of depressive and anxiety symptoms, it is encouraging that IPT-AST effectively reduces both types of symptoms immediately following the intervention. Thus, findings from these initial studies support IPT-AST's efficacy as a prevention program for both depressive and anxiety symptoms, although further modification of IPT-AST to address symptoms of social anxiety would be important and desirable.

Extending the IPT-AST Prevention Model to Address Issues of Social Anxiety

As noted in this chapter, adolescents with significant symptoms of social anxiety are characterized by having problematic interpersonal relationships, especially with peers (La Greca and Landoll 2011; La Greca and Lai 2013). Yet, only about a third of youth with anxiety disorders seek or receive treatment (Kataoka et al. 2002; Leaf et al. 1996; Merikangas et al. 2010). Thus, there is a need for preventive interventions for adolescent social anxiety and particularly for interventions that focus on adolescent peer relations.

At present, no evidence-based interventions have been developed specifically for preventing SAD in adolescents. It is notable that depression and social anxiety have a similar etiology, overlapping symptoms, and high comorbidity and consequently may benefit from the same treatment approach (Garber and Weersing 2010). Yet, with only a few exceptions, such as the *Unified Protocols for the Treatment of Emotional Disorders in Children and Adolescents* (Bilek and Ehrenreich-May 2012; Ehrenreich et al. 2008, 2009), interventions have been developed specifically for one diagnosis. Because similar interpersonal deficits and problems have been identified in both depressed and socially anxious youth (La Greca and Lai 2013), IPT-AST may be well suited to address these shared interpersonal risk factors and to prevent both social anxiety and depression in adolescents. Specifically, IPT-AST emphasizes interpersonal skill-building, enhancing social support, and dealing with interpersonal conflict; interpersonal problems are a common area of vulnerability for both socially anxious and depressed adolescents (see La Greca and Landoll 2011; La Greca et al. 2011).

At the same time, evidence also suggests that further enhancement or modification of IPT-AST may be useful to effectively target socially anxious youth. Thus, we briefly describe ongoing work that is aimed at adapting the IPT-AST preventive intervention to make it suitable for use with adolescents with elevated symptoms of social anxiety and/or depression and who also are experiencing some difficulties in their peer relationships. Specifically, we are developing and evaluating the PEERS/UTalk version of IPT-AST in order to address symptoms of SAD and depression in a unified manner and to emphasize adolescent peer relations and strategies for managing potential peer victimization experiences.

PEERS/UTalk Intervention. PEERS/UTalk targets adolescents in the 9th–11th grades, 13–18 years of age, who report subclinical symptoms of social anxiety and/or depression and who are also experiencing difficulties in their peer relations as reflected in elevated levels of interpersonal peer victimization (e.g., being left out or excluded by peers, being embarrassed by peers) (La Greca and Harrison 2005).

For the PEERS/UTalk intervention, we made several modifications to IPT-AST. To address strategies for social anxiety, we included psychoeducation about social anxiety and avoidance, and we stressed the importance of practicing skills in the group through role-plays, as an opportunity to overcome avoidance related to social anxiety; such treatment elements have been widely used for anxiety disorders in youth (Beidel et al. 2007; Ehrenreich et al. 2006; Silverman et al. 2008). We also added interpersonal work that addresses issues of "role insecurity" (similar to Lipsitz et al. 2008) that may be particularly relevant to youth with social anxiety. This work included helping adolescents feel more secure in their social roles, in approaching others, and in communicating their feelings more effectively and assertively. Further, we incorporated weekly monitoring of social anxiety symptoms (in addition to depressive symptoms) as well as adolescents' in-session ratings of social anxiety during role-plays, so that we could gauge adolescents' levels of social anxiety and see how they change during the course of the intervention. Finally, we expanded the IPT-AST intervention to incorporate many examples of and strategies for dealing with interpersonal peer victimization. This additional material extended the number of group sessions from 8 to 10, so that the current version of the PEERS/UTalk intervention is administered across 2 individual and 10 group sessions, over the span of 12-weeks (or one school semester).

To date, we have completed a Phase 1 Open Trial of the PEERS/UTalk intervention with 16 adolescents (ages 14–18 years; 69 % girls; 86 % Hispanic) (La Greca et al. 2014). All adolescents met initial eligibility criteria of elevated social anxiety (score $\geq$50 on the Social Anxiety Scale for Adolescents) and/or elevated depression (score $\geq$16 on the Center for Epidemiologic Studies Depression Scale) and elevated reports of peer victimization experiences; none met criteria for a clinical disorder based on a structured interview. Results revealed that the intervention was feasible and acceptable to adolescents (e.g., 86 % completion rate; adolescent satisfaction (100 %) and perceived quality (100 %) were high). Positive preliminary benefit was observed; in intent-to-treat analyses, adolescents showed significant pre- to post-intervention improvements for the Clinician Severity Ratings for SAD or depression ($p<.001$), Clinical Global Impression Scale-Severity ($p<.0001$), relational and reputational peer victimization (*p's*<*.05*), and adolescent report of social anxiety ($p<.01$) and depressive symptoms ($p<.05$). To our knowledge, this is the first school-based preventive intervention to take a unified approach to intervening with adolescents with subsyndromal SAD and/or depression. Further evaluation of PEERS/UTalk appears warranted, and a larger randomized controlled trial is currently in progress.

Summary/Conclusions

Research on risk factors, etiology, symptomatology, and comorbidity supports our work to develop an integrative approach to the treatment and/or prevention of SAD and depression in adolescents. There is significant evidence that youth with social anxiety and depression suffer from many of the same interpersonal difficulties and that these difficulties play an important role in the exacerbation and/or maintenance of the symptoms and disorders. The interpersonal approach to treating and preventing depression (IPT-A and IPT-AST) in youth has proven to be effective. Based on the shared pathways between depression and social anxiety, it also shows preliminary benefits for the treatment of the comorbid anxiety, although it appears to be less effective with social anxiety. Thus, it is important to assess whether the interpersonal approach could be extended to purposefully target the prevention of social anxiety along with depression.

Based on the studies of IPT-A and IPT-AST, modifications have been made to directly address social anxiety symptoms, especially those involving peer relationships, and to provide more psychoeducation about the interplay between social anxiety and avoidance of social interactions. The IPT-AST modification, called PEERS/UTalk, that is currently being studied is specifically targeted at adolescents who have also encountered peer victimization experiences that may place them at risk for both social anxiety and depression. Preliminary data suggests a potential benefit of this unified approach; more research is under way to further study the effectiveness of the PEERS/UTalk preventive intervention.

Acknowledgments We would like to thank Katherine Durham and Lauren Haliczer for their invaluable help conducting literature searches and preparing the chapter for publication.

References

Alden LE, Taylor CT (2004) Interpersonal processes in social phobia. Clin Psychol Rev 24:857–882. doi:10.1016/j.cpr.2004.07.006

Allen JP, Insabella G, Porter MR, Smith FD, Land D, Phillips N (2006) A social-interactional model of the development of depressive symptoms in adolescence. J Consult Clin Psychol 74:55–65. doi:10.1037/0022-006X.74.1.55

Barnett PA, Gotlib IH (1988) Psychosocial functioning and depression: distinguishing among antecedents, concomitants, and consequences. Psychol Bull 104(1):97–126. doi:10.1037/0033-2909.104.1.97

Beesdo K, Bittner A, Pine DS, Stein MB, Höfler M, Lieb R, Wittchen HU (2007) Incidence of social anxiety disorder and the consistent risk for secondary depression in the first three decades of life. Arch Gen Psychiatry 64(8):903–912. doi:10.1001/archpsyc.64.8.903

Beidel DC, Turner SM, Sallee FR, Ammerman RT, Crosby LA, Pathak S (2007) SET-C versus fluoxetine in the treatment of childhood social phobia. J Am Acad Child Adolesc Psychiatry 46(12):1622–1632. doi:10.1097/chi.0b013e318154bb57

Bilek EL, Ehrenreich-May J (2012) An open trial investigation of a transdiagnostic group treatment for children with anxiety and depressive symptoms. Behav Ther 43(4):887–897. doi:10.1016/j.beth.2012.04.007

Birmaher B, Ryan ND, Williamson DE, Brent DA, Kaufman J (1996) Childhood and adolescent depression: a review of the past 10 years. Part II. J Am Acad Child Adolesc Psychiatry 35(12):1575–1583. doi:10.1097/00004583-199612000-00008

Birmaher B, Brent DA, Chiappetta L, Bridge J, Monga S, Baugher M (1999) Psychometric properties of the Screen for Child Anxiety Related Emotional Disorders (SCARED): a replication study. J Am Acad Child Adolesc Psychiatry 38(10):1230–1236. doi:10.1097/00004583-199910000-00011

Blechman EA, McEnroe MJ, Carella ET, Audette DP (1986) Childhood competence and depression. J Abnorm Psychol 95(3):223–227. doi:10.1037/0021-843X.95.3.223

Borge F-M, Hoffart A, Sexton H, Clark DM, Markowitz JC, McManus F (2008) Residential cognitive therapy versus residential interpersonal therapy for social phobia: a randomized clinical trial. J Anxiety Disord 22:991–1010. doi:10.1016/j.janxdis.2007.10.002

Borge F-M, Hoffart A, Sexton H (2010) Predictors of outcome in residential cognitive and interpersonal treatment for social phobia: do cognitive and social dysfunction moderate treatment outcome? J Behav Ther Exp Psychiatry 41:212–219. doi:10.1016/j.jbtep.2010.01.005

Bosquet M, Egeland B (2006) The development and maintenance of anxiety symptoms from infancy through adolescence in a longitudinal sample. Dev Psychopathol 18:517–550. doi:10.1017/S0954579406060275

Bowlby J (1969) Attachment and loss, vol 1, Attachment. Basic Books, New York

Brent DA, Holder D, Kolko D, Birmaher B, Baugher M, Roth C, Iyengar S, Johnson BA (1997) A clinical psychotherapy trial for adolescent depression comparing cognitive, family, and supportive therapy. Arch Gen Psychiatry 54(9):877–885. doi:10.1001/archpsyc.1997.01830210125011

Brunstein-Klomek A, Marrocco F, Kleinman M, Schonfeld IS, Gould MS (2007) Bullying, depression, and suicidality in adolescents. J Am Acad Child Adolesc Psychiatry 46(1):40–49. doi:10.1097/01.chi.0000242237.84925.18

Chu BC, Harrison TL (2007) Disorder-specific effects of CBT for anxious and depressed youth: a meta-analysis of candidate mediators of change. Clin Child Fam Psychol Rev 10(4):352–372. doi:10.1007/s10567-007-0028-2

Clarke GN, Rohde P, Lewinsohn PM, Hops H, Seeley JR (1999) Cognitive-behavioral treatment of adolescent depression: efficacy of acute group treatment and booster sessions. J Am Acad Child Adolesc Psychiatry 38(3):272–279. doi:10.1097/00004583-199903000-00014

Coie JD, Dodge KA, Kupersmidt JB (1990) Peer group behavior and social status. In: Asher SR, Coie JD (eds) Peer rejection in childhood. Cambridge University Press, Cambridge, UK, pp 17–59

Costello EJ, Mustillo S, Erkanli A, Keeler G, Angold A (2003) Prevalence and development of psychiatric disorders in childhood and adolescence. Arch Gen Psychiatry 60(8):837–844. doi:10.1001/archpsyc.60.8.837

Costello EJ, Egger H, Copeland W, Erkanli A, Angold A (2011) The developmental epidemiology of anxiety disorders: phenomenology, prevalence, and comorbidity. In: Silverman WK, Field A (eds) Anxiety disorders in children and adolescents, 2nd edn. Cambridge University Press, New York, pp 56–75

Coyne JC (1976) Depression and the response of others. J Abnorm Psychol 85(2):186–193. doi:10.1037/0021-843X.85.2.186

Cuijpers P, Geraedts AS, van Oppen P, Andersson G, Markowitz JC, van Straten A (2011) Interpersonal psychotherapy for depression: a meta-analysis. Am J Psychiatry 168(6):581–592. doi:10.1176/appi.ajp.2010.10101411

Curry J, Silva S, Rohde P, Ginsburg G, Kratochvil C, Simons A, Kirchner J, May D, Kennard B, Mayes T, Feeny N, Albano AM, Lavanier S, Reinecke M, Jacobs R, Becker-Weidman E, Weller E, Emslie G, Walkup J, Kastelic E, Burns B, Wells K, March J (2011) Recovery and recurrence following treatment for adolescent major depression. Arch Gen Psychiatry 68(3):263–269. doi:10.1001/archgenpsychiatry.2010.150

Dalrymple KL, Zimmerman M (2011) Age of onset of social anxiety disorder in depressed outpatients. J Anxiety Disord 25(1):131–137. doi:10.1016/j.janxdis.2010.08.012

David-Ferdon C, Kaslow NJ (2008) Evidence-based psychosocial treatments for child and adolescent depression. J Clin Child Adolesc Psychology 37(1):62–104. doi:10.1080/15374410701817865

Davila J, Beck JG (2002) Is social anxiety associated with impairment in close relationships? A preliminary investigation. Behav Ther 33(3):427–446. doi:10.1016/S0005-7894(02)80037-5

Ehrenreich JT, Buzzella BA, Barlow DH (2006) General principles for the treatment of emotional disorders across the lifespan. In: Hofmann SG, Weinberger J (eds) The art and science of psychotherapy. Routledge/Taylor & Francis Group, New York, pp 191–209

Ehrenreich JT, Buzzella BA, Trosper SE, Bennett SM, Wright LA, Barlow DH (2008) Unified protocol for the treatment of emotional disorders in adolescents. Unpublished treatment manual, University of Miami and Boston University

Ehrenreich JT, Goldstein CR, Wright LR, Barlow DH (2009) Development of a unified protocol for the treatment of emotional disorders in youth. Child Fam Behav Ther 31(1):20–37. doi:10.1080/07317100802701228

Erikson E (1968) Identity, youth, and crisis. Norton, New York

Fergusson DM, Horwood LJ, Ridder EM, Beautrais AL (2005) Subthreshold depression in adolescence and mental health outcomes in adulthood. Arch Gen Psychiatry 62(1):66–72. doi:10.1001/archpsyc.62.1.66

Festa CC, Ginsburg GS (2011) Parental and peer predictors of social anxiety in youth. Child Psychiatry Hum Dev 42:291–306. doi:10.1007/s10578-011-0215-8

Galambos NL, Leadbeater BJ, Barker ET (2004) Gender differences in and risk factors for depression in adolescence: a 4-year longitudinal study. Int J Behav Dev 28:16–25. doi:10.1080/01650250344000235

Garber J, Weersing VR (2010) Comorbidity of anxiety and depression in youth: implications for treatment and prevention. Clin Psychol Sci Pract 17(4):293–306. doi:10.1111/j.1468-2850.2010.01221.x

Garber J, Clarke GN, Weersing VR, Beardslee WR, Brent DA, Gladstone TR, DeBar LL, Lynch FL, D'Angelo E, Hollon SD, Shamseddeen W, Iyengar S (2009) Prevention of depression in at-risk adolescents: a randomized controlled trial. J Am Med Assoc 301(21):2215–2224. doi:10.1001/jama.2009.788

Garcia-Lopez LJ, Olivares J, Turner SM, Beidel DC, Albano AM, Sánchez-Meca J (2002) Results at long-term among three psychological treatments for adolescents with generalized social phobia (II): clinical significance and effect size. Psicologia Conductual [Behav Psychol] 10:165–179

Garcia-Lopez LJ, Olivares J, Beidel D, Albano A, Turner S, Rosa AI (2006) Efficacy of three treatment protocols for adolescents with social anxiety disorder: a 5-year follow-up assessment. J Anxiety Disord 20:175–191. doi: 10.1016/j.janxdis.2005.01.003

Garcia-Lopez LJ, Ingles CJ, Garcia-Fernández JM (2008) Exploring the relevance of gender and age differences in the assessment of social fears in adolescence. Soc Behav Personal 36: 385–390

Garcia-Lopez LJ, Muela JA, Espinosa-Fernández L, Diaz-Castela MM (2009) Exploring the relevance of expressed emotion to the treatment of social anxiety disorder in adolescence. J Adolesc 32:1371–1376. doi: 10.1016/j.adolescence.2009.08.001

Garcia-Lopez LJ, Irurtia MJ, Caballo VE, Diaz-Castela MM (2011) Ansiedad social y abuso psicológico [Social anxiety and psychological abuse]. Behav Psychol 19:223–236

Garcia-Lopez LJ, Diaz-Castela MM, Muela-Martinez JA, Espinosa-Fernandez L (2014) Can parent training for parents with high levels of expressed emotion have a positive effect on their child's social anxiety improvement? J Anxiety Disord 28:812–822. doi: 10.1016/j.janxdis.2014.09.001

Gazelle H, Ladd GW (2003) Anxious solitude and peer exclusion: a diathesis-stress model of internalizing trajectories in childhood. Child Dev 74:257–278. doi:10.1111/1467-8624.00534

Ginsburg GS, La Greca AM, Silverman WK (1998) Social anxiety in children with anxiety disorders: relation with social and emotional functioning. J Abnorm Child Psychol 26(3):175–185. doi:10.1023/A:1022668101048

Glickman AR, La Greca AM (2004) The Dating Anxiety Scale for Adolescents: scale development and associations with adolescent functioning. J Clin Child Adolesc Psychol 33(3): 566–578. doi:10.1207/s15374424jccp3303_14

Goodyer I, Dubicka B, Wilkinson P, Kelvin R, Roberts C, Byford S, Breen S, Ford C, Barrett B, Leech A, Rothwell J, White L, Harrington R (2007) Selective serotonin reuptake inhibitors (SSRIs) and routine specialist care with and without cognitive behaviour therapy in adolescents with major depression: randomised controlled trial. Br Med J 335(7611):142. doi http://dx.doi.org/10.1136/bmj.39224.494340.55. PMCID: PMC1925185

Gotlib IH, Hammen CL (1992) Psychological aspects of depression: toward a cognitive-interpersonal integration. Wiley, Oxford, UK

Grant BF, Hasin D, Blanco C, Stinson FS, Chou SP, Goldstein RB, Dawson DA, Smith S, Saha TD, Huang B (2005) The epidemiology of social anxiety disorder in the United States: results from the national epidemiologic survey on alcohol and related conditions. J Clin Psychiatry 66(11):1351–1361. doi:10.4088/JCP.v66n110

Grant DM, Beck JG, Farrow SM, Davila J (2007) Do interpersonal features of social anxiety influence the development of depressive symptoms? Cogn Emotion 21:646–663. doi:10.1080/02699930600713036

Hammen C (1991) Generation of stress in the course of unipolar depression. J Abnorm Psychol 100(4):555–561. doi:10.1037/0021-843X.100.4.555

Hammen C (1999) The emergence of an interpersonal approach to depression. In: Joiner T, Coyne JC (eds) The interactional nature of depression: advances in interpersonal approaches. American Psychological Association, Washington, DC, pp 21–35

Hammen C, Brennan PA (2001) Depressed adolescents of depressed and nondepressed mothers: tests of an interpersonal impairment hypothesis. J Consult Clin Psychol 69(2):284–294. doi:10.1037/0022-006X.69.2.284

Hankin BL, Mermelstein R, Roesch L (2007) Sex differences in adolescent depression: stress exposure and reactivity models. Child Dev 78(1):279–295. doi:10.1111/j.1467-8624.2007.00997.x

Hebert KR, Fales J, Nangle DW, Papadakis AA, Grover RL (2013) Linking social anxiety and adolescent romantic relationship functioning: indirect effects and the importance of peers. J Youth Adolesc 42:1708–1720. doi:10.1007/s10964-012-9878-0

Heerey EA, Kring AM (2007) Interpersonal consequences of social anxiety. J Abnorm Psychol 116(1):125–134. doi:10.1037/0021-843X.116.1.125

Heimberg RG, Horner KJ, Juster HR, Safren SA, Brown EJ, Schneier FR (1999) Psychometric properties of the Liebowitz social anxiety scale. Psychol Med 29(1):199–212. doi:10.1017/S0033291798007879

Hoagwood K, Olin SS (2002) The NIMH blueprint for change report: research priorities in child and adolescent mental health. J Am Acad Child Adolesc Psychiatry 41(7):760–767. doi:10.1097/00004583-200207000-00006

Hogan MF (2003) New freedom commission report: the president's new freedom commission: recommendations to transform mental health care in America. Psychiatr Serv 54(11):1467–1474. doi:10.1176/appi.ps.54.11.1467

Kataoka SH, Zhang L, Wells KB (2002) Unmet need for mental health care among U.S. children: variation by ethnicity and insurance status. Am J Psychiatry 159(9):1548–1555. doi:10.1176/appi.ajp.159.9.1548

Kingery JM, Erdley CA, Marshall KC, Whitaker KG, Reuter TR (2010) Peer experiences of anxious and socially withdrawn youth: an integrative review of the developmental and clinical literature. Clin Child Fam Psychol Rev 13:91–128. doi:10.1007/s10567-009-0063-2

Kobak RR, Sudler N, Gamble W (1991) Attachment and depressive symptoms during adolescence: a developmental pathways analysis. Dev Psychopathol 3(04):461–474. doi:10.1017/S095457940000763X

La Greca AM, Harrison HM (2005) Adolescent peer relations, friendships, and romantic relationships: do they predict social anxiety and depression? J Clin Child Adolesc Psychol 34(1):49–61. doi:10.1207/s15374424jccp3401_5

La Greca AM, Lai B (2013) Peer influences. In: Chu B, Ehrenreich-May J (eds) Transdiagnostic mechanisms and treatment of youth psychopathology. Guilford Press, New York

La Greca AM, Landoll RR (2011) Peer influences in the development and maintenance of anxiety disorders. In: Silverman WK, Field A (eds) Anxiety disorders in children and adolescents: research, assessment, and intervention, 2nd edn. Cambridge University Press, London, pp 323–348

La Greca AM, Lopez N (1998) Social anxiety among adolescents: linkages with peer relations and friendships. J Abnorm Child Psychol 26(2):83–94. doi:10.1023/A:1022684520514

La Greca AM, Mackey ER (2007) Adolescents' anxiety in dating situations: the potential role of friends and romantic partners. J Clin Child Adolesc Psychol 36(4):522–533. doi:10.1080/15374410701662097

La Greca AM, Davila J, Siegel R (2009) Peer relations, friendships, and romantic relationships: implications for the development and maintenance of depression in adolescents. In: Allen NB, Sheeber LB (eds) Adolescent emotional development and the emergence of depressive disorders. Cambridge University Press, New York, pp 318–336

La Greca AM, Davila J, Landoll RR, Siegel R (2011) Dating, romantic relationships and social anxiety in young people. In: Alfano CA, Biedel DC (eds) Social anxiety disorder in adolescents and young adults: translating developmental research into practice. American Psychological Association, Washington, DC, pp 93–105

La Greca AM, Mufson L, Ehrenreich-May J, Girio-Herrera E, Chan S (2014) Developing an evidence-based preventive intervention for peer victimized adolescents at risk for social anxiety disorder and/or depression. Presented at the biennial meeting of the International Society for Affective Disorders, Berlin, Apr 2014

Leaf PJ, Alegria M, Cohen P, Goodman SH, Horwitz SM, Hoven CW, Narrow WE, Vaden-Kiernan M, Regier DA (1996) Mental health service use in the community and schools: results from the four-community MECA study. J Am Acad Child Adolesc Psychiatry 35(7):889–897. doi:10.1097/00004583-199607000-00014

Lewinsohn PM, Clarke GN, Seeley JR, Rohde P (1994) Major depression in community adolescents: age at onset, episode duration, and time to recurrence. J Am Acad Child Adolesc Psychiatry 33(6):809–818. doi:10.1097/00004583-199407000-00006

Lewinsohn PM, Rohde P, Klein DN, Seeley JR (1999) Natural course of adolescent major depressive disorder: I. Continuity into young adulthood. J Am Acad Child Adolesc Psychiatry 38(1):56–63. doi:10.1097/00004583-199901000-00020

Lewinsohn PM, Solomon A, Seeley JR, Zeiss A (2000) Clinical implications of "subthreshold" depressive symptoms. J Abnorm Psychol 109(2):345–351. doi:10.1037/0021-843X.109.2.345

Lipsitz JD (2012) Interpersonal psychotherapy for social anxiety disorder. In: Markowitz JC, Weissman MM (eds) Casebook of interpersonal psychotherapy. Oxford University Press, New York, pp 169–184

Lipsitz J, Markowitz J (2006) Interpersonal psychotherapy for social phobia. Unpublished treatment manual, Columbia University

Lipsitz JD, Markowitz JC, Cherry S, Fyer AJ (1999) Open trial of interpersonal psychotherapy for the treatment of social phobia. Am J Psychiatry 156(11):1814–1816

Lipsitz JD, Gur M, Vermes D, Petkova E, Cheng J, Miller N, Laino J, Liebowitz MR, Fyer AJ (2008) A randomized trial of interpersonal psychotherapy versus supportive therapy for social anxiety disorder. Depress Anxiety 25:542–553. doi:10.1002/da.20364

Markowitz JC, Lipsitz J, Milrod BL (2014) Critical review of outcome research on interpersonal psychotherapy for anxiety disorders. Depress Anxiety 31(4):316–325. doi:10.1002/da.22238

Masia-Warner C (2009) CBT for social anxiety disorder delivered by school counselor. Retrieved from: http://projectreporter.nih.gov/project_info_description.cfm?aid=8033730&icde=10353496&ddparam=&ddvalue=&ddsub=

Masia-Warner C, Klein R, Dent H, Fisher PH, Alvir J, Albano AM, Guardino M (2005) School-based intervention for adolescents with social anxiety disorder: results of a controlled study. J Abnorm Child Psychol 33(6):707–722. doi:10.1007/s10802-005-7649-z

Masia-Warner C, Fisher PH, Shrout PE, Rathor S, Klein RG (2007) Treating adolescents with social anxiety disorder in school: an attention control trial. J Child Psychol Psychiatry 48(7):676–686. doi:10.1111/j.1469-7610.2007.01737.x

Masia CL, Klein RG, Storch E, Corda B (2001) School-based behavioral treatment for social anxiety disorder in adolescents: results of a pilot study. J Am Acad Child Adolesc Psychiatry 40:780–86

Meredith LS, Stein BD, Paddock SM, Jaycox LH, Quinn VP, Chandra A, Burnam A (2009) Perceived barriers to treatment for adolescent depression. Med Care 47(6):677–685. doi:10.1097/MLR.0b013e318190d46b

Merikangas KR, He JP, Brody D, Fisher PW, Bourdon K, Koretz DS (2010) Prevalence and treatment of mental disorders among US children in the 2001–2004 NHANES. Pediatrics 125(1):75–81. doi:10.1542/peds. 2008-2598

Meyer A (1957) Psychobiology: a science of man. Charles C. Thomas, Oxford, UK

Mufson L, Weissman MM, Moreau D, Garfinkel R (1999) Efficacy of interpersonal psychotherapy for depressed adolescents. Arch Gen Psychiatry 56(6):573–579. doi:10.1001/archpsyc.56.6.573

Mufson L, Dorta KP, Moreau D, Weissman MM (2004a) Interpersonal psychotherapy for depressed adolescents, 2nd edn. Guilford Publications, New York

Mufson L, Dorta KP, Wickramaratne P, Nomura Y, Olfson M, Weissman MM (2004b) A randomized effectiveness trial of Interpersonal Psychotherapy for depressed adolescents. Arch Gen Psychiatry 61:577–584. doi:10.1001/archpsyc.61.6.577

Nolan SA, Flynn C, Garber J (2003) Prospective relations between rejection and depression in young adolescents. J Pers Soc Psychol 85:745–755. doi:10.1037/0022-3514.85.4.745
Plasencia ML, Alden LE, Taylor CT (2011) Functional implications of safety behaviour subtypes in social anxiety disorder. Behav Res Ther 49:665–675. doi:10.1016/j.brat.2011.07.005
Prinstein MJ, Aikins JW (2004) Cognitive moderators of the longitudinal association between peer rejection and adolescent depressive symptoms. J Abnorm Child Psychol 32(2):147–158. doi:10.1023/B:JACP.0000019767.55592.63
Puig-Antich J, Kaufman J, Ryan ND, Williamson DE, Dahl RE, Lukens E, Todak G, Ambrosini P, Rabinovich H, Nelson B (1993) The psychosocial functioning and family environment of depressed adolescents. J Am Acad Child Adolesc Psychiatry 32(2):244–253. doi:10.1097/00004583-199303000-00003
Puklek ML, Berce J (2012) Social anxiety, social acceptance and academic self perceptions in High School Students. Soc Res J Gen Soc Issues (Društvena istraživanja Časopis za opća društvena pitanja) 2:405–419, on www.ceeol.com
Ranta K, Kaltiala-Heino R, Pelkonen M, Marttunen M (2009) Associations between peer victimization, self-reported depression and social phobia among adolescents: the role of comorbidity. J Adolesc 32:77–93
Ranta K, Kaltiala-Heino R, Fröjd S, Marttunen M (2013) Peer victimization and social phobia: a follow-up study among adolescents. Soc Psychiatry Psychiatr Epidemiol 48:533–44
Rapee RM, Schniering CA, Hudson JL (2009) Anxiety disorders during childhood and adolescence: origins and treatment. Annu Rev Clin Psychol 5(1):311–341
Rosselló J, Bernal G (1999) Efficacy of cognitive-behavioral and interpersonal treatments for depression in Puerto Rican adolescents. J Couns Clin Psychol 67(5):734–745. doi:10.1037/0022-006X.67.5.734
Rosselló J, Bernal G, Rivera-Medina C (2008) Individual and group CBT and IPT for Puerto Rican adolescents with depressive symptoms. Cultur Divers Ethnic Minor Psychol 14(3):234–245. doi:10.1037/1099-9809.14.3.234
Rudolph KD, Hammen C, Burge D, Lindberg N, Herzberg D, Daley SE (2000) Toward an interpersonal life-stress model of depression: the developmental context of stress generation. Dev Psychopathol 12:215–234. doi:10.1017/S0954579400002066
Sanders MR, Dadds MR, Johnston BM, Cash R (1992) Childhood depression and conduct disorder: I. Behavioral, affective and cognitive aspects of family problem-solving interactions. J Abnorm Psychol 101(3):495–504. doi:10.1037/0021-843X.101.3.495
Sheeber L, Allen N, Davis B, Sorenson E (2000) Regulation of negative affect during mother-child problem-solving interactions: adolescent depressive status and family processes. J Abnorm Child Psychol 28(5):467–479. doi:10.1023/A:1005135706799
Sheeber L, Hops H, Davis B (2001) Family processes in adolescent depression. Clin Child Fam Psychol Rev 4:19–35. doi:10.1023/A:1009524626436
Sheeber LB, Davis B, Leve C, Hops H, Tildesley E (2007) Adolescents' relationships with their mothers and fathers: associations with depressive disorder and subdiagnostic symptomatology. J Abnorm Psychol 116(1):144–154. doi:10.1037/0021-843X.116.1.144
Siegel R, La Greca AM, Harrison HM (2009) Peer victimization and social anxiety in adolescents: prospective and reciprocal relationships. J Youth Adolesc 38:1096–1109
Silverman W, Pina AA, Viswesvaran C (2008) Evidence-based psychosocial treatments for phobic and anxiety disorders in children and adolescents. J Clin Child Adolesc Psychol 37(1):105–130. doi:10.1080/15374410701817907
Stader SR, Hokanson JE (1998) Psychosocial antecedents of depressive symptoms: an evaluation using daily experiences methodology. J Abnorm Psychol 107(1):17. doi:10.1037/0021-843X.107.1.17
Stangier U, Schramm E, Heidenreich T, Berger M, Clark DM (2011) Cognitive therapy vs interpersonal psychotherapy in social anxiety disorder: a randomized controlled trial. Arch Gen Psychiatry 68(7):692–700. doi:10.1001/archgenpsychiatry.2011.67
Stein MB, Fuetsch M, Müller N, Höfler M, Lieb R, Wittchen HU (2001) Social anxiety disorder and the risk of depression: a prospective community study of adolescents and young adults. Arch Gen Psychiatry 58(3):251–256. doi:10.1001/archpsyc.58.3.251

Steinberg L (1990) Autonomy, conflict, and harmony in the family relationship. In: Feldman S, Elliot G (eds) At the threshold: the developing adolescent. Harvard University Press, Cambridge, MA, pp 255–276

Stice E, Rohde P, Seeley JR, Gau JM (2008) Brief cognitive-behavioral depression prevention program for high-risk adolescents outperforms two alternative interventions: a randomized efficacy trial. J Consult Clin Psychol 76(4):595–606. doi:10.1037/a0012645

Storch EA, Masia-Warner C (2004) The relationship of peer victimization to social anxiety and loneliness in adolescent females. J Adolesc 27(3):351–362. doi:10.1016/j.adolescence.2004.03.003

Storch EA, Masia-Warner C, Crisp H, Klein RG (2005) Peer victimization and social anxiety in adolescence: a prospective study. Aggress Behav 31(5):437–452. doi:10.1002/ab.20093

Sullivan HS (1953) The interpersonal theory of psychiatry. WW Norton, New York

van Hees ML, Rotter T, Ellermann T, Evers SM (2013) The effectiveness of individual interpersonal psychotherapy as a treatment for major depressive disorder in adult outpatients: a systematic review. BMC Psychiatry 13(1):22–33. doi:10.1186/1471-244X-13-22

Vernberg EM (1990) Psychological adjustment and experiences with peers during early adolescence: reciprocal, incidental, or unidirectional relationships? J Abnorm Child Psychol 18(2):187–198. doi:10.1007/BF00910730

Vernberg EM, Abwender DA, Ewell KK, Beery SH (1992) Social anxiety and peer relationships in early adolescence: a prospective analysis. J Clin Child Psychol 21(2):189–196. doi:10.1207/s15374424jccp2102_11

Weissman MM (2006) A brief history of interpersonal psychotherapy. Psychiatr Ann 36(8): 553–557

Weissman MM, Paykel ES (1974) The depressed woman: a study of social relationships. University Chicago Press, Oxford, UK

Weissman MM, Markowitz JC, Klerman GL (2000a) Comprehensive guide to interpersonal psychotherapy. Basic Books, New York

Weissman MM, Wickramaratne P, Adams P, Wolk S, Verdeli H, Olfson M (2000b) Brief screening for family psychiatric history: the family history screen. Arch Gen Psychiatry 57(7):675–682, doi: 10-1001/pubs.Arch Gen Psychiatry-ISSN-0003-990x-57-7-yoa8214

Weisz JR, Jensen-Doss A, Hawley KM (2006) Evidence-based youth psychotherapies versus usual clinical care: a meta-analysis of direct comparisons. Am Psychol 61(7):671–689. doi:10.1037/0003-066X.61.7.671

Young JF, Mufson L (2006) Interpersonal psychotherapy: adolescent skills training manual. Unpublished treatment manual, Columbia University

Young JF, Mufson L, Davies M (2006a) Efficacy of interpersonal psychotherapy-adolescent skills training: an indicated preventive intervention for depression. J Child Psychol Psychiatry 47(12):1254–1262. doi:10.1111/j.1469-7610.2006.01667.x

Young JF, Mufson L, Davies M (2006b) Impact of comorbid anxiety in an effectiveness study of interpersonal psychotherapy for depressed adolescents. J Am Acad Child Adolesc Psychiatry 45(8):904–912. doi:10.1097/01.chi.0000222791.23927.5f

Young JF, Mufson L, Gallop R (2010) Preventing depression: a randomized trial of Interpersonal Psychotherapy-Adolescent skills training. Depress Anxiety 27:426–433. doi:10.1002/da.20664

Young JF, Kranzler A, Gallop R, Mufson L (2012a) Interpersonal psychotherapy-adolescent skills training: effects on school and social functioning. Sch Ment Health 4:254–264. doi:10.1007/s12310-012-9078-9

Young JF, Makover HB, Cohen JR, Mufson L, Gallop RJ, Benas JS (2012b) Interpersonal psychotherapy-adolescent skills training: anxiety outcomes and impact of comorbidity. J Clin Child Adolesc Psychol 41(5):640–653. doi:10.1080/15374416.2012.704843

School-Based Interventions for Adolescents with Social Anxiety Disorder

12

Carrie Masia Warner, Daniela Colognori, Chad Brice, and Amanda Sanchez

Social anxiety disorder (*SAD*) is the most impairing anxiety disorder among adolescents, impacting an estimated 9.1 % during their lifetime (Merikangas et al. 2010). The social discomfort and avoidance experienced by youngsters with *SAD* is associated with limited friendships, missed social opportunities (e.g., school clubs and sports teams), peer victimization (Garcia-Lopez et al. 2011; Ranta et al. 2013, 2009), and hardship executing class requirements (e.g., verbal presentations, class participation). These difficulties can lead to loneliness, academic difficulties, dysphoric mood, and an overall lower quality of life (Beidel et al. 1999; Grover et al. 2007; Katzelnick et al. 2001; Wittchen et al. 1999).

Given the high prevalence and impairment associated with *SAD*, several clinic-based efficacious psychological (Beidel et al. 1998; Heimberg and Becker 2002; Ledley et al. 2009) and pharmacological (Walkup et al. 2008) treatments have been

Author Note This work was supported by an NIMH grant awarded to Dr. Masia Warner, Grant R01MH081881.

C. Masia Warner, PhD (✉)
Department of Psychology, William Paterson University, Wayne, NJ 07470, USA

Nathan Kline Institute for Psychiatric Research, Orangeburg, NY, USA

Department of Child and Adolescent Psychiatry, NYU Langone Medical Center, New York, NY, USA
e-mail: masiac@wpunj.edu

D. Colognori, PsyD
Department of Advanced Studies in Psychology, Kean University, Union, NJ, USA

C. Brice, PhD
Cognitive and Behavioral Consultants, White Plains, NY, USA

A. Sanchez, BA
Department of Child and Adolescent Psychiatry, NYU Langone Medical Center, New York, NY, USA

K. Ranta et al. (eds.), *Social Anxiety and Phobia in Adolescents: Development, Manifestation and Intervention Strategies*, DOI 10.1007/978-3-319-16703-9_12

developed and evaluated (see Chap. 9 by Guerry et al.). Yet, the majority of socially anxious adolescents remain unlikely to receive mental health services (Colognori et al. 2012; Kashdan and Herbert 2001; Wittchen et al. 1999). A large epidemiological study found that only 12 % of adolescents with *SAD* received treatment (Merikangas et al. 2010). Excepting substance use, this was the lowest rate of service utilization among psychiatric disorders in adolescents.

Unfortunately, this problem is indicative of a larger public health crisis regarding the failure to provide mental health services to affected youngsters. Common barriers to care include stigma, cost, and transportation. In addition, families are often unaware of where to seek treatment, and not surprisingly, fewer than 20 % obtaining services receive evidence-based intervention (Collins et al. 2004; Lim et al. 2012; Wahl 2012). Schools play a central role in addressing the unmet mental health needs of youth. Providing intervention within schools minimizes the considerable burdens associated with accessing treatment in the community. In a study of 2,488 ninth graders, students referred for school services were twice as likely to receive help as those referred to community providers (Husky et al. 2011). In addition, there is considerable evidence that school-based services enhance access for minority and economically disadvantaged youth (Angold et al. 2002; Catron et al. 1998; Juszczak et al. 2003; Kataoka et al. 2007). Clearly, the educational sector provides an avenue for reaching the majority of children in need of intervention.

Beyond these advantages, schools are uniquely poised to address challenges specific to treating *SAD*. First, worries about stigma (e.g., being labeled as having a "problem") are likely magnified in socially anxious youth because of their severe sensitivity to negative evaluation. Thus, they may have heightened reluctance to disclose social difficulties. For example, Colognori and colleagues (2012) found that, of 270 adolescents reporting elevated social anxiety, 40 % had never informed an adult about their distress. Unlike externalizing disorders, which are clearly observable without self-disclosure, parents and school personnel often have difficulty identifying anxiety (Horwitz et al. 1998; Layne et al. 2006; Wren et al. 2003; Wu et al. 1999). In addition, even when key adults recognize that teenagers are extremely shy, their behaviors may be misunderstood as a personality style that does not require intervention. Schools can readily address these barriers to improve the recognition of *SAD*. For example, a brief *SAD* questionnaire could be added to routine school screenings, or students might be educated about anxiety in health classes and provided a chance to self-refer. (For more details on screening and assessment in SAD, refer to Chap. 6 by Garcia-Lopez, Salvador and De Los Reyes.) Further supporting identification, teachers and school counselors could receive training to enhance detection of more subtle avoidance behaviors.

In addition to facilitating increased recognition and referral, implementing intervention in schools affords opportunities to enrich treatment quality for *SAD*. For one, given that social evaluation fears are at the core of *SAD*, group treatment is particularly suitable and has been shown to be efficacious (Heimberg and Becker 2002). Supporting this notion, recent research has shown that, relative to other anxiety disorders in youth, *SAD* is less likely to respond to individual cognitive-behavioral therapy (CBT) (Ginsburg et al. 2011). Moreover, it is becoming increasingly accepted that social skills training may be necessary for maximal treatment benefits (Alfano et al. 2006; Kendall et al. 2012; Mesa et al. 2014). Learning new social skills is more feasible in a group format that includes peers for practicing skills and providing feedback. Whereas forming groups in clinics is challenging because of limited numbers of clients with similar diagnoses and varying schedules, schools are conducive to developing groups and routinely implement group programs. For these reasons, group interventions for *SAD* fit well into the school environment.

Finally, because many feared situations occur at school, school-based interventions provide an ecologically valid context for treatment. That is, implementing intervention at school affords opportunities to help adolescents enter into commonly avoided situations (e.g., eating in cafeteria, speaking with school personnel) and to practice skills in realistic contexts with a variety of individuals (e.g., teacher, coach). Thus, intervention delivered in school blends the treatment setting with the natural environment, which may improve the effectiveness of existing empirically based clinic treatments.

Based on the potential advantages of delivering treatment for *SAD* within the school environment, two interventions for adolescents have been specifically designed for school-based implementation and evaluated in schools. These include a program developed in Spain, the original *Intervención en Adolescentes con Fobia Social: Therapy for Adolescents with Social Phobia* (*IAFS;* Garcia-Lopez 2000, 2007), and one in the United States, *Skills for Academic and Social Success* (*SASS;* Masia et al. 1999). Both *IAFS* and *SASS* were developed from empirically supported, clinic-based treatments. *IAFS* was adapted from the adolescent Spanish version (*SET-Asv*; Olivares et al. 1998) of *Social Effectiveness Therapy (SET;* Turner et al. 1994) and *Cognitive-Behavioral Group Therapy for Adolescents* (*CBGT-A*; Albano et al. 1991). *SASS* was primarily based on the child format of *SET (SET-C;* Beidel et al. 2000), which emphasizes behavioral exposure and social skills training. A full description of these clinic-based treatments and their empirical support can be found in Chap. 13.

Considerations in Conducting School-Based Interventions for *SAD* in Adolescents

Due to the complexity of disseminating evidence-based treatments to community settings, several implementation frameworks have been developed (see Damschroder et al. 2009; Fixsen et al. 2005; Han and Weiss 2005; Meyers et al. 2012), all of which highlight the importance of ensuring fit between the intervention and the setting. *SET-Asv*, *SET-C*, and *CBGT-A* are intensive treatments, consisting of numerous sessions of long duration. For example, *SET-C* involves 24 sessions lasting 90 min each (12 social skills groups followed by planned social activities and 12 individual exposure sessions). Therefore, adapting clinic-based treatments to fit into the school environment required extensive changes.

Addressing School Priorities

When adapting a clinic-based intervention for the school setting, modifications are necessary to improve the program's acceptability to school administrators and staff. Naturally, the top priorities for schools are academic instruction and student performance. Although school personnel understand the potential benefit of addressing *SAD*, they are concerned about the loss of instructional time associated with implementing the intervention. In order to address this, the potential benefits of each session must be carefully weighed against the cost of lost instructional time. Minimizing individual sessions may be one valuable approach. Consistent with this, *SASS* contains only two brief individual meetings, and weekly individual sessions in *IAFS* are optional. Instead, *SASS* and *IAFS* rely primarily on a group format because of its clinical relevance for treating *SAD* and routine use in schools (e.g., clubs, drug prevention, peer leadership; Foster et al. 2005; Kelly and Lueck 2011). In addition, it is helpful for the length of school-based interventions to fit within one academic semester without excessive class absences. Accordingly, length of the original *IAFS* is 12, 90-min group sessions that are scheduled using one school hour (60 min) and a break period (30 min). *SASS* includes 12 group meetings shortened to fit within one academic period or approximately 40 min. To avoid repeated disruption of any single academic subject, *SASS* group times (e.g., class periods) are rotated so that students never miss the same class more than twice throughout the program.

To further address the schools' main objectives, it is essential that school-based programs explicitly target social avoidance that interferes with academic performance or engagement in the school community. The original *IAFS* contains a social skills module using unknown peers to practice initiating and maintaining conversations with same and opposite-sex teenagers. *IAFS* also has an intensive focus on public speaking, a skill essential to school performance. Similarly, *SASS* emphasizes improving skills such as participating in class, asking teachers for help, joining school activities, and speaking to school personnel such as principals, teachers, and counselors. In addition, school personnel are enlisted to assist students as they practice skills, and thus they readily observe treatment effects. Clearly, these situations are central to treating *SAD*, but targeting them directly in schools has the added benefit of facilitating collaboration and support from school administrators and personnel.

Delivery of the Intervention by School Personnel

Schools are more likely to adopt interventions that benefit their students and can be implemented and sustained utilizing the schools' existing resources (Atkins et al. 2003; Shediac-Rizkallah and Bone 1998). In the United States, frontline school practitioners (e.g., school psychologists and social workers) and school guidance counselors are key providers of services for youth (Lyon et al. 2011a, b; Ryan and Masia Warner 2012). In addition, school counselors' familiarity with the student population, school culture, and available school resources may enable them to easily relate to the students, anticipate concerns, and use the school environment effectively to optimize treatment gains. Therefore, our aim for *SASS* was to develop an intervention that could be feasibly delivered by school counselors. A group format was considered more viable for school counselors given their time burdens. In addition, the *SASS* manual was written to accommodate individuals without specialized training in CBT. Specifically, we used nontechnical language whenever possible and included detailed session scripts, as well as session outlines and checklists to help with executing groups and prioritizing session tasks.

Capitalizing on the School Environment

Given the severe reduction in treatment dose necessary to facilitate school delivery, *SASS* and *IAFS* aim to enhance their clinical impact by capitalizing on the natural advantages of treating *SAD* in the school community, namely, increased accessibility to parents and school peers (Ryan and Masia Warner 2012). *SASS* involves parents by holding two parent meetings at school. Garcia-Lopez et al. (2014) have developed a parent module, *Intervención en Familias & Adolescentes con Fobia Social; Therapy for Families and Adolescents with Social Phobia* (*IFAFS*; Garcia-Lopez et al. 2011b), to accompany the *IAFS* school-based treatment. In addition, both programs utilize school peers to assist with the implementation of exposures, and peer assistants also attend *SASS* social events with group members in the community. Finally, school-based exposures are designed to take advantage of the school context by utilizing real-life school situations (e.g., meeting with a teacher for clarification of academic material, approaching a peer in the library or cafeteria).

Developmental Adaptations for Adolescents

To create interventions appropriate for adolescents in schools, modifications to the core skills were required. Given that negative self-talk is more frequent among teenagers than children with *SAD* (Alfano et al. 2006), both *IAFS* and *SASS* added cognitive restructuring or realistic thinking. In addition, the social skills curriculum was adapted to include more advanced content (e.g., extending invitations, assertiveness) and include typical adolescent social challenges at school (e.g., joining a group in the school cafeteria).

Several of the considerations that have been discussed clearly shaped the development and implementation of the school-based programs for *SAD*. In the next section of this chapter, we describe *IAFS* and *SASS* and their treatment outcome data.

Evidence-Based School Interventions for *SAD*

Intervención en Adolescentes con Fobia Social: Therapy for Adolescents with Social Phobia (IAFS)

The original *IAFS* (Garcia-Lopez 2000, 2007) consists of 12 weekly group sessions, each 90 min in length in approximately 4 months (due to vacations and exams). Groups vary from 4 people to 8 people. Techniques include psychoeducation, self-esteem bibliotherapy, cognitive restructuring, social skills, exposure, and relapse prevention. During group sessions, exposures are carried out utilizing unknown school peers as co-therapists who interact with the participants. Targeted social situations include beginning and maintaining conversations with persons of the same or opposite sex and speaking in public in front of group members and therapists. A feature unique to *IAFS* is that exposure tasks are video recorded. Video feedback is then used to help students learn from exposures, detect safety behaviors, and establish a more realistic self-image. Participants and other group members provide feedback on speeches that is compared with students' objective performance from video recordings. Along with group sessions, weekly individual counseling sessions are offered in which a range of issues can be discussed. These optional individual meetings can be used to prepare exposure practice or review concepts presented during group sessions.

Evaluating *IAFS*

The original *IAFS* (Garcia-Lopez 2000, 2007) has been compared to the Spanish translations of two efficacious clinic-based treatments for *SAD*, *SET-Asv* (Olivares et al. 1998), and *CBGT-A* (Albano et al. 1991). Fifty-nine adolescents (mean age = 15.92, range 15–17 years) with a diagnosis of *SAD* received *IAFS* (n = 15), *CBGT-A* (n = 15), or *SET-Asv* (n = 14). Treatment groups were compared to a no-treatment control (n = 15) that included a random sample of students who refused intervention. The program was conducted during the school day by two therapists with a minimum of 2 years' experience who received supervision by a licensed psychologist.

Immediately following intervention, results showed superiority of all treatments relative to the no-treatment control. Students who received intervention reported decreased social anxiety and avoidance, reduced fear of public speaking, improved self-esteem, and a decrease in the number of feared social situations. Clinical improvements were largely maintained one year following treatment completion, with some possible advantages to *IAFS* on outcomes pertaining to social avoidance using self-reports (Olivares et al. 2002) and Corpus Linguistics methodology (Garcia-Lopez et al. 2011a). Effect sizes were large for all interventions compared to the no-treatment control immediately after treatment at one year follow-up. (Garcia-Lopez et al. 2002). To understand long-term impact, Garcia-Lopez and colleagues (2006) also conducted a 5-year follow-up of 25 participants who had received an active treatment in the initial study (n = 44). Although the study had a modest sample size, results demonstrated that treatment gains were maintained equally across interventions over 5 years. Clinical and effect size significance suggest the possibility of *IAFS* may have more robust long-term durability (see Garcia-Lopez et al. 2006).

In a second trial, Garcia-Lopez and colleagues (2014) evaluated the clinical benefits of including parents in the treatment of adolescents with *SAD*. The original *IAFS* was compared with *IAFS* plus a parent module (*IFAFS*) (Garcia-Lopez et al. 2011b) in a sample of 52 families. *IFAFS* consists of five, two-hour group sessions for parents that target expressed emotion (EE), as a previous study revealed that high EE is associated with less positive treatment outcomes in adolescents with social phobia (Garcia-Lopez et al. 2009). Parent sessions include psychoeducation about *SAD* and the role of expressed emotion in their children's symptomatology, communication skills to replace the use of rejection, criticism and hostile verbal comments, and contingency management training aimed at teaching strategies to better manage children's *SAD*. Parent sessions were conducted by two clinical psychologists with extensive experience in parent training. Adolescents aged 14–18 years (mean age = 15.92) with parents exhibiting high EE were randomly assigned to either *IAFS* (n = 32) or *IAFS* plus *IFAFS* (n = 20). Findings revealed that adding a parent component to *IAFS* enhanced its clinical benefits and may be a promising approach for treating adolescents with *SAD* if parents exhibit high levels of EE. Taken together, these trials support the efficacy of *IFAFS* when delivered by trained psychologists in the school setting.

Skills for Academic and Social Success (SASS)

The *SASS* intervention (Masia et al. 1999) consists of 12 weekly group sessions, two group booster sessions, and two brief individual meetings. Additionally, four weekend social events that include prosocial peers, called peer assistants, provide real-world exposures and skills generalization. Parents attend two group meetings during which they receive psychoeducation regarding *SAD* and learn techniques to address their child's anxiety. Teachers can participate in two optional meetings in which they learn about *SAD* and the program and receive instruction to help students practice classroom exposures. The program is designed to be flexible to accommodate the school calendar (e.g., vacations and exams) and typically spans about 3 months. Treatment groups are small (4–6 students) and can be facilitated by one or two group leaders. Each *SASS* component is discussed in the sections that follow, with an emphasis on how to capitalize on the school environment to implement and practice skills.

School Group Sessions

The 12 groups last one class period or about 40 min. They cover five core components: (a) psychoeducation, (b) realistic thinking, (c) social skills training, (d) exposure, and (e) relapse prevention.

Psychoeducation

The first group informs students about the structure of the program and provides an overview of the cognitive-behavioral model of *SAD*. Given socially anxious adolescents' heightened social evaluative concerns coupled with specific worries about attending a group with classmates that is run by a school counselor, considerable time is dedicated to confidentiality.

Realistic Thinking

The second group session focuses on realistic thinking, primarily adapted from Ronald Rapee's (1998) book *Overcoming Shyness and Social Phobia*. Students are taught to identify negative expectations (e.g., I will sound boring) and to use specific questions to evaluate them more realistically (e.g., How many times has this happened in the past? How do I feel when I see others in similar situations?). Engaging in this process with school peers can be valuable because students' negative predictions are often related to school situations that they may have in common (e.g., certain teachers or coaches). These strategies of identifying and challenging thoughts are practiced and revisited throughout the program.

Social Skills Training

Compared to 12 social skills sessions in *SET-C*, *SASS* contains four. Of the 12, we chose four skills we considered most essential for enhancing adolescent social experiences including: (a) initiating conversations, (b) maintaining conversations and establishing friendships, (c) listening and remembering, and (d) assertiveness. In the initiating conversations session, students learn how to identify opportunities for interactions and tips for starting a conversation (e.g., comment on something you have in common or on something going on around you). Conducting these groups in schools with school peers often creates natural opportunities for conversation starters about well-known eccentric teachers, cafeteria food, or frustrating locker assignments. In the second skills group, students are taught strategies to sustain conversations as well as how to appropriately switch topics. This session also teaches group members how to invite peers to get together outside of school (e.g., to go to a movie, hang out). Group members often express interfering beliefs about the need to know peers very well before an invitation is considered acceptable. Having other teenagers challenge these assumptions can be valuable in providing more realistic socially acceptable norms. In addition, it is valuable to have other group members generate ideas for extending social invitations that are relevant to their school culture (e.g., school performances, sporting events).

The third skills session is listening and remembering. Some of the difficulty that socially anxious individuals have maintaining conversations is due to limitations in fully attending to the conversation at hand. Such impairment may be partially related to worries about what to say next or evaluative concerns (e.g., I will sound boring). This session trains students to fully engage in conversations by attending to what others are saying and how to use this information to maintain conversations. The final social skills session focuses on how to be assertive with others. Working on these behaviors at school can be particularly potent because relevant situations often arise in the school environment. For example, we may facilitate having students speak with teachers about various classroom difficulties (e.g., getting an unfair grade). Group members may also be asked to make complaints about school policies or schedules to school administrators or staff. Finally, group participants often support each other and problem-solve typical school incidents such as other students requesting to copy homework or cheat on an exam. These are just a few of the examples that make integrating this treatment into the school setting so compelling.

There are a few specific recommendations for teaching social skills to socially anxious teenagers. First, shy students often look unfriendly or unapproachable because of their nonverbal behaviors (e.g., tense expressions, avoidance of eye contact). Therefore, all skills groups focus on shaping and reinforcing behaviors consistent with appearing friendly and confident (e.g., engaged and relaxed body positioning, smiling). The majority of session time should be dedicated to helping students incorporate constructive feedback such as speaking louder or smiling and role-playing the skill repeatedly until improvement is observed. In addition, because socially anxious individuals often depend on a single way to initiate conversations (e.g., commenting on the weather), we attempt to train conversational flexibility. Through repeated practice, students are asked to generate different statements in similar situations. Other group members are encouraged to offer alternatives.

Facing Your Fears

Whereas *SET-C* contains 12 individual, 90-min exposures, *SASS* was reduced to five group exposure sessions, referred to as facing-your-fear sessions. Given the personalized nature of fear hierarchies, we recommend that they be completed during an individual session (see below). Hierarchies should include some exposure situations that can be readily executed in the school environment. Students are often sent to public areas (e.g., cafeteria, library) to interact with peers or school staff. For example, they may ask a teacher for help or make school announcements on the loudspeaker. In addition, the school auditorium can be used for students to practice speeches with school personnel attending as an audience. Students may also practice intentionally dropping their books in a crowded hallway or entering a classroom late. Conducting exposure within various parts of the school environment also reduces typical resistance, because leaders are available to provide real-time coaching and immediate feedback. In addition, performing realistic tasks in the school environment can produce natural positive consequences (e.g., a student is invited to sit with a peer in the library after initiating a conversation) that may result in more immediate gains and generalization of treatment effects.

Relapse Prevention

The final group is designed to help students consolidate gains and create a realistic plan for continuing progress. Each group member gives a speech about his or her experience in the program, which serves as an exposure exercise and termination activity.

Booster Sessions

Two group booster sessions occur monthly for 2 months after termination. The purpose is to monitor progress, discuss barriers to continued improvement, and highlight additional ways to strengthen peer relationships and engagement in social activities. Additional exposures can also be conducted during boosters.

Social Events

SASS includes four 90-min social events, reduced from 12 in *SET-C*, that are held on weekends in community settings. Group leaders, participants, and peer assistants from the students' schools (see next section) attend these events. Activities include bowling, a picnic, laser tag, board games, billiards, miniature golf, rollerblading, ceramics, cooking, and rock climbing. These events provide unique benefits because they offer opportunities to partake in social activities without close friends, practice conversational skills, and perform in front of others. We also use these events to challenge students to take risks in a safer social environment, such as ordering food for the group or asking to be on a peer's team. In planning social events, we start with structured activities such as bowling and progress to unstructured ones (e.g., a pizza party) that require more self-reliance to engage with others.

Peer Assistants

Similar to *SET-C*, prosocial peers are recruited to attend the social events with group participants. The *SASS* program benefits from the ability to enroll school peers to assist with social events. The primary role of peer assistants is to create a positive climate at social events by engaging group members in conversation and integrating reluctant participants into activities. In addition, peer assistants may help encourage resistant students to attend the initial social event by coordinating arrival times. However, because peer assistants are in the same schools as program participants, careful selection is essential. The optimal strategy is to use students who have previously completed the *SASS* program because they are sensitive to the concerns of group members. When this method is not feasible, we recommend asking school counselors for nominations of good-natured, mature, and friendly students.

Individual Sessions

SASS includes two brief individual sessions about 20 min in length. Often the first meeting is used to develop an individualized fear hierarchy. These meetings also allow for tailored cognitive restructuring, review of specific social skills, or individual exposures. Finally, group leaders try to better understand personal issues that may be interfering with group participation or program progress.

Parent Meetings

Two meetings were added to *SASS* to provide parents with psychoeducation about *SAD*, orient them to the program, and offer strategies to support their child's participation and progress. The first parent meeting occurs within the first 3 weeks of *SASS*. Group leaders provide psychoeducation about *SAD* and information about the rationale and structure of the program. Presenting *SASS* as a way to prevent long-term difficulties such as transitioning to college can increase buy-in from parents. The second meeting is more directive, highlighting common yet unhelpful parental reactions to children's anxiety and providing suggestions for more constructive strategies (Rapee et al. 2008). Parents are encouraged to foster their children's autonomy and self-efficacy by supporting them to approach anxiety-provoking situations.

Evaluating *SASS*

SASS was first evaluated in an open pilot study to demonstrate the feasibility of conducting the program in schools (Masia et al. 2001). Based on its potential benefits, this pilot work was followed by two randomized controlled trials evaluating the efficacy of *SASS* for adolescents, ages 13–17, with *SAD*. The first study ($n=35$) comparing *SASS* to a waiting list demonstrated that *SASS* was superior in reducing the rate and severity of *SAD* and enhancing functioning as noted by blinded evaluator, as well as parent and adolescent ratings (Masia Warner et al. 2005). To test the specific efficacy of *SASS*, a second trial ($n = 36$) compared *SASS* to a credible control that omitted its core components (e.g., social skills training, exposure) but was matched in its overall structure including four social events without peer assistants. The attention control consisted of psychoeducation about *SAD*, relaxation, and support. Immediately after treatment, only 7 % in the attention control versus 82 % of participants in *SASS* were rated as treatment responders by blind independent evaluators. In addition, 59 % of the *SASS* group no longer had a diagnosis of *SAD* relative to 0 % of the control. *SASS* was also superior to the attention control 6 months following the end of the program (Masia Warner et al. 2007).

Findings of both studies support the efficacy of *SASS* when delivered by clinical psychologists with training in CBT. As described above, other studies of school-based intervention for *SAD* have shown positive effects when implemented by research psychologists (Garcia-Lopez et al. 2002; Olivares et al. 2002). This work has been important in enhancing access to evidence-based treatments and demonstrating effectiveness in community settings. However, reliance on specialized psychologists to implement interventions in schools will ultimately limit wide-scale dissemination and implementation. To achieve sustainable school-based programs, responsibility must be transferred to school personnel. However, it is uncertain whether treatment delivery by community providers will be effective.

To this aim, studies have evaluated whether school-based providers (e.g., social workers, counselors) can effectively implement evidence-based interventions for various anxiety disorders (e.g., Ginsburg et al. 2008; Rapee 2000). Specific to *SAD*, a recent Canadian study by Miller and colleagues (2011) trained teachers and adolescent peer counselors to conduct *SASS* with 27 socially anxious high school students who were nominated by school personnel or self-referred. Students showed a reduction in anxiety and depression symptoms as well as behavioral avoidance following *SASS*. Masia Warner and colleagues (2014) recently completed a randomized controlled trial of 136 adolescents with *SAD* that compared *SASS* delivered by school counselors to *SASS* delivered by psychologists and to a nonspecific school counseling program (NIMH R01MH081881). Preliminary results reveal that students receiving *SASS* led by school counselors or specialized psychologists, relative to those who participated in the nonspecific intervention, showed significant reductions in *SAD* severity and higher rates of treatment response (Masia Warner et al. 2014). Based on this limited research, the approach of training school-based providers appears promising but raises questions about the types of delivery models that will support competent treatment implementation in schools.

Future Directions

School-based intervention has been shown to be an effective approach for treating *SAD* in adolescents in several countries. However, a main challenge to the success of school-based treatments is their sustainability following the removal of external support from highly specialized psychologists or grant funding. Thus, the next crucial step for our field is to obtain a better understanding of how to support competent implementation of school-based interventions utilizing resources that already exist within schools. Identifying feasible solutions will likely vary by country based on societal values, differing school structures, and availability and educational backgrounds of various school professionals. The Canadian study (Miller et al. 2011), for example, used teachers and adolescent peers to implement the *SASS* program, while the American trial (Masia Warner et al. 2014) used school counselors. From our perspective, it would be challenging to convince school administrators in the United States to permit teachers to devote resources to implementing a program like *SASS*, given the current political climate that evaluates schools based on students' achievement on national standardized tests. When selecting appropriate school personnel to deliver an intervention, it is important to consider competing demands that will take priority over mental health programming. Schools that can commit to protecting identified personnel's time for providing socio-emotional programming like *SASS* or *IAFS*, and possibly reducing administrative (e.g., making student schedules) or other nonessential responsibilities, will likely have greater success in long-term sustainability of these interventions.

Central to supporting services provided by existing school personnel will be gaining a clearer understanding of the training and consultation strategies required to promote robust program quality, although strategies may vary based on the diverse backgrounds and roles of school professionals identified as potential implementers. Overall, previous efforts to train community-based clinicians have shown that providing manuals, expert workshops, or Web-based training improves therapists' attitudes and knowledge but has minimal impact on actual skill (Beidas et al. 2009; Chagnon et al. 2007; Dimeff et al. 2009; Sholomskas and Carroll 2006). For skill acquisition, ongoing feedback and coaching is essential (Mannix et al. 2006; Miller et al. 2004; Sholomskas et al. 2005). Han and Weiss (2005) suggest a rigorous consultation model to promote high-quality implementation skills that include (1) direct observation of implementation, (2) feedback and partnering on resolving issues, (3) modeling of program techniques, and (4) attending to student improvements and connecting them to program use. Our previously mentioned controlled trial of *SASS* implemented by school counselors (Masia Warner et al. 2014) was among the initial attempts to train school personnel to independently conduct a specialized treatment; therefore, we developed a comprehensive training and consultation approach consistent with Han and Weiss' (2005) recommendations. *SASS* training consisted of (1) receipt of a treatment manual, (2) attendance at a five-hour interactive workshop coled by the treatment developer and a postdoctoral level psychologist, and (3) coleading a twelve-session *SASS* training group with a CBT-trained postdoctoral fellow with ongoing performance feedback. This initial training was followed by independent implementation of the *SASS* program with weekly individual consultation for one school period (40 min). While this training and consultation model yielded promising results (Masia Warner et al. 2014), it may be too resource intensive to be sustainable and cost-effective in the long term. On the other hand, this model may be necessary for school personnel who tend to have minimal mental health training, such as teachers. The field is in its infancy regarding how to support and sustain high-quality implementation of evidence-based interventions by school providers and would benefit from further research in this area across countries and cultures.

Another avenue for identifying feasible methods of training frontline school professionals involves evidence-based decision making about the program content and quality of implementation necessary to produce positive student outcomes. Most *SAD* interventions contain multiple treatment components (e.g., cognitive reappraisal, exposure, multiple social skills), yet we have not examined which of these are essential. Identifying active ingredients will inform which strategies should receive emphasis when training school personnel. This approach would also likely reduce program length by eliminating time spent on nonessential skills, an advancement that would further enhance intervention fit with the school environment. Information is also lacking regarding what level of treatment quality is sufficient to produce positive student outcomes. Examining links between treatment elements, program quality, and clinical outcomes will help determine critical treatment features and priorities for training (Masia Warner et al. 2013). Such research advances have the potential to result in more empirically informed approaches to training and consultation that may be effective, yet less labor intensive.

Finally, we must address methods to support the maintenance of skills over time as well as ways to train new school personnel. One option may be a "train the trainer" or pyramid model (Demchak and Browder 1990), in which one school personnel would be intensively trained to deliver the intervention and then provide training and consultation to his or her colleagues. Other variations might include initial training by experts followed by on-site consultation by school personnel with program experience or peer group supervision. Maintaining support for the program and protecting against turnover of trained staff may also be strengthened by the development of Learning Collaboratives (Cohen and Mannarino 2008). Such learning collaboratives would consist of trained school personnel across school districts with the goal of supporting training and supervisory capabilities as well as the viability and effectiveness of the program.

Conclusion

SAD is highly prevalent and impairing in adolescents, yet severely undertreated. Schools play an important role in addressing the unmet mental health needs of socially anxious youth. School-based intervention may be particularly beneficial to adolescents with *SAD* because the school environment supports a group modality and provides a rich context for practicing skills and conducting exposures. Based on these positive features, two *SAD* interventions *(IAFS and SASS)* have been specifically designed for the school setting and have demonstrated effectiveness when implemented by specialized psychologists. *SASS* has also shown to be effective when delivered by school counselors with rigorous training and consultation. This approach appears promising, yet we know little about the type of training and consultation necessary to sustain high-quality treatment delivery by school-based providers with varying educational background and resources. A better understanding of crucial intervention ingredients, as well as streamlining program content, should allow for more efficient procedures such as training school providers intensively in fewer core techniques. These strategies may be a better fit for the time constraints of the educational sector while still promoting quality delivery of efficacious interventions by school personnel to the many youngsters in need of services.

References

Albano AM, Marten PA, Holt CS (1991) Therapist's manual for cognitive-behavioral group therapy for adolescent social phobia. Unpublished manuscript

Alfano CA, Beidel DC, Turner SM (2006) Cognitive correlates of social phobia among children and adolescents. J Abnorm Child Psychol 34:189–201. doi:10.1007/s10802-005-9012-9

Angold A, Erkanli A, Farmer EMZ, Fairbank JA, Burns BJ, Keeler G, Costello EJ (2002) Psychiatric disorder, impairment, and service use in rural African American and white youth. Arch Gen Psychiatry 59:893–901. doi:10.1001/archpsyc.59.10.893

Atkins MS, Graczyk PA, Frazier SL, Jaleel AA (2003) Toward a new model for promoting urban children's mental health: accessible, effective, and sustainable school-based mental health services. Sch Psychol Rev 32:503–514

Beidas RS, Barmish AJ, Kendall PC (2009) Training as usual: can therapist behavior change after reading a manual and attending a brief workshop on cognitive behavioral therapy for youth anxiety? Behav Ther 32(5):97–101

Beidel DC, Turner SM, Morris TL (1998) Social effectiveness therapy for children: a treatment manual. Medical University of South Carolina, Charleston

Beidel DC, Turner SM, Morris TL (1999) Psychopathology of childhood social phobia. J Am Acad Child Adolesc Psychiatry 38:643–650. doi:10.1097/00004583-199906000-00010

Beidel DC, Turner SM, Morris TL (2000) Behavioral treatment of childhood social phobia. J Consult Clin Psychol 68:1072–1080. doi:10.1037//0022-006X.68.6.1072

Catron T, Harris VS, Weiss B (1998) Posttreatment results after 2 years of services in the Vanderbilt school-based counseling project. In: Epstein MH, Kutash K, Duchnowski A (eds) Outcomes for children and youth with emotional and behavioral disorders and their families: programs and evaluation best practices. PRO-ED, Austin, pp 633–656

Chagnon F, Houle J, Marcoux I, Renaud J (2007) Control-group study of an intervention training program for youth suicide prevention. Suicide Life Threat Behav 37:135–144. doi:10.1521/suli.2007.37.2.135

Cohen J, Mannarino AP (2008) Disseminating and implementing trauma-focused CBT in community settings. Trauma Violence Abuse 9:214–226. doi:10.1177/1524838008324336

Collins KA, Westra HA, Dozois DJ, Burns DD (2004) Gaps in accessing treatment for anxiety and depression: challenges for the delivery of care. Clin Psychol Rev 24:583–616. doi:10.1016/j.cpr.2004.06.001

Colognori D, Esseling P, Stewart CE, Reiss P, Lu F, Case B, Masia Warner C (2012) Self-disclosure and mental health service use in socially anxious adolescents. Sch Ment Health 4:219–230. doi:10.1007/s12310-012-9082-0

Damschroder LJ, Aron DC, Keith RE, Kirsch SR, Alexander JA, Lowery JC (2009) Fostering implementation of health services research findings into practice: a consolidated framework for advancing implementation science. Implement Sci 4:50. doi:10.1186/1748-5908-4-50

Demchak M, Browder DM (1990) An evaluation of the pyramid model of staff training in group homes for adults with severe handicaps. Educ Train Ment Retard 25:150–163

Dimeff LA, Koerner K, Woodcock EA, Beadnell B, Brown MZ, Skutch JM, Paves AP, Bazinet A, Harned MS (2009) Which training method works best? A randomized controlled trial comparing three methods of training clinicians in dialectical behavior therapy skills. Behav Res Ther 47:921–930. doi:10.1016/j.brat.2009.07.011

Fixsen DL, Naoom SF, Blase KA, Friedman RM, Wallace F (2005) Implementation research: a synthesis of the literature (FMHI #231). Tampa: University of South Florida, Louis de la Parte Florida Mental Health Institute, The National Implementation Research Network. Retrieved December 15, 2012 from http://nirn.fpg.unc.edu/resources/implementation-research-synthesis-literature

Foster S, Rollefson M, Doksum T, Noonan D, Robinson G, Teich J (2005) School mental health services in the United States, 2002–2003. DHHS Pub. No. (SMA) 05–4068. Center for Mental Health Services, Substance Abuse and Mental Health Services Administration, Rockville

Garcia-Lopez LJ (2000, 2007) Examining the efficacy of three cognitive-behavioural treatments aimed at overcoming social anxiety in adolescents. University of Murcia: Publication Service, Spain

Garcia-Lopez LJ, Irurtia MJ, Caballo VE, Diaz-Castela MM (2011) Ansiedad social y abuso psicológico [Social anxiety and psychological abuse]. Behav Psychol 19:223–236

Garcia-Lopez LJ, Olivares J, Turner SM, Beidel DC, Albano AM, Sánchez-Meca J (2002) Results at long-term among three psychological treatments for adolescents with generalized social phobia (II): clinical significance and effect size. Psicología Conductual [Behav Psychol] 10:371–385

Garcia-Lopez LJ, Olivares J, Beidel D, Albano AM, Turner S, Rosa AI (2006) Efficacy of three treatment protocols for adolescents with social anxiety disorder: a 5-year follow-up assessment. J Anxiety Disord 20:175–191. doi:10.1016/j.janxdis.2005.01.003

Garcia-Lopez LJ, Muela JA, Espinosa-Fernández L, Diaz-Castela MM (2009) Exploring the relevance of expressed emotion to the treatment of social anxiety disorder in adolescence. J Adolesc 32:1371–1376. doi:10.1016/j.adolescence.2009.08.001

Garcia-Lopez LJ, Diez-Bedmar MB, Perez-Paredes P, Tornero E (2011a) Treatment change in adolescents with social anxiety disorder: insights from corpus linguistics. Ansiedad y Estress [Anxiety Stress] 17:149–155

Garcia-Lopez LJ, Espinosa-Fernandez L, Muela JA, Diaz-Castela MM (2011b) IFAFS: Intervención en Familias & Adolescentes con Fobia Social [Therapy for Families and Adolescents with Social Phobia]. Unpublished manuscript

Garcia-Lopez LJ, Diaz-Castela MM, Muela-Martinez JA, Espinosa-Fernandez L (2014) Can parent training for parents with high levels of expressed emotion have a positive effect on their child's social anxiety improvement? J Anxiety Disord 28:812–822. doi:10.1016/j.janxdis.2014.09.001

Ginsburg GS, Becker KD, Kingery JN, Nichols T (2008) Transporting CBT for childhood anxiety disorders into inner-city school-based mental health clinics. Cogn Behav Pract 15:148–158. doi:10.1016/j.cbpra.2007.07.001

Ginsburg GS, Kendall PC, Sakolsky D, Compton SN, Piacentini J, Albano AM, Walkup JT, Sherrill J, Coffey KA, Rynn MA, Keeton CP, McCracken JT, Bergman L, Iyengar S, Birmaher B, March J (2011) Remission after acute treatment in children and adolescents with anxiety disorders: findings from the CAMS. J Consult Clin Psychol 79:806–813. doi:10.1037/a0025933

Grover RL, Ginsburg GS, Ialongo N (2007) Psychosocial outcomes of anxious first graders: a seven-year follow-up. Depress Anxiety 24:410–420. doi:10.1002/da. 20241

Han SS, Weiss B (2005) Sustainability of teacher implementation of school-based mental health programs. J Abnorm Child Psychol 33:665–679. doi:10.1007/s10802-005-7646-2

Heimberg RG, Becker RE (2002) Cognitive-behavioral group therapy for social phobia: basic mechanisms and clinical strategies. Guilford Press, New York

Horwitz SM, Leaf PJ, Leventhal JM (1998) Identification of psychosocial problems in pediatric primary care: do family attitudes make a difference? Arch Pediatr Adolesc Med 152:367–371. doi:10.1001/archpedi.152.4.367

Husky MM, Sheridan M, McGuire L, Olfson M (2011) Mental health screening and follow-up care in public high schools. J Am Acad Child Adolesc Psychiatry 50:881–891. doi:10.1016/j.jaac.2011.05.013

Juszczak L, Melinkovich P, Kaplan D (2003) Use of health and mental health services by adolescents across multiple delivery sites. J Adolesc Health 32(6S):108–118. doi:10.1016/S1054-139X(03)00073-9

Kashdan TB, Herbert JD (2001) Social anxiety disorder in childhood and adolescence: current status and future directions. Clin Child Fam Psychol Rev 4:37–61. doi:10.1023/A:1009576610507

Kataoka SH, Stein BD, Nadeem E, Wong M (2007) Who gets care? Mental health service use following a school-based suicide prevention program. J Am Acad Child Adolesc Psychiatry 46:1341–1348. doi:10.1097/chi.0b013e31813761fd
Katzelnick DJ, Kobak KA, DeLeire T, Henk HJ, Greist JH, Davidson JR, Schneier FR, Stein MB, Helstad CP (2001) Impact of generalized social anxiety disorder in managed care. Am J Psychiatry 158:1999–2007. doi:10.1176/appi.ajp.158.12.1999
Kelly MS, Lueck C (2011) Adopting a data-driven public health framework in schools: results from a multi-disciplinary survey on school-based mental health practice. Adv Sch Ment Health Promot 4(4):5–12. doi:10.1080/1754730X.2011.9715638
Kendall PC, Settipani CA, Cummings CM (2012) No need to worry: the promising future of child anxiety research. J Clin Child Adolesc Psychol 41:103–115. doi:10.1080/15374416.2012.632352
Layne AE, Bernstein GA, March JS (2006) Teacher awareness of anxiety symptoms in children. Child Psychiatry Hum Dev 36:383–392. doi:10.1007/s10578-006-0009-6
Ledley DR, Heimberg RG, Hope DA, Hayes SA, Zaider TI, Van Dyke M, Turk CL, Kraus C, Fresco DM (2009) Efficacy of a manualized and workbook-driven individual treatment for social anxiety disorder. Behav Ther 40:414–424. doi:10.1016/j.beth.2008.12.001
Lim SW, Chhabra R, Rosen A, Racine AD, Alderman EM (2012) Adolescents' views on barriers to health care: a pilot study. J Prim Care Community Health 3:99–103. doi:10.1177/2150131911422533
Lyon AR, Charlesworth-Attie S, Vander Stoep A, McCauley E (2011a) Modular psychotherapy for youth with internalizing problems: implementation with therapists in school-based health centers. Sch Psychol Rev 40:569–581
Lyon AR, McCauley E, Vander Stoep A (2011b) Toward successful implementation of evidence-based practices: characterizing the intervention context of counselors in school-based health centers. Emot Behav Disord Youth 11:19–25
Mannix KA, Blackburn IM, Garland A, Gracie J, Moorey S, Reid B, Standart S, Scott J (2006) Effectiveness of brief training in cognitive behaviour therapy techniques for palliative care practitioners. Palliat Med 20:579–584. doi:10.1177/0269216306071058
Masia Warner C, Klein RG, Dent HC, Fisher PH, Alvir J, Albano AM, Guardino M (2005) School-based intervention for adolescents with social anxiety disorder: results of a controlled study. J Abnorm Child Psychol 33:707–722. doi:10.1007/s10802-005-7649-z
Masia Warner C, Fisher PH, Shrout PE, Rathor S, Klein RG (2007) Treating adolescents with social anxiety disorder in school: an attention control trial. J Child Psychol Psychiatry 48:676–686. doi:10.1111/j.1469-7610.2007.01737.x
Masia Warner C, Brice C, Esseling PG, Stewart CE, Mufson L, Herzig K (2013) Consultants' perceptions of school counselors' ability to implement an empirically-based intervention for adolescent social anxiety disorder. J Admin Pol Ment Health Ment Health Serv Res 40:541–554. doi:10.1007/s10488-013-0498-0
Masia Warner C, Brice C, Moceri DC, Mufson L, Lynch C, Klein R, Sanchez A (2014). CBT for social anxiety disorder delivered by school counselors: Preliminary results of a randomized controlled trial. Paper presented at the Association for Behavioral and Cognitive Therapies 48th Annual Convention, Philadelphia, Nov 2014
Masia C, Beidel DC, Albano AM, Rapee RM, Turner SM, Morris TL, Klein RG (1999) Skills for Academic and Social Success. Available from Carrie Masia Warner, PhD, United States,
Masia C, Klein RG, Storch E, Corda B (2001) School-based behavioral treatment of social anxiety disorder: results of a pilot study. J Am Acad Child Adolesc Psychiatry 40:780–786. doi:10.1097/00004583-200107000-00012
Merikangas KR, He JP, Burnstein M, Swanson SA, Avenevoli S, Cui L, Benjet C, Georgiades K, Swendsen J (2010) Lifetime prevalence of mental disorders in U.S. adolescents: results from the national comorbidity survey replication-adolescent supplement (NCS-A). J Am Acad Child Adolesc Psychiatry 49:980–989. doi:10.1016/j.jaac.2010.05.017
Mesa F, Beidel DC, Bunnell BE (2014) An examination of psychopathology and daily impairment in adolescents with social anxiety disorder. PLoS One 9(4):e93668. doi:10.1371/journal.pone.0093668

Meyers DC, Durlak JA, Wandersman A (2012) The quality implementation framework: a synthesis of critical steps in the implementation process. Am J Community Psychol 50:462–480. doi:10.1007/s10464-012-9522-x
Miller WR, Yahne CE, Moyers TB, Martinez J, Pirritano M (2004) A randomized trial of methods to help clinicians learn motivational interviewing. J Consult Clin Psychol 72:1050–1062. doi:10.1037/0022-006X.72.6.1050
Miller LD, Laye-Gindhu A, Liu Y, March JS, Thordarson DS, Garland EJ (2011) Evaluation of a preventive intervention for child anxiety in two randomized attention-control school trials. Behav Res Ther 49:315–323. doi:10.1016/j.brat.2011.02.006
Olivares J, Garcia-Lopez LJ, Beidel DC, Turner SM (1998) Social effectiveness therapy for adolescents—Spanish version. Unpublished manuscript
Olivares J, Garcia-Lopez LJ, Beidel DC, Turner SM, Albano AM, Hidalgo MD (2002) Results at long-term among three psychological treatments for adolescents with generalized social phobia (I): statistical significance. Psicologia Conductual [Behav Psychol] 10:147–164
Ranta K, Kaltiala-Heino R, Pelkonen M, Marttunen M (2009) Associations between peer victimization, self-reported depression and social phobia among adolescents: the role of comorbidity. J Adolesc 32:77–93. doi:10.1016/j.adolescence.2007.11.005
Ranta K, Kaltiala-Heino R, Fröjd S, Marttunen M (2013) Peer victimization and social phobia: a follow-up study among adolescents. Soc Psychiatry Psychiatr Epidemiol 48:533–544. doi:10.1007/s00127-012-0583-9
Rapee RM (1998) Overcoming shyness and social phobia: a step-by-step guide. First Rowman & Littlefield, Lanham
Rapee RM (2000) Group treatment of children with anxiety disorders: outcome and predictors of treatment response. Aust J Psychol 52:125–129. doi:10.1080/00049530008255379
Rapee R, Wignall A, Spence S, Lyneham H, Cobham V (2008) Helping your anxious child: a step-by-step guide for parents. New Harbinger, Oakland
Ryan JL, Masia Warner C (2012) Treating adolescents with social anxiety disorders in schools. Child Adolesc Psychiatr Clin N Am 21:105–118. doi:10.1016/j.chc.2011.08.011
Shediac-Rizkallah MC, Bone LR (1998) Planning for the sustainability of community-based health programs: conceptual frameworks and future directions for research, practice, and policy. Health Educ Res 13:87–108. doi:10.1093/her/13.1.87
Sholomskas DE, Carroll KM (2006) One small step for manuals: computer-assisted training in twelve-step facilitation. J Stud Alcohol 67:939–945
Sholomskas DE, Syracuse-Siewert G, Rounsaville BJ, Ball SA, Nuro KF, Carroll KM (2005) We don't train in vain: a dissemination trial of three strategies of training clinicians in cognitive-behavioral therapy. J Consult Clin Psychol 73:106–115. doi:10.1037/0022-006X.73.1.106
Turner SM, Beidel DC, Cooley MR (1994) Social effectiveness therapy: a program for overcoming social anxiety and social phobia. Turndel, Mt. Pleasant
Wahl OF (2012) Stigma as a barrier to recovery from mental illness. Trends Cogn Sci 16:9–10. doi:10.1016/j.tics.2011.11.002
Walkup JT, Albano AM, Piacentini J, Birmaher B, Compton SN, Sherrill JT, Ginsburg GS, Rynn MA, McCracken J, Waslick B, Iyengar S, March JS, Kendall PC (2008) Cognitive behavioral therapy, sertraline, or a combination in childhood anxiety. N Engl J Med 359:2753–2766. doi:10.1056/NEJMoa0804633
Wittchen HU, Stein MB, Kessler RC (1999) Social fears and social phobia in a community sample of adolescents and young adults: prevalence, risk factors, and co-morbidity. Psychol Med 29:309–323. doi:10.1017/S0033291798008174
Wren FJ, Scholle SH, Heo J, Comer DM (2003) Pediatric mood and anxiety syndromes in primary care: who gets identified? Int J Psychiatry Med 33:1–16. doi:10.2190/UT6D-RDFG-LBT7-G39N
Wu P, Hoven CW, Bird HR, Moore RE, Cohen P, Alegria M, Dulcan MK, Goodman SH, Horwitz SM, Lichtman JH, Narrow WE, Rae DS, Regier DA, Roper MT (1999) Depressive and disruptive disorders and mental health service utilization in children and adolescents. J Am Acad Child Adolesc Psychiatry 38:1081–1090. doi:10.1097/00004583-199909000-00010

Social Skill-Based Treatment for Social Anxiety Disorder in Adolescents

13

Franklin Mesa, Thien-An Le, and Deborah C. Beidel

Social Skill Deficits

Adolescents with social anxiety disorder (SAD) exhibit anxious behaviors and social withdrawal across many social situations (e.g., public speaking, interacting with groups, or initiating conversations; Beidel et al. 2007b; Mesa et al. 2014; Mesa et al. 2011). In many instances, the pervasive shyness displayed by adolescents with this disorder leads to reduced opportunities to develop, practice, and refine skills necessary for effective social interaction (Albano et al. 1995a; Albano 1995). A growing body of empirical evidence indicates that underlying social skill deficits are a common feature of SAD in adolescents (Alfano et al. 2008; Beidel and Turner 2007; Inderbitzen-Nolan et al. 2007). Often, these deficits remain unaffected despite a significant decrease in anxiety following psychosocial or psychopharmacological treatment (Beidel and Turner 2007; Compton et al. 2014; Spence et al. 1999; Spence 2003).

Broadly defined, social skills are the behaviors necessary for effective social communication and effective social functioning. Definitions of social skill vary but typically include molecular behaviors that are verbal or nonverbal in nature. Nonverbal skills include eye contact, physical posture, and facial gaze, whereas verbal behaviors include the specific words spoken as well as what are known as paralinguistic features such as voice volume and vocal tone. All of these behaviors combine to result in more complicated (sometimes known as molar) social behaviors such as initiating and maintaining conversations, assertiveness, and joining groups. Deficits in both molecular and molar social skills have been found in adolescents with SAD.

F. Mesa, MS • T.-A. Le • D.C. Beidel, PhD (✉)
Department of Psychology, University of Central Florida,
4111 Pictor Lane, Orlando, FL 32816, USA
e-mail: franklin.mesa@knights.ucf.edu; an.le@knights.ucf.edu; deborah.beidel@ucf.edu

K. Ranta et al. (eds.), *Social Anxiety and Phobia in Adolescents: Development, Manifestation and Intervention Strategies*, DOI 10.1007/978-3-319-16703-9_13

Commensurate with observations of children and adults with SAD, adolescents with SAD exhibit social skill deficits during various social tasks. Beidel's group utilized two tasks: a read-aloud task and a role-play social interaction. During the read-aloud task, participants read an age-appropriate story aloud for 10 min with the assessor and a same-age peer as an audience. The role-play task consisted of five role-play scenes, each introduced by the assessor and followed by two standardized statements from a same-age peer. Participants were instructed to respond to the peer as if they were actually in the situation. Independent evaluators blinded to diagnostic group rate adolescents with SAD as less effective (i.e., less skilled) during the read-aloud and role-play social interaction tasks (Alfano et al. 2008; Beidel et al. 2007b). Adolescents with SAD also display significantly longer speech latencies when interacting with a same-aged peer (Alfano et al. 2008; Beidel et al. 2007b). When compared to preadolescent children with SAD, however, adolescents with SAD exhibit more skill and less anxiety during these social tasks (Rao et al. 2007). Inderbitzen-Nolan and colleagues (2007) examined social skill using tasks with less structure. Participants were given 3 min to prepare a 10-min speech from a list of potential topics and then delivered the speech before a small audience. Additionally, adolescents engaged in an unstructured conversation with an unfamiliar same-sex and same-age peer for 10 min. Socially anxious adolescents rated themselves as less skilled during both tasks relative to the self-ratings of adolescents with no psychiatric disorder. A similar speech task was paired with a novel social interaction task in a recent study (Mesa et al. 2014). During the novel task, adolescents played a video game with an unfamiliar same-sex confederate for 10 min. Confederates were instructed to deliver standardized questions every 2 min if the participant had not spoken in the previous 2 min. Adolescents with SAD appeared less engaged socially while playing the video game with a confederate. Specifically, they asked fewer questions and initiated conversation less frequently relative to adolescents with no psychiatric disorder. Adolescents with SAD also exhibited poorer skill while delivering the speech, as they spoke for a shorter duration despite discussing a similar number of topics than adolescents with no psychiatric disorder. Therefore, the speeches delivered by adolescents with SAD appeared to be devoid of details and substance, which will result in poorer evaluations by listeners.

Unfortunately, peer interactions in adolescence demand refined abilities (e.g., maintain lengthy conversations or initiate spontaneous conversations) that many adolescents with SAD are unable to practice (Englund et al. 2000; Obradovic et al. 2006). The combination of elevated anxiety, avoidance, and social skills in adolescents with SAD deficits makes it difficult to socialize appropriately and hinders the achievement of typical development milestones (e.g., establishing a social network; Ballenger et al. 1998; Eder and Nenga 2003; Inderbitzen et al. 1997). In turn, social skill deficits in this group may contribute to decreased social functioning and support, particularly among girls (Inderbitzen et al. 1997; LaGreca and Lopez 1998; Vernberg et al. 1992).

These data highlight the importance of addressing social skill deficits in adolescents with SAD. Social skills are malleable and may be significantly improved in individuals with SAD, including adolescents (Albano 1995). The procedures for enhancing skills entail behavioral strategies for teaching and refining skills, often through some combination of instruction, modeling, behavioral rehearsals, positive reinforcement, and therapist feedback. Many successful interventions for SAD use these strategies.

One conceptualization of social skill deficits, acquisition deficits, posits that an individual does not have a particular social skill in their behavioral repertoire and therefore does not demonstrate the skill (Gresham 1997). An alternative conceptualization, performance deficit, refers to situations where the individual possesses the skill but fails to demonstrate the skill in one or more social situations. Empirical evidence indicates that both of these skill deficit processes likely contribute to the difficulties observed in adolescents with SAD (Spence et al. 1999). Thus, social skill-based interventions for youth with SAD are founded on these underlying assumptions (Gresham 1997). While extant studies support the use of social skill training (SST) to increase effective social interaction in adolescents with mild to moderate social withdrawal (Christoff et al. 1985; Jupp and Griffiths 1990), it is unlikely that SST alone will yield an optimal treatment outcome in adolescents with SAD (Beidel and Turner 2007). Rather, SST is an important component of successful interventions for SAD. Below, we discuss current interventions for SAD that include a SST component.

Current Social Skill-Based Interventions

Cognitive-Behavioral Group Therapy

Cognitive-Behavioral Group Therapy for Adolescents (CBGT-A; Albano et al. 1991; 1995b) was the first treatment program developed specifically for adolescents with SAD. CBGT-A combines established methods for treating SAD in adults (Heimberg et al. 1985, 1990, 1993) with early models of SST (Christoff et al. 1985). The intervention is delivered in a group format over 16 sessions, each approximately 1.5 h in duration. CBGT-A is organized into two phases: (a) psychoeducation and skills building and (b) behavioral exposure. During the psychoeducational and skill-building phase, patients are provided with psychoeducation about social anxiety and participate in SST, problem-solving training, assertiveness training, and cognitive restructuring over 7 sessions. Therapists emphasize modeling, shaping, and role-playing scenarios to help adolescents acquire and master necessary social skills. Session 8 is spent preparing parents and adolescents for the behavioral exposure phase (sessions 9 through 16) during which structured and graduated in vivo exposure therapy is conducted. Each adolescent works through an individualized fear hierarchy comprised of situations that produce varying levels of distress. Group members also receive additional exposure by participating in the exposure situations of other members. Participants are encouraged to utilize the coping strategies learned in the skill-building phase during exposure to regulate their anxiety. Additionally, participants are instructed to complete in vivo exposures between sessions.

Two studies examining the efficacy of CBGT-A for SAD have been published. In a small pilot study, four of five adolescents treated with CBGT-A evidenced SAD in partial remission 3 months after treatment (Albano et al. 1995b). At 3-months after completion of treatment, SAD decreased to subclinical levels for four out of five adolescents. At 12-month follow-up, four adolescents did not meet diagnostic criteria for any psychiatric disorder, while the fifth was diagnosed with SAD in partial remission. Participants also reported reduced ratings of distress and fewer negative cognitions during an impromptu speech and an oral reading task. A subsequent controlled trial of CBGT-A in female adolescents with SAD found that 45 % of individuals treated with CBGT-A no longer met diagnostic criteria for SAD, whereas only 4 % of individuals in the wait-list control group lost their SAD diagnosis at posttreatment (Hayward et al. 2000). One year following the conclusion of the study, however, treatment gains in the CBGT-A group had disappeared and no group differences were observed in the rate of SAD. Collectively, these studies support the short-term efficacy of CBGT-A for SAD; however, it is unclear whether this intervention produces long-term improvement reliably without booster sessions. CBGT-A has also been compared to other active treatments for adolescents with social anxiety disorder. These comparative trials are discussed later in the chapter.

Spence's Integrated Cognitive-Behavioral Treatment Program

Another efficacious treatment for social anxiety disorder combines traditional CBT with social skills training. A randomized, controlled trial examined the efficacy of a comprehensive treatment program for children and adolescents (aged 7–14; $M = 10.64$) with SAD (Spence et al. 2000). The program included group-based SST, relaxation training, social problem-solving, positive self-instruction, cognitive challenging, and graduated exposure therapy given over 12 sessions held once per week. Booster sessions occur 3 months and 6 months posttreatment. Each session was 60 min in duration, followed by a 30-min play period during which participants prompted to and reinforced for practicing their social skills. Weekly homework assignments encouraged participants to practice social skills outside of session and include a graduated exposure task. Additionally, some youth in the study were randomized to a parent involvement condition in which parents observed the treatment sessions and were provided with instruction in prompting, encouraging, modeling, and reinforcing appropriate proactive social behavior in their children.

While adolescents were not targeted specifically in this trial, a group of children aged 12–14 years (i.e., early adolescence) was included. At posttreatment, both treatment groups significantly reduced the severity and rate of SAD relative to the wait-list control condition. Furthermore, parents rated the children and young adolescents who were treated in one of the active treatment conditions as having improved social skills. These outcomes were maintained at 6- and 12-month follow-up. Although there was a trend toward a lower rate of SAD diagnosis in the parent involvement condition, no significant differences were found between treatment conditions. Finally, a significant correlation was reported between parent-rated social skill improvements and youth-reported social anxiety reductions from pretreatment to 12-month follow-up. These findings support the utility of SST in treatment paradigms for SAD.

Social Effectiveness Therapy for Children

Social Effectiveness Therapy for Children (SET-C; Beidel et al. 2000b) is a behavioral, group-based intervention for youth aged 8–17 with SAD. SET-C was adapted from a successful treatment program for adults with SAD. Participants complete two sessions each week for 12 weeks. One session consists of individual graduated exposure therapy, typically 60 min in duration. The second session contains two components. Participants first complete group-based SST. The content of the training sessions focuses on general interpersonal skills and identified as specifically problematic for adolescents with SAD, such as listening skills and topic transitioning. Strategies used to teach and reinforce appropriate social behavior include instruction, modeling, behavior rehearsal, feedback, and social reinforcement. SET-C targets 6 major topic areas: nonverbal social skills (eye contact, smiles), initiating and maintaining conversations, joining groups of children, friendship establishment and maintenance, positive assertion, and negative assertion. SST groups are held once per week and consist of 4–5 children. Homework assignments are given for participants to practice the social skill learned in SST outside of session.

Unique to SET-C is the peer generalization component, designed to provide practice of social skills in community settings (bowling alleys, pizza parlors, museums) with same-aged friendly (non-anxious) peers. These 90-min generalization sessions occur immediately following group SST. The friendly peers are trained to engage the socially anxious youth frequently. Generalization sessions provide SET-C participants the opportunity to practice their social skills in situations where they may actually interact with peers.

The initial trial of SET-C did not include youth in the adolescent age range. Nevertheless, 67 % of the individuals who received SET-C relative to 5 % of the individuals who received an active, nonspecific anxiety intervention no longer met diagnostic criteria for SAD at posttreatment (Beidel et al. 2000a). Furthermore, children who received SET-C reported significantly less social anxiety and evidenced greater global functioning at posttreatment. Treatment gains in the SET-C group were maintained or improved at a 6-month follow-up assessment for all but one child. This sample was examined again, along with two adolescents treated with SET-C, at 3 years (Beidel et al. 2005) and 5 years following treatment (Beidel et al. 2006). By the 5-year posttreatment assessment, all youth in the sample were of adolescent age. Participants continued to evidence maintenance of treatment gains through 5-year follow-up in self-reported social anxiety, social interaction and read-aloud tasks, clinician ratings of anxiety, and loss of SAD diagnosis. At 5-year follow-up, global functioning in the adolescent treatment responders who received SET-C was comparable to adolescents with no psychiatric disorder.

In a subsequent RCT (Beidel et al. 2007a), SET-C was compared to fluoxetine and pill placebo in children and adolescents aged 7–17 ($M = 11.61$). SET-C and fluoxetine significantly reduced social distress and behavioral avoidance and increased social functioning relative to pill placebo; however, only youth who received SET-C displayed significantly improved social skill as rated by independent evaluators relative to youth in the fluoxetine and pill placebo conditions. Furthermore, treatment gains among those who received SET-C continued through the entire 12-week program, whereas the maximum effect for fluoxetine was observed by 8 weeks of treatment. SET-C further demonstrated superiority at 1-year follow-up, where youth treated with SET-C demonstrated a lower relapse rate (10.3 %) than youth treated with fluoxetine (17 %). Thus, SET-C demonstrates efficacy in producing reduced social anxiety and improved social skill, outcomes which are maintained long after treatment is completed. These outcomes again highlight the importance of a SST component in SAD interventions. SET-C has now been adapted for school (Skills for Academic and Social Success; Masia et al. 2001; see Chap. 12) and community settings (Baer and Garland 2005).

A Spanish version of SET-C adapted for adolescents, SET-Asv (Social Effectiveness Therapy for Adolescents-Spanish version; Olivares et al. 1998), eliminated the peer generalization sessions in an effort to streamline the treatment. In a series of studies, Garcia-Lopez, Olivares, and their colleagues (2002, 2006; Olivares et al. 2002) compared SET-Asv to CBGT-A and Therapy for Adolescents with Generalized Social Phobia (Intervención en Adolescentes con Fobia Social: Therapy for Adolescents with Social Phobia (IAFS); Garcia-Lopez 2000, 2007).

Therapy for Adolescents with (Generalized) Social Phobia

The original Therapy for Adolescents with Generalized Social Phobia (Intervencion en Adolescentes con Fobia Social; IAFS) is a school-based program that consists of 12 90-min group sessions. It includes psychoeducation, social skills training, exposure, and cognitive restructuring techniques. In particular, sessions 1 and 2 focus on psychoeducation, cognitive therapy (realistic thinking), and bibliotherapy. During sessions 3–8, adolescents are trained in social skills included in the SET protocols (initiating and maintaining conversations, attending and remembering, being assertive, giving and receiving compliments, establishing and maintaining friendships). In addition, sessions 6 and 8 include the use of unknown peer assistants of same and opposite sex to assist in initiating and maintaining conversations. Sessions 9–12 deal with public speaking training and relapse prevention. Speeches are video recorded and followed by a discussion of the participant's performance first from the perspective of the participant and then from additional group members. These discussions are followed by a review of the video recording. Similar to social skills sessions, additionally to speaking in front of their group mates and the therapist, sessions 11 and 12 include the use of assistants, which took place in the conference hall of each school. Weekly individual sessions in IAFS are optional and address a range of social skill-related issues. In a comparative study, results at posttreatment and at 1- and 5-year follow-up

(Garcia-Lopez et al. 2002, 2006; Olivares et al. 2002), participants in all three groups (SET-Asv, CBGT-A and IAFS) were significantly and clinically improved and maintained that improvement even 5 years later. Some of the social situations usually treated during therapy can be found in Garcia-Lopez (2013). Further, Garcia-Lopez et al. (2009) explored whether high levels of expressed emotion (EE) in parents could be associated with lower treatment outcome in adolescents with social phobia. Findings revealed the parents' level of EE moderated the treatment outcome of their adolescents. To further examine the role of EE, Garcia-Lopez et al. (2014) have conducted a RCT to examine the IAFS with an added parent training component (named as IFAFS), and the original IAFS, focused solely on intervening with the adolescent (no parental involvement). Posttreatment and 12-month follow-up findings showed that school-based intervention with parent training (IFAFS) was superior to the adolescent-specific program, yielding significant reductions in diagnosis remission, social, and depressive symptomatology, particularly when the EE status of parents changed. Overall, the findings suggest that high-EE parents of children with social anxiety need to be involved in their child's therapy. This is in line with Wei and Kendall's (2014) finding suggesting there is potential in the assessment of parent/family factors prior to treatment followed by a target-oriented implementation of parent training.

An adaptation of SET-C for adolescents is Skills for Social and Academic Success (SASS; Fisher et al. 2004). SASS is a school-based intervention that includes social skills training, in vivo exposure, and weekend peer generalization sessions. As an entire chapter of this volume is devoted to school-based interventions, including SASS, we will not discuss it further here (see also Chap. 12).

Future Directions

Despite the success of SET-C and other social skill-based interventions in treating adolescent SAD, these interventions are often difficult to implement in treatment settings outside of a university setting for two primary reasons (Wong-Sarver et al. 2013). First, these interventions depend on skill practice outside of sessions to promote skill generalization. In the past, many SST programs have failed to generalize outside of the clinic setting (Spence 2003). In other words, children and adolescents become very socially skilled in the therapist's office but never use the skills in community settings. SET-C attempts to address this limitation by including peer generalization sessions as part of the treatment protocol. However, generalization sessions require the assistance of peers from the community, and recruitment of a cadre of peers without psychiatric disorders is probably not feasible for clinicians in community settings. There is also a substantial monetary and time cost to organizing and financing generalization sessions.

Second, poor homework compliance is reported often by therapists. Homework assignments are integral to SST paradigms, providing patients with necessary additional practice in varied situations outside of the treatment group setting. Various factors contribute to poor homework compliance, including patient report of difficulty completing the assignment and failure by parents to provide patients the opportunity to complete homework (e.g., by taking the patient to a homework activity) or to assist patients in completing the homework. A promising solution to these two limitations to dissemination is a virtual environment-based intervention (Wong-Sarver et al. 2013). A virtual environment (VE) may provide numerous virtual characters and settings to which patients may generalize social skill and allow patients to practice at home without parental assistance.

The Pegasys-VR™ system (Beidel et al. 2011) allows providers in non-research settings to provide peer generalization experiences without the need for same-age peers. The VE allows clinicians to (a) provide practice with a variety of interpersonal partners, (b) use a dose-controlled strategy to control the pace of the training and practice, and (c) assure acquisition of basic skills before proceeding to more advanced and challenging interactions. This saves clinician's time (i.e., recruiting, screening and training peers, coordinating, traveling, and supervising activities) and money (i.e., for social activities). The VE assures skill acquisition and increases the likelihood that skills acquired in the clinic are used in real-life interactions. With respect to homework assignments, *Pegasys-VR*™ allows children to have repeated behavioral practice with different people in a variety of social situations independent of parental involvement.

The first iteration of *Pegasys-VR*™ can be used with children ages 8–14 and consisted of multiple locations within a school setting and had six avatars: two classroom teachers, a school principal, a gym teacher, a bully, a "cool girl," and a "smart girl." Four social skill areas were targeted in the prototype, including greetings and initiating conversations, maintaining conversations, and assertiveness. Each skill area had three skill levels that allowed the therapist to modulate the difficulty of the interaction for patients. The characters had preconstructed responses that varied by skill level, allowing therapists to promote skill generalization by creating dozens of unique situations. Using a Wizard of Oz interface, the therapist controls the avatar's response, thereby controlling the flow of the conversation.

The initial investigation of the *Pegasys-VR*™ prototype (Wong-Sarver et al. 2013) examined feasibility and acceptability of the VE. The preliminary data indicated that families were enthusiastic about the VE, found it easy to use, and believed that it was helpful. Clinicians found the program easy to use and a valuable tool for intervention. There were insufficient data to examine efficacy in the aforementioned VE trial and adolescents were not included. Furthermore, adjustments are necessary to increase interest and compliance in the homework component of this intervention and expanded product development, including avatars that will represent older adolescents, is underway. Even so, by potentially circumventing the shortcomings of traditional social skill-based interventions, the VE-modified SET-C represents a promising advancement in social skill-based interventions for SAD, particularly for clinicians working outside of a university setting. The data presented here clearly support the inclusion of SST in psychosocial interventions for SAD; therefore, improving the feasibility of delivering SST for all clinicians increases the likelihood that adolescents with SAD will receive this important training.

Summary

There is a growing literature that suggests that social skills training may be a necessary element to optimize treatment for adolescents with SAD. Typically, most individuals acquire social skills through social interactions – they observe others (modeling and information transfer) and they receive feedback (positive or negative) as they interact. However, anxiety in social settings leads to avoidance, thereby denying individuals with SAD the opportunity to observe others interact and model appropriate social behavior. Given the documented chronic nature of this condition, it is highly likely that years of social isolation prevented opportunities to learn and practice social skills through social interaction with others. Therefore, it should not be surprising that at least some adolescents with SAD lack the skills necessary for successful social engagement. If one does not know the mechanics of downhill skiing, anxiety-reduction procedures alone would not produce a successful run down the mountain.

SST interventions designed by different research groups have adopted SST as one component in the efficacious treatment programs for adolescents with SAD, and these programs appear to be equally effective when implemented in clinical or school settings. Furthermore, treatment gains are maintained at least 5 years later. The major challenges for optimal utilization of SST in adolescents are the same as they are for other any other group: homework compliance and skill generalization. Innovative strategies, including the use of non-anxious peers, school classmates, and VEs hold significant promise of optimization and dissemination.

References

Albano AM (1995) Treatment of social anxiety in adolescents. Cogn Behav Pract 2:271–298

Albano AM, Marten PA, Holt CS (1991) Cognitive-behavioral group treatment of adolescent social phobia: therapist's manual. Unpublished manuscript, State University of New York at Albany

Albano AM, DiBartolo PM, Heimberg RG, Barlow DH (1995a) Children and adolescents: assessment and treatment. In: Heimberg RG, Liebowitz MR, Hope DA, Schneier FR (eds) Social phobia: diagnosis, assessment and treatment. Guilford Press, New York

Albano AM, Marten PA, Holt CS, Heimberg RG, Barlow DH (1995b) Cognitive-behavioral group treatment for social phobia in adolescents: a preliminary study. J Nerv Ment Dis 183: 649–656

Alfano CA, Beidel DC, Turner SM (2008) Negative self-imagery among adolescents with social phobia: a test of an adult model of the disorder. J Clin Child Adolesc Psychol 37:327–336

Baer S, Garland J (2005) Pilot study of community-based cognitive behavioral group therapy for adolescents with social phobia. J Am Acad Child Adolesc Psychiatry 44:258–264

Ballenger JC, Davidson J, Lecrubrier Y, Nutt D, Bobes J, Beidel DC et al (1998) Consensus statement on social anxiety disorder from the international consensus group on depression and anxiety. J Clin Psychiatry 59:54–60

Beidel DC, Spitalnick JS, Wong-Sarver N (2011) Pegasys-VR: development of a virtual environment for childhood social phobia. University of Central Florida. Unpublished manuscript

Beidel DC, Turner SM (2007) Shy children, phobic adults: the nature and treatment of social anxiety disorder. American Psychological Association, Washington, DC

Beidel DC, Turner SM, Morris TL (2000a) Behavioral treatment of childhood social phobia. J Consult Clin Psychol 68:1072–1080
Beidel DC, Turner SM, Morris TL (2000b) Social effectiveness therapy for children and adolescents (SET-C). Multi-Health Systems, Toronto
Beidel DC, Turner SM, Young B, Paulson A (2005) Social effectiveness therapy for children: three-year follow-up. J Consult Clin Psychol 17:721–725
Beidel DC, Turner SM, Young BJ (2006) Social effectiveness therapy for children: five years later. Behav Ther 37:416–425
Beidel DC, Turner SM, Sallee FR, Ammerman RT, Crosby LA, Pathak S (2007a) SET-C versus fluoxetine in the treatment of childhood social phobia. J Am Acad Child Adolesc Psychiatry 46(12):1622–1632
Beidel DC, Turner SM, Young BJ, Ammerman RT, Sallee FR, Crosby L (2007b) Psychopathology of adolescent social phobia. J Psychopathol Behav Assess 29:47–54
Christoff KA, Scott WO, Kelley ML, Schlundt D, Baer G, Kelly JA (1985) Social skills and social problem-solving training for shy young adolescents. Behav Ther 16:468–477
Compton SN, Peris TS, Almirall D, Birmaher B, Sherrill J et al (2014) Predictors and moderators of treatment response in childhood anxiety disorders: results from the CAMS trial. J Consult Clin Psychol. doi:10.1037/a0035458
Eder D, Nenga SK (2003) Socialization in adolescence. In: Delamater J (ed) Handbook of social psychology. Kluwer Academic/Plenum Publishers, New York
Englund MM, Levy AK, Hyson DM, Sroufe LA (2000) Adolescent social competence: effectiveness in a group setting. Child Dev 71:1049–1060
Fisher PH, Masia-Warner C, Klein RG (2004) Skills for social and academic success: a school-based intervention for social anxiety disorder in adolescents. Clin Child Fam Psychol Rev 7:241–249
Garcia-Lopez LJ (2000, 2007). Examining the efficacy of three cognitive-behavioural treatments aimed at overcoming social anxiety in adolescents. University of Murcia: Publication Service. Murcia, Spain
Garcia-Lopez LJ (2013) Tratando…trastorno de ansiedad social [Treating…social anxiety disorder]. Piramide, Madrid
Garcia-Lopez LJ, Olivares J, Turner SM, Beidel DC, Albano AM, Sanchez-Meca J (2002) Results at long-term among three psychological treatments for adolescents with generalized social phobia (II): clinical significance and effect size. Psicol Conduct (Behav Psychol) 10:165–179
Garcia-Lopez LJ, Olivares J, Beidel D, Albano AM, Turner S, Rosa AI (2006) Efficacy of three treatment protocols for adolescents with social anxiety disorder: a 5-year follow-up assessment. J Anxiety Disord 20:175–191. doi:10.1016/j.janxdis.2005.01.003
Garcia-Lopez LJ, Muela JA, Espinosa-Fernández L, Diaz-Castela MM (2009) Exploring the relevance of expressed emotion to the treatment of social anxiety disorder in adolescence. J Adolesc 32:1371–1376. doi:10.1016/j.adolescence.2009.08.001
Garcia-Lopez LJ, Diaz-Castela MM, Muela-Martinez JA, Espinosa-Fernandez L (2014) Can parent training for parents with high levels of expressed emotion have a positive effect on their child's social anxiety improvement? J Anxiety Disord. doi:10.1016/j.janxdis.2014.09.001
Gresham FM (1997) Social competence and students with behavior disorders: where we've been, where we are, and where we should go. Educ Treat Child 20:233–249
Hayward C, Varady S, Albano AM, Theinemann M, Henderson L, Schatzberg AF (2000) Cognitive-behavioral group therapy for social phobia in female adolescents: results of a pilot study. J Am Acad Child Adolesc Psychiatry 39:721–726
Heimberg RG, Becker RE, Goldfinger K, Vermilyea JA (1985) Treatment of social phobia by exposure, cognitive restructuring, and homework assignments. J Nerv Ment Dis 173:236–245
Heimberg RG, Dodge CS, Hope DA, Kennedy CR, Zollo LJ, Becker RE (1990) Cognitive behavioral group treatment for social phobia: comparison with a credible placebo control. Cogn Ther Res 14:1–23
Heimberg RG, Salzman DG, Holt CS, Blendell KA (1993) Cognitive-behavioral group treatment for social phobia: effectiveness at five year follow up. Cogn Ther Res 17:325–339

Inderbitzen H, Walters K, Bukowski A (1997) The role of social anxiety in adolescent peer relations: differences among sociometric status groups and rejected subgroups. J Clin Child Psychol 26:338–348

Inderbitzen-Nolan HM, Anderson ER, Johnson HS (2007) Subjective versus objective behavioral ratings following two analogue tasks: a comparison of socially phobic and non-anxious adolescents. J Anxiety Disord 21:76–90

Jupp JJ, Griffiths MD (1990) Self-concept changes in shy, socially isolated adolescents following social skills training emphasizing role-plays. Aust Psychol 25:165–177

La Greca AM, Lopez N (1998) Social anxiety among adolescents: linkages with peer relations and friendships. J Abnorm Child Psychol 26:83–94

Masia CL, Klein RG, Storch E, Corda B (2001) School-based behavioral treatment for social anxiety disorder in adolescents: results of a pilot study. J Am Acad Child Adolesc Psychiatry 40:780–786

Mesa F, Nieves MM, Beidel DC (2011) Clinical presentation of social anxiety disorder in adolescents and young adults. In: Alfano CA, Beidel DC (eds) Social anxiety disorder in adolescent and young adults. American Psychological Association Press, Washington, DC

Mesa F, Beidel DC, Bunnell BE (2014) An examination of psychopathology and daily impairment in adolescents with social anxiety disorder. PLoS One 9:e93668. doi:10.1371/journal.pone.0093668

Obradovic J, van Dulman MH, Yates TM, Carlson EA, Egeland B (2006) Developmental assessment of competence from early childhood to middle adolescence. J Adolesc 29:857–889

Olivares J, Garcia-Lopez LJ, Beidel DC, Turner SM (1998) Social effectiveness therapy for adolescents—Spanish version. Unpublished manuscript

Olivares J, Garcia-Lopez LJ, Beidel DC, Turner SM, Albano AM, Hidalgo MD (2002) Results at long-term among three psychological treatments for adolescents with generalized social phobia (I): statistical significance. Psicol Conduct (Behav Psychol) 10:147–164

Rao PA, Beidel DC, Turner SM, Ammerman RT, Crosby LE, Sallee FR (2007) Social anxiety disorder in childhood and adolescence: descriptive psychopathology. Behav Res Ther 45:1181–1191

Spence SH (2003) Social skills training with children and young people: theory, evidence and practice. Child Adolesc Mental Health 8(2):84–96

Spence SH, Donovan C, Brechman-Toussaint M (1999) Social skills, social outcomes, and cognitive features of childhood social phobia. J Abnorm Psychol 108:211–221

Spence SH, Donovan C, Brechman-Toussaint M (2000) The treatment of childhood social phobia: the effectiveness of a social skills training-based, cognitive-behavioural intervention, with and without parental involvement. J Child Psychol Psychiatry 41:713–726

Vernberg E, Abwender D, Ewell K, Beery S (1992) Social anxiety and peer relationships in early adolescence: a prospective analysis. J Clin Child Psychol 21:189–196

Wei C, Kendall PC (2014) Parental involvement: contribution to childhood anxiety and its treatment. Clin Child Fam Psychol Rev 17(4):319–339

Wong-Sarver N, Beidel DC, Spitalnick JS (2013) The feasibility and acceptability of virtual environments in the treatment of childhood social anxiety disorder. J Clin Child Adolesc Psychol 43(1):63–73

Pharmacotherapy for Adolescent Social Phobia

14

Michael Van Ameringen, Jasmine Turna, Beth Patterson, and Chloe Lau

Introduction

Social anxiety disorder (SAD), formerly known as social phobia, is an anxiety disorder characterized by excessive fear of exposure to situations that involve potential scrutiny by others. SAD is a common psychiatric problem in children and adolescents, often presenting with comorbid anxiety and mood disorders. Although the onset of SAD is typically in late childhood or early adolescence, most afflicted individuals go undiagnosed for years, not seeking treatment until adulthood (Mancini et al. 2005).

In the past, SAD or social phobia was considered to be a temporary condition ("shyness"), which children would outgrow, and as a consequence was infrequently diagnosed in childhood (Stein et al. 2001). However, with a lifetime prevalence rate of 12.1 % in the US adult population (Kessler et al. 2005), SAD has been found to be the third most prevalent psychiatric disorder in the community in the adult population (Kessler et al. 2005). In adolescents, lifetime prevalence of SAD has been estimated to be 8.6 % according to the adolescent supplement of the National Comorbidity Survey (NCS-A) (Burstein et al. 2011), 11.2 % in girls and 7 % in boys aged 13–18 years (Merikangas et al. 2010). According to this data, SAD is the second most prevalent anxiety disorder (specific phobia being the highest) and the fourth most common adolescent mental disorder, behind specific phobia (19.3 %), major depressive disorder (11.7 %), and oppositional defiant disorder (12.6 %) (Merikangas et al. 2010).

The diagnosis of SAD in DSM-5 was modified in several key areas. Firstly, the name was officially changed to SAD from social phobia. In addition, the definition of the fear in SAD was significantly broadened such that "the individual fears that he or she will act in a way or show anxiety symptoms that will be negatively evaluated (i.e., will be humiliating or embarrassing; will lead to rejection or offend

M. Van Ameringen, MD, FRCPC (✉) • J. Turna, BSc • B. Patterson, MSc, BEd • C. Lau
Department of Psychiatry and Behavioural Neurosciences, McMaster University, MacAnxiety Research Centre, 1057 Main Street West, Hamilton L8S 1B7, ON, Canada
e-mail: vanamer@mcmaster.ca

K. Ranta et al. (eds.), *Social Anxiety and Phobia in Adolescents: Development, Manifestation and Intervention Strategies*, DOI 10.1007/978-3-319-16703-9_14

others)" [1, p. 202, APA 2013]. For children and young adolescents, behaviors such as extreme clinging, crying tantrums, and not being able to speak in social situations are included as potential expressions of social anxiety. The social situations are either avoided or endured with distress, and the clinician must determine whether or not the fear is out of proportion to the actual threat and the sociocultural context. Other diagnostic criteria determined by the clinician include a symptom duration of at least 6 months, significant distress or impairment in at least one area of functioning, and symptoms not attributable to the effects of a substance or other medical condition or be better explained by another mental or medical disorder. In DSM-5, a performance-only specifier has been added to characterize individuals whose anxiety is limited to speaking or performing in public (APA 2013).

As it is in adulthood, SAD in adolescence is associated with significant comorbidity, particularly with other anxiety and mood disorders such as generalized anxiety disorder (GAD), specific phobia, and depression (Beidel et al. 1999; Coyle 2001; Burstein et al. 2011). In the majority of cases, SAD appears to precede the onset of other psychiatric disorders (Chavira et al. 2004). In the NCS-A, over one-fifth of adolescents diagnosed with SAD met the criteria for another anxiety disorder in their lifetime (20.1 %), and 18.6 % of adolescents diagnosed with SAD met the criteria for a lifetime mood disorder (Burstein et al. 2011). Specific disorders in the NCS-A demonstrating high rates of comorbidity with SAD included agoraphobia (32.4 %), GAD (32 %), separation anxiety disorder (27.4 %), and panic disorder (27.2 %) (Burstein et al. 2011).

Selective mutism (SM) is a disorder of childhood characterized by a persistent refusal to speak in one or more major social situations, despite having the ability to speak and comprehend spoken language (APA 2013). Selective mutism is thought to be either an extreme variant of SAD in children where intense fear and panic may lead to the inability to speak in certain social settings or to be a co-occurring disorder (Stein et al. 2001; Yeganeh et al. 2006). Examinations of comorbidity between SM and SAD have revealed rates as high as 90–100 % (Black and Uhde 1995; Kristensen 2000; Yeganeh et al. 2006). Although there is an obvious relationship between SAD and SM, the exact nature of that relationship remains unclear. Few studies have directly compared youth with SM and SAD to children with SAD alone (Manassis et al. 2003; Yeganeh et al. 2003, 2006). In the limited literature, children with both SAD and SM did not endorse higher levels of social anxiety than children with SAD alone on self-report measures (Manassis et al. 2003; Yeganeh et al. 2003, 2006); however, clinicians rated those with both disorders as having more severe SAD symptoms (Yeganeh et al. 2003, 2006). It is possible that clinicians and parents may be misattributing the degree of anxiety associated with the social silence or that SM may be a form of avoidance behavior, similar to school refusal, and not a separate disorder (Yeganeh et al. 2006).

Avoidant personality disorder (APD) is another diagnosis where there is significant conceptual overlap with SAD and may lead to confusion for clinicians. Evidence has supported APD as a distinct personality disorder as it has consistent state and trait characteristics (Reich 2009), and it has been included in DSM-5 (APA 2013). In a review of empirical studies comparing social phobia and avoidant personality disorder, Reich (2009) reported that rates of comorbidity between the two disorders ranged from 22 to 89 %, with an average rate of 56 %, and symptoms overlapped almost completely. Both disorders have a similar chronic course and appear to respond to similar pharmacological (SSRIs, benzodiazepines, other antidepressants) and psychological treatments (CBT), leading some to conclude that they are different forms of the same disorder (Reich 2009). It may be that APD is the more severe form of the disorder, signified by its grouping with the personality disorders, which are also less responsive to treatment, and by SAD classified as an anxiety disorder.

For both adults and adolescents, first-line, evidence-based treatments include cognitive–behavioral therapy (CBT) and pharmacotherapy. In general, CBT for the treatment of pediatric anxiety disorders is supported by a large body of evidence and has been shown to be at least as effective as pharmacotherapy (Mohatt et al. 2014). According to a recent meta-analysis (Reynold et al. 2012), the effect size of disorder-specific group CBT in youth with SAD was –0.79 (95% CI –1.39 to –0.19). Individual CBT has also demonstrated strong efficacy. Although some studies have reported improved response with individual CBT for youth with SAD (Crawley et al. 2008), other studies have found group and individual modalities to be equally effective (Wergeland et al. 2014). Advantages of CBT include enduring long-term effects – some studies have reported maintenance of treatment gains lasting for 19 years (Benjamin et al. 2013; Wergeland et al. 2014) as well as the avoidance of side effects associated with pharmacotherapy. Drawbacks include the availability of skilled therapists who have experience treating teens with SAD as well as the cost of treatment. In addition, many teens are reluctant to put in the requisite time and effort in order to make CBT successful. The practice guidelines of both the American Academy of Child and Adolescent Psychiatry (AACAP guidelines 2007) and the National Institute for Health and Care Excellence (NICE guidelines 2013) highlighted the importance of CBT in youth with mild to moderate anxiety. Although in the past, it appeared that combination treatment with CBT and pharmacotherapy did not offer any additional benefits, there is now emerging evidence supporting the efficacy of combination pharmacotherapy and CBT in youth with SAD (Walkup et al. 2008). However, further randomized controlled trial evidence is warranted for a recommendation.

In adults with SAD, pharmacological interventions supported by meta-analytic evidence include SSRIs, particularly escitalopram, fluvoxamine, fluvoxamine CR and sertraline, as well as the SNRI venlafaxine XR (Fedoroff & Taylor 2001; van der Linden et al. 2000; Canton et al. 2012; Stein et al. 2004; Hedges et al. 2007). The anticonvulsant pregabalin has also demonstrated efficacy over placebo in several RCTs and could be considered a first-line treatment. Cognitive–behavioral therapy (CBT) and exposure therapy alone are also considered effective first-line options for the treatment of SAD in adults. Although CBT and pharmacotherapy appear to have similar efficacy for the acute treatment of adult SAD, there is some evidence which suggests that following treatment discontinuation, gains achieved with CBT may persist longer than those achieved with pharmacotherapy (Liebowitz et al. 1999; Haug et al. 2003).

This chapter will focus primarily on pharmacotherapy as treatment for adolescents with social anxiety disorder. Similar to adults, the first-line pharmacological treatment for social anxiety disorder in this population includes antidepressants.

More specifically selective serotonin reuptake inhibitors remain the most frequently researched compounds in terms of their efficacy and tolerability, although evidence is emerging for the serotonin noradrenalin reuptake inhibitors (SNRIs). In addition to being the most widely researched, these compounds are also favorable treatment options due to their efficacy, safety, and tolerability as compared to other antidepressant medications. SSRIs and SNRIs used in this population include fluoxetine, sertraline, fluvoxamine, paroxetine, escitalopram, citalopram, and venlafaxine. The benzodiazepines have not been evaluated in SAD in youth.

When compared to the adult SAD literature, the studies in adolescent populations are much smaller in number. In addition, instead of including "pure SAD" adolescents, many studies have examined the "anxiety triad" of symptoms and disorders, which is the combination of separation anxiety disorder, generalized anxiety disorder, and social anxiety disorder (Strawn et al. 2012). When possible, we have reported the outcome measures specific to SAD for each study. Open-label studies are also summarized in Table 14.1; randomized controlled trials (RCTs) are summarized in Table 14.2.

Selective Serotonin Reuptake Inhibitors (SSRIs)

Fluoxetine

The SSRI fluoxetine has been shown to be effective in one open-label trial (Fairbanks et al. 1997), a naturalistic retrospective study (Masi et al. 2012), as well as three RCTs (Birmaher et al. 2003; Beidel et al. 2007; da Costa et al. 2013). The open-label study involved a sample of 16 adolescent outpatients with mixed anxiety disorders, including SAD (mean dose 40 mg/day) (Fairbanks et al. 1997). A naturalistic, retrospective study also reported efficacy of fluoxetine (Masi et al. 2012).

Birmaher et al. (2003) conducted a 12-week study of fluoxetine in 59 children and adolescents (7–17 years) meeting DSM-IV criteria for either generalized anxiety disorder (63 %), separation anxiety disorder (47 %), or SAD (54 %). Children with significant impairment in their functioning, as dictated by a Children's Global Assessment Scale [CGAS] $\leq$60, were randomly assigned to a double-blind treatment of fluoxetine (10 mg/day for 1 week, increased to 20 mg/day for the remainder of the trial) or placebo. Using the intent-to-treat (ITT) analysis, patients treated with fluoxetine (61 %) showed a greater clinical improvement than those treated with a placebo (35 %) as per a CGI-I $\leq$2 (p=0.03). Improvements gained by the group receiving fluoxetine were visible by week 4; however, these were not statistically significant until week 9. SAD patients randomized to fluoxetine (n=21) also had significantly better clinical outcome (CGI $\leq$2) (76 %) than SAD patients treated with placebo (n=19) (21 %) (χ^2=12.13, p=.001, ES=0.55). This effect was significantly greater than the treatment effect for patients without SAD. (Test of interaction, $\chi^2 1$=8.28, p=.004).

These response rates also mirrored better functional outcome following treatment (CGAS $\geq$70) (45.5 % vs. 10.5 %, respectively; χ^2=6.01, p=.01, ES=0.38). Overall, patients tolerated the medicine well with a few occurrences of mild,

Table 14.1 Open-label trials of pharmacotherapy in adolescents with social anxiety disorder

Drug and study	Sample	*N*	Weeks	Design	Efficacy	Effect size
Selective serotonin reuptake inhibitors (SSRIs)						
Escitalopram Isolan et al. (2007)	Ages 10–17	**N_{total} = 20**	12	ESC (5–20 mg/day)	Posttreatment > Pre-treatment	0.9–1.9
	Mean age = 15 ± 1.5	**$N_{adolescent}$ = Not reported**				
	Primary SAD					
	60 % comorbid anxiety disorders					
Fluoxetine Fairbanks et al. (1997)	Ages 9–18	N_{total} = 16	6–9	FLU (5–80 mg/day) vs. pretreatment	Posttreatment > pre-treatment	None reported
	Mean = 13 ± 2.9	**$N_{adolescent}$ = 11 (12 years old or over)**				
	Mixed anxiety disorders SEP, SAD, SPEC, PDAg, BDD, GAD					
Citalopram Chavira and Stein (2002)	Ages 8–17	N_{total} = 12	12	Psychoeducation and CIT (10–40 mg/day) vs. pretreatment	Psychoeducation and CIT > pretreatment	0.49–1.66
	Mean = 13.42 ± 3.03	**$N_{adolescent}$ = 8 (age range not defined for children and** *adolescents)*				
	Primary SAD + comorbidity					
	33 % had comorbid anxiety disorder					
Sertraline Compton et al. (2001)	Ages 10–17	N_{total} = 14	8	SERT (50–200 mg/day) vs. pretreatment	Posttreatment > Pre-treatment	None reported
	Mean age = 13.57 ± 1.60	**$N_{adolescent}$ = not reported**				
	Primary SAD + comorbidity					
	43 % had comorbid anxiety disorder					

(continued)

Table 14.1 (continued)

Drug and study	Sample	N	Weeks	Design	Efficacy	Effect size
Sertraline and tandospirone Huang et al. (2013)	Ages 17–21	N_{total} = **71**	8	SERT (25–200 mg/day) vs. TAN (20–60 mg/day)	SERT = TAN	None reported
	Median age reported = 18.25. (mean age TAN: 17.66 ± 2.07, SERT = 18.25 ± 2.10)	$N_{adolescent}$ = **not reported**				
	SAD only					
Tricyclic antidepressants						
Mirtazapine Mrakotsky et al. (2008)	Ages 8–17	N_{total} = **18**	8	MIR (15–30 mg/day)	Posttreatment > Pre-treatment	None reported
	Mean age = 12.06 ± 2.78	$N_{adolescent}$ = **not reported**				
	Primary SAD + comorbidity					
	67 % had comorbid anxiety or depressive disorder					

BDD body dysmorphic disorder, *CIT* citalopram, *ESC* escitalopram, *FLU* fluoxetine, *GAD* generalized anxiety disorder, *MIR* mirtazapine, *PDAg* panic disorder ± agoraphobia, *SAD* social anxiety disorder, *SEP* separation anxiety disorder, *SERT* sertraline, *SPEC* specific phobia

Table 14.2 Randomized controlled trials of pharmacotherapy in adolescents with social anxiety disorder

Study	Sample	*N*	Weeks	Design	Efficacy	Treatment condition effect size	Treatment condition NNT
Selective serotonin reuptake inhibitors (SSRIs)							
Fluoxetine							
Birmaher et al. (2003)	Ages 7–17	**N_{total}=74**	12	FLU (20 mg/day) vs. PBO	FLU > PBO	*Overall* = 0.26	*All Dx* = 3.85
	Mean age = 11.8 ± 2.8	**$N_{adolescent}$=31 (ages 12 and up)**				*SAD only* =0.55	*SAD only* = 1.82
	GAD, SAD, and/or SEP						
	54 % SAD						
	70 % had comorbid anxiety disorder						
Beidel et al. (2007)	Ages 7–17	**N_{total}=122**	12	SET-C vs. FLU (40 mg/day) vs. PBO	SET-C, FLU > PBO	Cramer's V:	*SET-C* =1.38
	Mean age = 11.61 ± 2.6	**$N_{adolescent}$= not reported**			SET-C > FLU (social skills)	*Overall* = 0.61	*FLU* = 3.32
	Primary SAD					*SET-C vs. PBO* = 0.70	
	53 % had a comorbid anxiety disorder, DYS, or ADHD					*FLU vs. PBO* = 0.37	

(continued)

Table 14.2 (continued)

Study	Sample	*N*	Weeks	Design	Efficacy	Treatment condition effect size	Treatment condition NNT
da Costa et al. (2013)	Ages 7–17	**N_{total}=30**	12	FLU (10–60 mg/day) vs. CLO (25–225 mg/day) vs. PBO	CLO=FLU=PBO	Unable to compute	*Total sample:*
	Mean age FLU=11.6. Mean PBO=11.4. Mean CLOM=11.2	**$N_{adolescent}$=not reported**					*CLO*=10.2
	GAD, SEP, and/or						*FLU*=4.48
	SAD+≥ 1 comorbid anxiety disorder						
Paroxetine							
Wagner et al. (2004)	Ages 8–17	**N_{total}=322**	16	PAR (10–50 mg) vs. PBO	PAR>PBO	*Total sample:* 0.47	*Total sample:*
	Mean age=13.1±2.77	**$N_{adolescent}$=228 (ages 12–17)**				*Adolescents*: 0.49	*PAR*=2.55
	Primary SAD						
	53 % had a comorbid anxiety disorder						
Sertraline							
Walkup et al. (2008) (CAMS)	Ages 7–17	**N_{total}=488**	12	SERT (25–200 mg/day)+CBT vs. CBT vs. SERT (25–200 mg/day) vs. PBO	CBT+SERT, CBT, SERT>PBO	*Total sample:*	*Total sample:*
	Mean age=10.7±2.8	**$N_{adolescent}$=126 (13–17 years old)**			CBT+SERT >CBT, SERT	*CBT+SERT: 0.86* (95 % CI, 0.56–1.15)	*CBT+SERT*=1.7
	SEP, GAD, or SAD				SERT=CBT	*SERT: 0.45* (95 % CI, 0.17–0.74)	*SERT*=3.2
						CBT: 0.31 (95 % CI, 0.02–0.59)	*CBT*=2.8

Fluvoxamine							
Walkup et al. (2001) (RUPP)	Ages 6–17	**N_{total}=128**	8	FVX (50–300 mg/day) vs. PBO	FVX>PBO	Unable to compute	*Total sample:*
	Mean PBO age=10.3±3.1; mean FVX age=10.4±2.8	**$N_{adolescent}$=33 (13–17 years old)**					*FVX*=2.12
	SAD, SEP, or GAD+comorbidities						
Selective noradrenaline reuptake inhibitors (SNRIs)							
Venlafaxine ER							
March et al. (2007)	Ages 8–17	**N_{total}=293**	16	VEN (37.5–225 mg/day) vs. PBO	VEN>PBO	*Total sample*:	*Total sample:*
	Mean age PBO=13.6±2.63. Mean age of VEN=13.6±2.46	**$N_{adolescent}$ =not reported**				Hedge's g=0.46	*VEN*=5.26
	Primary SAD						

ADHD attention deficit hyperactivity disorder, *CAMS* Child–Adolescent Anxiety Multimodal Study, *CBT* cognitive–behavioral therapy, *CLO* clomipramine, *DYS* dysthymic disorder, *FLU* fluoxetine, *FVX* fluvoxamine, *GAD* generalized anxiety disorder, *NNT* number needed to treat, *PAR* paroxetine, *PBO* placebo, Research Unit on Pediatric Psychopharmacology, *SAD* social anxiety disorder, *SEP* separation anxiety disorder, *SERT* sertraline, *SET-C* Social Effectiveness Therapy for Children, *VEN* venlafaxine ER transient headaches and gastrointestinal symptoms. However, there were also 20 incidences of excitement, giddiness, or disinhibition in 11 patients (7 on fluoxetine and 4 on placebo p=NS), of whom, five randomized to fluoxetine were removed from the study. Nevertheless, the lack of statistical significance between placebo and active treatment was interpreted to suggest that not all episodes were due to the SSRI.

In another randomized controlled trial, Beidel et al. (2007) evaluated the efficacy of fluoxetine, placebo, and a behavioral program (Social Effectiveness Therapy for Children [SET-C]) in youth with primary SAD (ages 7–17). Of the 139 subjects randomized, 57 received SET-C, 33 received fluoxetine, and 32 received placebo. The fluoxetine and identical pill placebo were started at 10 mg/day, and the dosage was titrated by 10 mg/day every 2 weeks. Once a dose of 40 mg/day was reached at week 7, it was held constant through week 12. The SET-C intervention involved one group and one individual session per week for 12 weeks. The SET-C sessions focused on social skills training, peer generalizations, and in vivo exposure. Primary efficacy was measured via the CGI-I. Although a larger proportion of the SET-C group (79 %) were classified as responders than either fluoxetine (36.4 %; χ^2 [df=1]=16.32; $p<.001$) or placebo (6.3 %; χ^2 [df=1]=43.46; $p<.001$), fluoxetine showed superiority over placebo (χ^2 [df=1]=8.72; $p<.005$). At study end point, significantly greater proportions of the SET-C (53 %) and fluoxetine (21.2 %) conditions no longer met the criteria for SAD than those receiving placebo (3.1 %). In addition, significant differences in high end-state functioning were found in favor of the SET-C condition (46 %) versus 21 % achieved by fluoxetine ($p<0.025$) and 3.1 % for placebo ($p<0.001$). The difference between fluoxetine was also significantly higher than placebo ($p<0.05$) in terms of high end-state functioning. From weeks 8 to 12, the severity ratings for SET-C decreased significantly when compared to placebo ($p<0.001$); however, this was not seen for fluoxetine. At the 1-year follow-up, treatment gains were maintained and both groups had continued to improve; relapse rates were 17 % for fluoxetine and 10.3 % for SET-C.

In a randomized trial comparing clomipramine, fluoxetine, and placebo, $N=30$ youth aged 7–17 with generalized anxiety disorder, separation anxiety disorder, and/or social phobia were entered into a 12-week study (da Costa et al. 2013). All medication was flexibly dosed: fluoxetine 10 mg to 60 mg/day or clomipramine 25 mg to 5 mg/kg/day up to 150 mg/day. Although the results of the social phobic patients were not presented separately, significant improvement in global symptom severity from baseline to end point was found across all three treatment conditions according to the CGI-S ($p<.001$) and Children's Global Assessment Scale (CGAS) ($p<.01$); however, no treatment condition was superior to placebo. Significant differences were found on week 12 scores of the social anxiety subscale of the Multidimensional Anxiety Scale for Children (MASC) between fluoxetine and placebo ($p=.039$) but not between clomipramine and placebo or between clomipramine and fluoxetine. Of note, the rate of placebo response in this study was quite high: 77.7 % compared to 100 % for fluoxetine and 87.5 % for clomipramine, as defined by a CGI-I score of ≤2 (da Costa et al. 2013).

Sertraline

This agent has been examined in two open label (Compton et al. 2001; Huang et al. 2013) and one RCT (Walkup et al. 2008) in anxious adolescents. An 8-week open-label trial by (Compton et al. 2001) suggested efficacy of sertraline (50–200 mg/day, mean dose 123.21 ± 37.29 mg/day) in a sample of youths aged 10–17 years. At completion, 36 % of the sample were classified as responders and 29 % as partial responders, as per CGI-I ratings. A significant clinical response appeared at week 6. Efficacy of sertraline was also shown in a case study (Mancini et al. 1999).

Another 8-week randomized, open-label trial (Huang et al. 2013) compared sertraline (25–200 mg/day) to tandospirone (20–60 mg/day), a serotonin 1A partial agonist. Primary end points included HAM-A scores at week 8 and changes from baseline as per CGI-I scores. Although sertraline was used as an active comparator, both treatments reduced HAM-A scores significantly from baseline ($p < 0.0001$). In this adolescent sample, response rates were 55.6 % based on CGI-I and 41.7 % as per a ≥50 % reduction in HAM-A score in the group treated with sertraline.

The Child/Adolescent Anxiety Multimodal Study (CAMS) study was a 12-week, randomized controlled trial comparing CBT treatment and sertraline as monotherapies and as a combination treatment to placebo (Walkup et al. 2008). The sample included 488 youths, ages 7–17, with separation anxiety disorder, generalized anxiety disorder, or social anxiety disorder. CBT involved 14, 60-min sessions based on the Coping Cat program which was adapted for the subjects' age. Patients also received training in anxiety management skills and behavioral exposure to anxiety-provoking situations. Sertraline and placebo were administered in a fixed–flexible schedule, beginning at 25 mg/day, and adjusted up to 200 mg/day by week 8. Overall, results suggested that the combination treatment was shown as superior ($p < 0.001$) to either monotherapy alone or placebo. As per the CGI-I ratings, 80.7 % of patients were rated as either very much or much improved. Such ratings were achieved by 59.7 and 54.9 % of patients receiving CBT and sertraline monotherapies, respectively. All treatments were superior to placebo ($p < 0.001$). Results of the Pediatric Anxiety Rating Scale documented a similar pattern with the combination treatment demonstrating superiority over either monotherapy or placebo; there was no significant difference between CBT and sertraline monotherapies. It was noted that sertraline was well tolerated and adverse events, including suicidal and homicidal ideations, were no more frequent in the sertraline group than placebo.

Following completion of the main study (Walkup et al. 2008), the CAMS sample was offered ongoing treatment for 6 months. At weeks 24 and 36, the combined condition maintained steady response rates; however, both monotherapies (sertraline and CBT) showed steady improvement such that the previous superiority demonstrated by the combined condition no longer applied. This pattern was evident only by the CGI-I remission criteria; however, for remission based on the absence of ADIS diagnosis criteria, there was no difference between treatment groups from week 12 to week 36. Of the responders during the acute phase, 83 % of the combination group, 82 % of sertraline group, and 80 % of CBT group maintained the same response.

Ginsburg et al. (2011) reported that remission rates in the CAMS study sample were lower than reported response rates for all definitions of remission (loss of anxiety disorder diagnosis ($p<0.0001$), CGI-S ≤ 2 ($p<0.0001$), and CGI-I=1 ($p<0.0001$)). Using diagnostic status as a definition of remission, patients randomized to the combined condition had significantly higher remission rates than other treatment conditions. Furthermore, children and adolescents treated with either monotherapy had similar remission rates; yet they were both higher than those achieved by the placebo group. As per CGI-I and CGI-S models, it was seen that patients in the combined treatment were more likely to remit than those in the CBT condition. Despite this, no active treatment group exhibited significantly different CGI-I/CGI-S remission rates than the placebo.

Fluvoxamine

Fluvoxamine has been examined in one RCT (Anxiety Study Group 2001). The Research Unit on Pediatric Psychopharmacology Anxiety Study Group (2001) conducted an 8-week randomized controlled trial evaluating the efficacy of fluvoxamine (50–300 mg/day) as compared to placebo. One-hundred and twenty-eight patients (ages 6–17) were randomized to receive fluvoxamine or placebo, all of whom were previously unresponsive to 3 weeks of psychotherapy. This sample included youths with a primary diagnosis of separation anxiety, generalized anxiety disorder, or SAD. The dose of fluvoxamine was increased by approximately 50 mg/week to a maximum of 300 mg/day in adolescents. After 8 weeks of treatment, patients receiving fluvoxamine (including 63 % with separation anxiety disorder, 54 % with generalized anxiety disorder, and 62 % with SAD) showed greater reductions in symptoms of anxiety and higher rates of clinical response than those in the placebo group (including 55 % with separation anxiety disorder, 63 % with generalized anxiety disorder, and 69 % with SAD) as indicated by the CGI-I and change in score from baseline on the Pediatric Anxiety Rating Scale (PARS). Significant differences ($p<0.001$) in the fluvoxamine group were detectable by week 3 of treatment as per the PARS with scores indicative of only mild anxiety; the ratings in the placebo group remained high. A robust treatment effect was noted with a 76 % response to fluvoxamine treatment while only 29 % did in the placebo group ($p<0.001$). Although well tolerated, fluvoxamine was associated with significantly more gastrointestinal symptoms. However, only 5/63 children discontinued treatment as a result of adverse events.

Following completion of the 8-week trial, participants were categorized into three groups (fluvoxamine responders, fluvoxamine nonresponders, and placebo nonresponders) and invited to begin 6 months of open-label treatment (RUPP 2002). Not all participants from the double-blind trial chose to continue into the extension trial; however, 94 % of the sample who initially responded to fluvoxamine (CGI-S ≤ 2 and CGI-I ≤ 3) sustained remission while continuing 24 weeks of open-label fluvoxamine. Statistically significant decreases were found in mean scores on all measures (PARS ($p=0.02$), CGAS ($p<0.0001$), Multidimensional Anxiety Scale for Children (MASC) ($p=0.04$), and Screen for Child Anxiety Related Emotional Disorders (SCARED) ($p=0.02$)). Fluvoxamine nonresponders were switched to fluoxetine, where anxiety symptoms improved in 71 % of the sample; however, improvements were only noted in clinician ratings and not child/parent ratings. Finally 56 % of placebo nonresponders showed clinically significant improvement in anxiety after being given open-label fluvoxamine.

Paroxetine

The SSRI paroxetine was shown to be effective in one case series (Mancini et al. 1999) and was also examined in one RCT (Wagner et al. 2004).

In the only randomized controlled trial looking at the efficacy of paroxetine (Wagner et al. 2004), 322 children and adolescents with primary SAD received either flexibly dosed paroxetine (10–50 mg/day) or placebo for 16 weeks. The mean end point dose for adolescent patients was 35.0 mg/day. The intent-to-treat (ITT) sample ($n=319$) included 71.5 % adolescents (12–17 years of age). In the overall ITT group, 77.6 % of patients randomized to paroxetine were defined as CGI-I responders (CGI-I ≤ 2) as compared to 38.3 % of the placebo group ($p<0.001$), a difference which was significant over both age groups. Moreover, paroxetine-treated patients also demonstrated greater improvements from baseline on all secondary measures including the LSAS-CA, where a greater proportion of individuals achieved remission (47.2 % vs. 13.3 %), as per a ≥ 70 % reduction in LSAS-CA score. The benefit of paroxetine was apparent within the first 4 weeks of treatment. In the adolescent subgroup of the ITT sample, the drop in LSAS-CA score was –20.62 points in favor of paroxetine (95 % CI, –28.10—13.14; $p<.001$). For both children and adolescents, the median difference in CGI-S scores between paroxetine and placebo at week 16 last observation carried forward (LOCF) end point in change from baseline was–1.0 ($p<.001$). More than 4 times as many patients randomized to paroxetine met both remission criteria (>70 % LSAS reduction and CGI-I of 1). The most common adverse events included insomnia, decreased appetite, and vomiting. Emotional lability was reported by 2.5 % of the paroxetine versus 1.3 % of the placebo group ($p=0.12$); one subject in the paroxetine group also exhibited self-harm behavior.

Escitalopram

There is only one open-label study assessing the efficacy and safety of escitalopram in a sample of children and adolescents with primary SAD (Isolan et al. 2007) and no RCTs. Following a 1-week, single-blind placebo run-in period, patients began 12 weeks of treatment at a dose of 5 mg/day. During subsequent visits, dosages were increased at 5 mg intervals to a maximum of 20 mg/day. At week 12, 65 % of the sample achieved response criteria (CGI-I ≤ 2) and all symptomatic measures (self-reports and parent reports) showed significant differences from baseline. The end point dose was 13 ± 4.1 mg/day.

Citalopram

Evidence for the SSRI citalopram is also limited to one open-label trial (Chavira and Stein 2002) with no RCTs. Chavira and Stein (2002) conducted a 12-week open-label study of citalopram treatment in children and adolescents with SAD. Patients were started at 10 mg/day and increased by 10 mg intervals to a maximum of 40 mg/day. Pharmacological treatment was supplemented with 15–20 min of psychoeducation sessions about SAD, and behavioral recommendations were made to both parent and child. Based on CGI-I ratings, 41.7 % of participants were very much improved and 41.7 % were much improved.

Serotonin–Norepinephrine Reuptake Inhibitors (SNRIs)

Venlafaxine

To date, one multicenter, randomized controlled trial has been conducted evaluating the efficacy of the SNRI venlafaxine extended release (ER) (March et al. 2007), and to our knowledge, there are no open-label trials. March et al. (2007) examined the efficacy of 16 weeks of venlafaxine treatment in SAD patients aged 8–17 years. Venlafaxine ER was flexibly dosed from 37.5 to 225 mg/day, with dose increases determined by the subject's weight. Primary efficacy measures included the Social Anxiety Scale (child and adolescent versions SASC-R and SAS-A, respectively) and the CGI-I for the responder analysis. Responders were classified as individuals with CGI-I ≤ 2 at week 16; response rates were 56.0 % for venlafaxine ER and 37.0 % for placebo. Further comparisons to placebo, ITT random regression analyses revealed a statistically significant advantage for venlafaxine ER ($p<0.001$) on the SASC-R/SAS-A.

Other Antidepressants

Mirtazapine

Mirtazapine has been examined in one open-label trial only. Mrakotsky et al. (2008) conducted an 8-week open-label trial of flexibly dosed mirtazapine (15–30 mg/day) in patients with SAD and comorbid conditions. Primary efficacy measures included the LSAS-CA and CGI-SP GI (CGI-Social Phobia Global Improvement). Overall, mirtazapine was associated with improvements in SAD and comorbid symptoms, with a 56 % response as per the Global Improvement ratings. Using the LSAS-CA ratings, 39 % reached remission of SAD symptoms, and 22 % had full remission of all anxiety symptoms.

Azapirones

This drug class has been examined in the form of tandospirone in one open-label study only. Huang and colleagues (2013) reported on an 8-week, randomized open trial of sertraline versus the specific serotonin 1A partial agonist, tandospirone citrate in 71 adolescents, aged 17–21 years. Medication was flexibly dosed: 20–60 mg/day of tandospirone, mean 35.14 ± 7.75, and 25–200 mg/day sertraline, mean 89.58 ± 30.47 mg/day. The results of the study revealed significant differences in baseline to end point scores on both primary outcome measures (HAM-A and CGI-I) for each agent individually ($p < .0001$), although significant differences in scores between the agents were not found. In addition, rates of response (CGI-I) on both primary outcome measures did not differ from each other, although rates of response were slightly higher in the sertraline group (48.6 % tandospirone vs. 55.6 % sertraline).

Safety and Tolerability

Overall, SSRIs seem to be a well-tolerated treatment for social anxiety disorder in youths. In the studies examined in this chapter, the most common adverse events (AEs) were gastrointestinal symptoms, namely, abdominal discomfort and nausea. Other common, usually mild and transient, side effects of SSRIs include headaches, motor restlessness, and insomnia (Connolly et al. 2011). Less common AEs are disinhibition and behavioral activation. More uncommon side effects have included enuresis, tremor, tics, apathy, and sedation, which typically result in medication discontinuation (Murphy et al. 2008). Side effects commonly emerge earlier in the course of treatment or during dosage adjustments but may subside within days or weeks.

While most AEs reported in the RCTs treating adolescent social anxiety disorder did not reach statistical significance, Wagner et al. (2004) reported a few adverse events that were considered possibly treatment emergent in a 16-week RCT using paroxetine; however, insomnia was the only AE to occur significantly more frequently in youths receiving paroxetine than those receiving placebo. Insomnia appeared more frequently in the paroxetine-treated adolescents than in paroxetine-treated children. Although incidences of suicidal ideation or threatened suicide have been reported in some studies of depression (Henry et al. 2012; Isacsson and Rich 2014), the rates of such adverse events were not significantly greater in the SSRI treatment versus those receiving placebo in any of the studies of SAD reviewed in this chapter.

Nevertheless, the use of antidepressants particularly in patients younger than 18 years of age has been under scrutiny by regulatory authorities due to concerns of a possible increased risk of suicidal thinking, suicide attempts, and self-harm. There are currently no available pharmacological agents with regulatory approval in the treatment of social anxiety disorder in children and adolescents. In 2004, the US Food and Drug Administration (Food and Drug Administration 2004) issued a statement indicating that antidepressant manufacturers include a "black box warning" regarding antidepressant treatment and risk of suicide in children and adolescents. This warning followed an examination of 25 short-term clinical trials of antidepressant medications treating major depressive disorder (15 trials), obsessive–compulsive disorder (5 trials), generalized anxiety disorder (2 trials), attention deficit hyperactivity disorder (2 trials), and one social anxiety disorder trial. The resulting analysis revealed a greater risk of suicidality if patients were taking an antidepressant medication (4 % risk) than a placebo (2 % risk). Many have since contested this decision as the majority of trials in the sample analyzed by the FDA treated depression suggesting that the increased risk of suicidality is linked to MDD and not anxiety disorders (Isacsson and Rich 2014). In addition, there have been several reports from Sweden, the United States, and Denmark which have examined toxicological evidence from completed suicides in adolescents from 1999 to 2002. These reports found little evidence of antidepressants in the toxicology and, when present, were mostly in the form of tricyclic antidepressants. Isacsson et al. (2005) found that the relative risk of suicide associated with SSRIs versus non-SSRIs was 0.14 (95 % CI 0.05–0.43) after the examination of 14,857 adolescent suicide cases.

It should be noted that no youths have completed suicide in any RCT to date (Henry et al. 2012; Isacsson and Rich 2014). Three meta-analyses (Hammad et al. 2006; Bridge et al. 2007; Whittington et al. 2004) have examined suicidality in youths treated with antidepressant medications, only two of which included studies treating both depression and anxiety disorders (Bridge et al. 2007; Hammad et al. 2006). All three studies concluded that there is some risk of increased mood-related side effects, including suicide attempts, in youth treated with antidepressant medications.

Following the FDA's black box warning in 2003, an increase in completed suicides was reported the following year in individuals between the ages of 10–19 in the United States (from 2.83 per 100,000 to 3.23 per 100,000), in the Netherlands (from 0.86 per 100,000 to 1.28 per 100,000), and in Canada (0.04 per 1,000 to 0.15 per 1,000) (Katz et al. 2008). This increase corresponded with a decrease in SSRI prescriptions following the FDA warning (Gibbons et al. 2007) and a decrease in diagnosis of depression in the United States, United Kingdom, Canada, Australia, and Sweden (Isacsson and Rich 2014). The potential risks associated with SSRI use in adolescents are likely multifaceted issues and appear to be more of an issue in depressed versus anxious youth. The safety and suicide risk associated with antidepressants should be weighed against the potential benefits of therapy.

Discussion

Response and Long-Term Efficacy

Despite relatively high rates of response, pharmacological treatments have overall demonstrated a modest efficacy for the treatment of SAD in adolescents when compared to placebo. It is important to mention the high rates of placebo response, particularly noticeable in short-term studies which currently make up the majority of the RCTs investigating pharmacotherapy of social anxiety disorder in youth. In the studies included in this chapter, placebo response ranged from 6.3 to 77.7 % (Beidel et al. 2007; da Costa et al. 2013), while medication response ranged from 56 to 100 % (March et al. 2007; da Costa et al. 2013).

In the adult literature, placebo response rates in SAD treatment studies range from 9 to 50 % (Stein and Stein. 2008), while the response rates for medication are similar to those in adolescent studies. Response rates for escitalopram in adult SAD range from 54 to 71 %, while placebo response rates between 39 and 50 % have been reported (Stein and Stein 2008). The only single-blind, placebo-controlled study using escitalopram in adolescents demonstrated response in 65 % of the sample receiving active medication (Isolan et al. 2007). Studies evaluating sertraline as a treatment for adult SAD have produced response rates ranging from 40 to 53 % (Stein and Stein 2008), comparable to the response rate in one pediatric SAD RCT (Walkup et al. 2008). While both monotherapies demonstrated similar response rates, 54.9 % of the pediatric group receiving sertraline was considered responders to the treatment compared with 23.7 % in the placebo group. Adults receiving fluoxetine as SAD treatment have shown response rates between 40 and 51 % with 30–32 % responding to placebo (Stein and Stein 2008). In two RCTs using fluoxetine in sample of youths with mixed anxiety disorders and another pure SAD sample, response was quantified as a CGI-I ≤2, 36.4 and 61 %, respectively. An RCT comparing clomipramine and fluoxetine to a placebo presented response rates (CGI-I≤) of 87.5, 100 and 77.7 %, respectively (da Costa et al. 2013).

Results of the RUPP study showed that children (with mixed anxiety disorders, including SAD) treated with fluvoxamine had response rates of 76 % with only 29 % of the placebo group responding to treatment. However, it should be noted that this study used a less conservative definition of response, labeling responders as those with a CGI-I <4. This proportion of responders is considerably higher than the 43–48 % response rate reported in adult SAD trials (Stein and Stein 2008). Placebo response rates in fluvoxamine adult SAD trials range from 7 to 44 % (Stein and Stein 2008). The response rate in the lone paroxetine in youth RCT was 77.6 % with a placebo response of 38.3 %. Wagner et al. (2004) commented that the response rates in this sample were much higher than what was typical in socially anxious adults (55–72 %). Despite the larger response rate in the child/adolescent sample, patients were receiving a lower average dose (24.8 mg/day) compared to the average dose for adults (36.6 mg/day), leading the authors to comment that the disorder may be more difficult to treat in adulthood.

The SNRI venlafaxine in adults has revealed response rates ranging from 44 to 69 % (Stein and Stein 2008). March et al. (2007) reported a 56 % response in SAD youths treated with venlafaxine. The placebo response rate in this sample was 37 %, quite similar to the 30–36 % response rates reported in SAD adult trials (Stein and Stein 2008) of venlafaxine.

Response rates in pharmacological trials for other youth anxiety disorders are likely comparable to those in SAD; however, most studies of other anxiety disorders were based on the "anxiety triad" of disorders. That is, the studies included youth with GAD, separation anxiety disorder, and SAD. Overall rates of response in these studies have ranged from 54.9 to 76 %. We are not aware of any pharmacological RCTs of panic disorder in youth. Formerly classed as an anxiety disorder, but now in its own diagnostic category, obsessive–compulsive disorder is one of the few pediatric mental disorders having FDA approval for pharmacological treatment (Hamilton et al. 2007; Gleason et al. 2007; Reinblatt and Riddle 2007). Response rates for OCD range from 44 to 49 % for fluoxetine (Geller et al. 2001; Riddle et al. 1992), 42 % for sertraline (March et al. 1998), and 64 % for clomipramine (Leonard et al. 1989; Leonard et al. 1991). Placebo response rates for these trials ranged from 8 to 27 % (Franklin et al. 2011; Geller et al. 2004; Riddle et al. 2001).

In terms of long-term efficacy, only three follow-up studies have been conducted commenting on the long-term efficacy of sertraline (Piacentini et al. 2014), fluvoxamine (RUPP 2002), and fluoxetine (Clark et al. 2005) in adolescent populations. The majority of patients maintained treatment benefits during follow-up visits occurring between 24 weeks to 1 year between the three studies.

Few studies have directly examined functional improvement in adolescents with social phobia. Furthermore, significant methodological differences exist between studies. Isolan et al. (2007) reported that scores on the Youth Quality of Life Instrument-Research Version (Y-QOL-R) improved following open escitalopram treatment. Similarly, Wagner et al. 2004 found improvement in Global Assessment of Functioning (GAF) scores in patients treated with paroxetine compared to placebo. Studies using the Children's Global Assessment Scale (CGAS) also suggest that treatment results in significant functional improvement in patients treated with fluoxetine (Fairbanks et al. 1997; Birmaher et al. 2003).

Clinical Implications

Although there have been a relatively small number of double-blind, placebo-controlled studies evaluating the pharmacological treatment of SAD in adolescents, current data would support the use of SSRIs and potentially SNRIs as useful treatments for this disorder. These agents have demonstrated significant symptom improvement when compared to placebo and are generally well tolerated. Some adolescent studies of depression and anxiety have indicated a potential risk for the development of suicidality with SSRIs and SNRIs. Therefore, clinicians should be aware of the potential for the development of suicidality when using these helpful agents in youth SP.

The Canadian Journal of Psychiatry's Clinical Practice Guidelines (2006) recommend psychotherapy as the first-line treatment for adolescent anxiety disorders and that pharmacotherapy not be used alone in this population. However, they indicate that antidepressants may be important in children or adolescents with OCD or in those who are severely impaired by anxiety symptoms or less likely to respond to CBT (e.g., because of cognitive limitations). As such, while in milder cases psychological treatments should be the first-line treatment, current evidence does not support an increased risk of suicide in anxiety disordered youth. This coupled with the strong evidence supporting the use of antidepressants in youth with SAD would indicate that pharmacotherapy warrants strong consideration in moderate to severe adolescent SAD.

Future Directions

Although there is preliminary evidence for effective pharmacological treatments in adolescents with SAD, many unanswered questions remain. The evidence for the use of SSRIs and SNRIs in the treatment of youth SAD is promising but not conclusive. Most studies have used mixed populations, either including different disorders or including children and adolescents together. In order to adequately examine the efficacy of pharmacological treatments, in adolescents, it would be helpful if more studies included only specific disorders and limited study populations to individuals between 12 and 19. Future directions should examine the optimal duration of pharmacotherapy, given that SAD is a chronic condition. In addition, evaluation of other pharmacological agents such as anticonvulsants, which have been found to be beneficial in adults with SAD, may provide an alternative pharmacological treatment. The question of whether pharmacological interventions actually alter the course of SAD and/or prevent the development of comorbid conditions should also be addressed. Further attention needs to be given to potential treatment strategies that involve combining and sequencing pharmacological and psychological treatments and clear, updated guidelines as to when each strategy should be employed need to be established. Finally, we require more studies investigating predictors of response to current treatments as well as longitudinal studies to demonstrate the impact of early identification and treatment on reducing the significant burden and sequelae associated with adolescent SAD.

References

American Academy of Child and Adolescent Psychiatry (2007). Practice parameter for the assessment and treatment of children and adolescents with anxiety disorders. J Am Acad Child Adolesc Psychiatry 46(2):267–283.

American Psychiatric Association (2000) Diagnostic and statistical manual of mental disorders, fourth edition, text revision: DSM-IV-TR, 4th edn. American Psychiatric Pub, Washington, DC

American Psychiatric Association (2013) Diagnostic and statistical manual of mental disorders, 5th edn. American Psychiatric Pub, Arlington

Beidel DC, Turner SM, Morris TL (1999) Psychopathology of childhood social phobia. J Am Acad Child Adolesc Psychiatry 38(6):643–650

Beidel DC, Turner SM, Sallee FR, Ammerman RT, Crosby LA, Pathak S (2007) Sertraline in children and adolescents with social anxiety disorder: an open trial. J Am Acad Child Adolesc Psychiatry 46(12):1622–1632

Benjamin CL, Harrison JP, Settipani CA, Brodman DM, Kendall PC (2013) Anxiety and related outcomes in young adults 7 to 19 years after receiving treatment for child anxiety. J Consult Clin Psychol 81(5):865

Birmaher B, Axelson DA, Monk K, Kalas C, Clark DB, Ehmann M et al (2003) Fluoxetine for the treatment of childhood anxiety disorders. J Am Acad Child Adolesc Psychiatry 42(4): 415–423

Black B, Uhde TW (1995) Psychiatric characteristics of children with selective mutism: a pilot study. J Am Acad Child Adolesc Psychiatry 34(7):847–856

Bridge JA, Iyengar S, Salary CB, Barbe RP, Birmaher B, Pincus HA et al (2007) Clinical response and risk for reported suicidal ideation and suicide attempts in pediatric antidepressant treatment: a meta-analysis of randomized controlled trials. JAMA 297(15):1683–1696

Burstein M, He JP, Kattan G, Albano AM, Avenevoli S, Merikangas KR (2011) Social phobia and subtypes in the National Comorbidity Survey–adolescent supplement: prevalence, correlates, and comorbidity. J Am Acad Child Adolesc Psychiatry 50(9):870–880

Canadian Psychiatric Association (2006) Clinical practice guidelines. Management of anxiety disorders. Can J Psychiatry 51(8 Suppl 2):9S

Canton J, Scott KM, Glue P (2011) Optimal treatment of social phobia: systematic review and meta-analysis. Neuropsychiatr Dis Treat 8:203–215

Chavira DA, Stein MB (2002) Combined psychoeducation and treatment with selective serotonin reuptake inhibitors for youth with generalized social anxiety disorder. J Child Adolesc Psychopharmacol 12(1):47–54

Chavira DA, Stein MB, Bailey K, Stein MT (2004) Child anxiety in primary care: prevalent but untreated. Depress Anxiety 20(4):155–164

Clark DB, Birmaher B, Axelson D, Monk K, Kalas C, Ehmann M et al (2005) Fluoxetine for the treatment of childhood anxiety disorders: open-label, long-term extension to a controlled trial. J Am Acad Child Adolesc Psychiatry 44(12):1263–1270

Compton SN, Grant PJ, Chrisman AK, Gammon PJ, Brown VL, March JS (2001) Sertraline in children and adolescents with social anxiety disorder: an open trial. J Am Acad Child Adolesc Psychiatry 40(5):564–571

Connolly SD, Suarez L, Sylvester C (2011) Assessment and treatment of anxiety disorders in children and adolescents. Curr Psychiatry Rep 13(2):99–110

Coyle JT (2001) Fluvoxamine for the treatment of anxiety disorders in children and adolescents. N Engl J Med 344(17):1326–1327

Crawley SA, Beidas RS, Benjamin CL, Martin E, Kendall PC (2008) Treating socially phobic youth with CBT: differential outcomes and treatment considerations. Behav Cogn Psychother 36(4):379–389

da Costa CZG, de Morais RMCB, Zanetta DMT, Turkiewicz G, Neto FL, Morikawa M et al (2013) Comparison among clomipramine, fluoxetine, and placebo for the treatment of anxiety disorders in children and adolescents. J Child Adolesc Psychopharmacol 23(10):687–692

Food and Drug Administration, U.S. (2004) Suicidality in children and adolescents being treated with antidepressant medications. Available at: http://www.fda.gov/drugs/drugsafety/postmarketdrugsafetyinformationforpatientsandproviders/drugsafetyinformationforheathcareprofessionals/publichealthadvisories/ucm161679.htm. Accessed 13 June 2014

Fairbanks JM, Pine DS, Tancer NK, Dummit ES III, Kentgen LM, Martin J et al (1997) Open fluoxetine treatment of mixed anxiety disorders in children and adolescents. J Child Adolesc Psychopharmacol 7(1):17–29

Fedoroff IC, Taylor S (2001) Psychological and pharmacological treatments of social phobia: a meta-analysis. J Clin Psychopharmacol 21(3):311–324

Franklin ME, Sapyta J, Freeman JB, Khanna M, Compton S, Almirall D et al (2011) Cognitive behavior therapy augmentation of pharmacotherapy in pediatric obsessive-compulsive disorder: the Pediatric OCD Treatment Study II (POTS II) randomized controlled trial. JAMA 306(11):1224–1232

Geller DA, Hoog SL, Heiligenstein JH, Ricardi RK, Tamura R, Kluszynski S et al (2001) Fluoxetine treatment for obsessive-compulsive disorder in children and adolescents: a placebo-controlled clinical trial. J Am Acad Child Adolesc Psychiatry 40(7):773–779

Geller DA, Wagner KD, Emslie G, Murphy T, Carpenter DJ, Wetherhold E et al (2004) Paroxetine treatment in children and adolescents with obsessive compulsive disorder: a randomized, multicenter, double-blind, placebo-controlled trial. J Am Acad Child Adolesc Psychiatry 43(11):1387–1396

Gibbons RD, Brown CH, Hur K, Marcus SM, Bhaumik VK, Erkens JA (2007) Early evidence on the effects of regulators' suicidality warnings on SSRI prescriptions and suicide in children and adolescents. Am J Psychiatry 164:1356–1363

Ginsburg GS, Kendall PC, Sakolsky D, Compton SN, Piacentini J, Albano AM et al (2011) Remission after acute treatment in children and adolescents with anxiety disorders: findings from the CAMS. J Consult Clin Psychol 79(6):806–813

Gleason M, Egger HL, Emslie GJ, Greenhill LL, Kowatch RA, Lieberman AF et al (2007) Psychopharmacological treatment for very young children: contexts and guidelines. J Am Acad Child Adolesc Psychiatry 46(12):1532–1572

Hamilton BE, Minino AM, Martin JA, Kochanek KD, Strobino DM, Guyer B (2007) Annual summary of vital statistics: 2005. Pediatrics 119:345–360

Hammad TA, Laughren T, Racoosin J (2006) Suicidality in pediatric patients treated with antidepressant drugs. Arch Gen Psychiatry 63(3):332–339

Haug TT, Blomhoff S, Hellstrøm K, Holme I, Humble M, Madsbu HP et al (2003) Exposure therapy and sertraline in social phobia: 1-year follow-up of a randomised controlled trial. Br J Psychiatry 182(4):312–318

Hedges DW, Brown BL, Shwalb DA, Godfrey K, Larcher AM (2007) The efficacy of selective serotonin reuptake inhibitors in adult social anxiety disorder: a meta-analysis of double-blind, placebo-controlled trials. J Psychopharmacol 21(1):102–111
Henry A, Kisicki MD, Varley C (2012) Efficacy and safety of antidepressant drug treatment in children and adolescents. Mol Psychiatry 17(12):1186–1193
Huang X, Li C, Li WH, Luo YL, Wang B, Zhang W et al (2013) Clinical evaluation of the efficacy and safety of tandospirone versus sertraline monotherapy for social anxiety disorder: a randomized open label trial. Hum Psychopharmacol 28(6):594–599
Isacsson G, Rich CL (2014) Antidepressant drugs and the risk of suicide in children and adolescents. Pediatr Drugs 16(2):115–122
Isacsson G, Holmgren P, Ahlner J (2005) Selective serotonin reuptake inhibitor antidepressants and the risk of suicide: a controlled forensic database study of 14 857 suicides. Acta Psychiatr Scand 111(4):286–290
Isolan L, Pheula G, Salum GA Jr, Oswald S, Rohde LA, Manfro GG (2007) An open-label trial of escitalopram in children and adolescents with social anxiety disorder. J Child Adolesc Psychopharmacol 17(6):751–760
Katz LY, Kozyrskyj AL, Prior HJ, Enns MW, Cox BJ, Sareen J (2008) Effect of regulatory warnings on antidepressant prescription rates, use of health services and outcomes among children, adolescents and young adults. CMAJ 178(8):1005–1011
Kessler RC, Berglund P, Demler O, Jin R, Merikangas KR, Walters EE (2005) Lifetime prevalence and age-of-onset distributions of DSM-IV disorders in the National Comorbidity Survey Replication. Arch Gen Psychiatry 62(6):593–602
Kristensen H (2000) Selective mutism and comorbidity with developmental disorder/delay, anxiety disorder, and elimination disorder. J Am Acad Child Adolesc Psychiatry 39(2): 249–256
Leonard HL, Swedo SE, Rapoport JL, Koby EV, Lenane MC, Cheslow DL et al (1989) Treatment of obsessive compulsive disorder with clomipramine and desipramine in children and adolescents. A double-blind crossover comparison. Arch Gen Psychiatry 46(12):1088
Leonard HL, Swedo SE, Lenane MC, Rettew DC, Cheslow DL, Hamburger SD et al (1991) A double-blind desipramine substitution during long-term clomipramine treatment in children and adolescents with obsessive-compulsive disorder. Arch Gen Psychiatry 48(10):922–927
Liebowitz MR, Heimberg RG, Schneier FR, Hope DA, Davies S, Holt CS et al (1999) Cognitive-behavioral group therapy versus phenelzine in social phobia: long term outcome. Depress Anxiety 10(3):89–98
Manassis K, Fung D, Tannock R, Sloman L, Fiksenbaum L, McInnes A (2003) Characterizing selective mutism: is it more than social anxiety? Depress Anxiety 18(3):153–161
Mancini C, Van Ameringen M, Oakman JM, Farvolden P (1999) Serotonergic agents in the treatment of social phobia in children and adolescents: a case series. Depress Anxiety 10(1): 33–39
Mancini C, Van Ameringen M, Bennett M, Patterson B, Watson C (2005) Emerging treatments for child and adolescent social phobia: a review. J Child Adolesc Psychopharmacol 15(4):589–607
March JS, Biederman J, Wolkow R, Safferman A, Mardekian J, Cook EH et al (1998) Sertraline in children and adolescents with obsessive-compulsive disorder: a multicenter randomized controlled trial. JAMA 280(20):1752
March JS, Entusah AR, Rynn M, Albano AM, Tourian KA (2007) A randomized controlled trial of venlafaxine ER versus placebo in pediatric social anxiety disorder. Biol Psychiatry 62(10):1149–1154
Masi G, Pfanner C, Mucci M, Berloffa S, Magazù A, Parolin G et al (2012) Pediatric social anxiety disorder: predictors of response to pharmacological treatment. J Child Adolesc Psychopharmacol 22(6):410–414
Merikangas KR, He JP, Burstein M, Swanson SA, Avenevoli S, Cui L et al (2010) Lifetime prevalence of mental disorders in US adolescents: results from the National Comorbidity Study-Adolescent Supplement (NCS-A). J Am Acad Child Adolesc Psychiatry 49(10):980–989
Mohatt J, Bennett SM, Walkup JT (2014) Treatment of separation, generalized, and social anxiety disorders in youths. Am J Psychiatry 171(7):741–748
Mrakotsky C, Masek B, Biederman J, Raches D, Hsin O, Forbes P et al (2008) Prospective open-label pilot trial of mirtazapine in children and adolescents with social phobia. J Anxiety Disord 22(1):88–89

Murphy TK, Segarra A, Storch EA, Goodman WK (2008) SSRI adverse events: how to monitor and manage. Int Rev Psychiatry 20(2):203–208

National Institute for Health and Care Excellence (2013) Social anxiety disorder: recognition, assessment and treatment of social anxiety disorder. Clinical guideline 159. http://guidance.nice.org.uk/CG159

Piacentini J, Bennett S, Compton SN, Kendall PC, Birmaher B, Albano AM et al (2014) 24-and 36-week outcomes for the child/adolescent anxiety multimodal study (CAMS). J Am Acad Child Adolesc Psychiatry 53(3):297–310

Reich J (2009) Avoidant personality disorder and its relationship to social phobia. Curr Psychiatry Rep 11(1):89–93

Reinblatt SP, Riddle MA (2007) The pharmacological management of childhood anxiety disorders: a review. Psychopharmacology (Berl) 191(1):67–86

Research Units on Pediatric Psychopharmacology Anxiety Study Group (2001) Fluvoxamine for the treatment of anxiety disorders in children and adolescents. N Engl J Med 344(17):1279–1285

Research Units on Pediatric Psychopharmacology Anxiety Study Group (2002) Treatment of pediatric anxiety disorders: an open-label extension of the research units on pediatric psychopharmacology anxiety study. J Child Adolesc Psychopharmacol 12(3):175–188

Reynold S, Wilson, Austin J, Hooper L (2012) Effects of psychotherapy for anxiety in children and adolescents: a meta-analytic review. Clin Psychol Rev., 32:251–262

Riddle MA, Scahill L, King RA, Hardin MT, Anderson GM, Ort SI et al (1992) Double-blind, crossover trial of fluoxetine and placebo in children and adolescents with obsessive-compulsive disorder. J Am Acad Child Adolesc Psychiatry 32(6):1062–1069

Riddle MA, Reeve EA, Yaryura-Tobias JA, Yang HM, Claghorn JL, Gaffney G et al (2001) Fluvoxamine for children and adolescents with obsessive-compulsive disorder: a randomized, controlled, multicenter trial. J Am Acad Child Adolesc Psychiatry 40(2):222–229

Stein MB, Stein DJ (2008) Social anxiety disorder. Lancet 371(9617):1115–1125

Stein MB, Chavira DA, Jang KL (2001) Bringing up bashful baby. Psychiatr Clin North Am 24(4):661–675

Stein DJ, Ipser JC, Balkom AJ (2004) Pharmacotherapy for social phobia. Cochrane Database Syst Rev (4):CD001206

Strawn JR, Sakolsky DJ, Rynn MA (2012) Psychopharmacologic treatment of children and adolescents with anxiety disorders. Child Adolesc Psychiatr Clin N Am 21(3):527–539

Van der Linden GJ, Stein DJ, Van Balkom AJ (2000) The efficacy of the selective serotonin reuptake inhibitors for social anxiety disorder (social phobia): A meta-analysis of randomized controlled trials. Int Clin Psychopharmacol 15(2):15–23

Wagner KD, Berard R, Stein MB, Wetherhold E, Carpenter DJ, Perera P et al (2004) A multicenter, randomized, double-blind, placebo-controlled trial of paroxetine in children and adolescents with social anxiety disorder. Arch Gen Psychiatry 61(11):1153–1162

Walkup JT, Albano AM, Piacentini J, Birmaher B, Compton SN, Sherrill JT, Kendall PC (2008) Cognitive behavioral therapy, sertraline, or a combination in childhood anxiety. N Engl J Med 359(26):2753–2766

Wergeland GJH, Fjermestad KW, Marin CE, Haugland BSM, Bjaastad JF, Oeding K et al (2014) An effectiveness study of individual vs. group cognitive behavioral therapy for anxiety disorders in youth. Behav Res Ther 57:1–12

Whittington CJ, Kendall T, Fonagy P, Cottrell D, Cotgrove A, Boddington E (2004) Selective serotonin reuptake inhibitors in childhood depression: systematic review of published versus unpublished data. Lancet 343(9418):1341–1345

Yeganeh R, Beidel DC, Turner SM, Pina AA, Silverman WK (2003) Clinical distinctions between selective mutism and social phobia: an investigation of childhood psychopathology. J Am Acad Child Adolesc Psychiatry 42(9):1069–1075

Yeganeh R, Beidel DC, Turner SM (2006) Selective mutism: more than social anxiety? Depress Anxiety 23(3):117–123

Concluding Remarks

15

Klaus Ranta, Annette M. La Greca,
Luis Joaquin Garcia-Lopez, and Mauri Marttunen

This volume brings together several perspectives on the development, manifestations, and treatment of social anxiety and phobia in adolescence. Following the general outline of the volume, we present some concluding remarks on the field, with an emphasis on future challenges and directions.

Aetiology and Epidemiology

SAD is a common and highly comorbid disorder among adolescents that has high societal and personal burden. Improved understanding of factors that maintain and provide risk for this disorder is critical to help reduce its impact (Chaps. 2 and 3). Evidence suggests that risk factors such as genetic influence, temperament, parental variables (i.e., parental level of expressed emotion), and peer experiences play a major role in the onset of SAD during adolescence (Chaps. 2, 3, 4, 5, and 7), although efforts to evaluate other potential risk factors for SAD onset in

K. Ranta, MD, PhD (✉)
Department of Adolescent Psychiatry, Helsinki University Central Hospital, Helsinki, Finland

Department of Psychology, University of Turku, Turku, Finland
e-mail: klaus.ranta@hus.fi

A.M. La Greca, PhD
Department of Psychology, University of Miami, Coral Gables, FL, USA

L.J. Garcia-Lopez, PhD
Department of Psychology, University of Jaen, Jaen, Spain

M. Marttunen, MD, PhD
Department of Mental Health and Substance Abuse, National Institute for Health and Welfare, Helsinki, Finland

Department of Psychiatry, University of Helsinki, Helsinki, Finland

K. Ranta et al. (eds.), *Social Anxiety and Phobia in Adolescents: Development, Manifestation and Intervention Strategies*, DOI 10.1007/978-3-319-16703-9_15

adolescence are needed (Chap. 2). For example, relatively little is known about how the common developmental transitions of adolescence (in school settings, romantic relationships, biological transitions, individuation process) affect or exacerbate SAD in youth (Chap. 5).

Epidemiological research indicates that the onset of social anxiety symptoms severe enough to warrant a clinical diagnosis typically occurs during the second decade of life. This body of research signals a risk for youths' continued distress and impairment in social functioning well into young and middle adulthood as well as for the subsequent onset of depressive and substance use disorders. Although less studied, it is possible that the consequences of early SAD may even include such severe problems as personality disorders and even psychosis (Chap. 3). The differential maturation between the subcortical regions of the brain (e.g. amygdala) in combination with late development of the regulatory prefrontal cortical regions during adolescence, paired with the vulnerability brought about by increased sensitivity to social rewards in adolescent peer contexts, may act as precipitating factors to heighten social anxiety in this developmental period (Chaps. 2, 3, and 4).

The influence of problematic peer processes on social anxiety has been studied across a broad developmental age range, from childhood through adolescence, and the results reveal the stability of this negative effect (Chaps. 2, 3, 5, and 7). However, surprisingly little is known about the relative weight of family factors and interactions that may contribute to social anxiety during the adolescent period.

Recognition and Manifestations

Early detection of adolescents at risk for SAD is an important practice goal. Using a comprehensive, multidisciplinary perspective and focusing on evidence-based and culturally adapted screening protocols may facilitate the assessment of SAD in adolescents (Chap. 6). Studies conducted in ecological peer groups, such as among classmates, have begun to reveal the complex mechanisms by which socially anxiety may persist and worsen in school settings. For example, factors in youths' overt appearance, behaviour, and social skills may contribute to their being disliked or treated poorly, and their internalized negative expectations about their peer relations may also lead to further social withdrawal (Chap. 7).

Social anxiety has consequences for youths' social and emotional development, such as by causing distress and impairment in emerging romantic relationships and undermining the transition to more independent functioning outside of the family (Chaps. 5, 8, and 9). Adding to the evidence gained from population studies, clinical observations confirm the negative influence on adolescents' social anxiety of dysfunctional parental behaviours, such as modelling of shame, dependency of other's opinions, and low sociability and also stress the need to address family factors in clinical interventions (Chap. 9).

Treatment and Prevention

Social skills training and cognitive-behavioural treatments (CBT) are efficacious in treating SAD in adolescents (Chaps. 10, 12, and 13). CBT-based interventions have seen a gradual evolution towards advanced developmental sensitivity of the content (e.g. CBGT-LEAP for emerging adults; Chap. 9) and advanced ecological validity of the settings (e.g. school-based programmes such as the original IAFS, IFAFS and the SASS; Chap. 12). Also, treatment applications using new technology, such as computer-aided virtual environment social skills training programmes, allow gradual exposure and practising of socially adaptive behaviour (Chap. 13). Computer-based CBM protocols that train socially anxious youth to direct their attention away from threat or to construct benign interpretations of ambiguous social situations (Chap. 10) also hold promise. Efforts to assess and intervene in school settings may facilitate the identification and treatment of youth with SAD (or youth at risk for the disorder); as such youth are not likely to seek traditional clinical services (Chaps. 6, 11, and 12).

Interpersonal approaches to the treatment and prevention of SAD also appear promising and are currently being investigated. The most recent developments based on the interpersonal model acknowledge the significance of problematic peer relationships and peer victimization as risk factors for SAD and seek to prevent it by focusing on peer relationships, interpersonal skills, and assertiveness (Chap. 11). The pharmacological treatment of SAD has advanced during the last 10 years; however, most controlled studies have been performed in mixed child-adolescent samples and in samples consisting of mixed disorders. Future studies that specifically target adolescents aged 12–19 years with SAD are needed. Despite these drawbacks, evidence supports the use of SSRI, and possibly SNRI, at least in complex and treatment resistant cases (see Chap. 14).

Finally, in closing, significant developments have been made in recent years in the study of etiological and precipitating factors of adolescent social anxiety/SAD, their manifestations in both clinical and real-life contexts, and their treatment. We hope that the present volume will encourage further developmental research and clinical efforts that ultimately will lead to enhanced early detection and intervention of SAD and to better outcomes for youth who suffer from it.

MIX
Papier aus verantwortungsvollen Quellen
Paper from responsible sources
FSC® C105338

If you have any concerns about our products,
you can contact us on
ProductSafety@springernature.com

In case Publisher is established outside the EU,
the EU authorized representative is:
Springer Nature Customer Service Center GmbH
Europaplatz 3, 69115 Heidelberg, Germany

Printed by Libri Plureos GmbH
in Hamburg, Germany